Anxiety in Older People

T0201374

Anxiety in Older People

Clinical and Research Perspectives

Edited by

Gerard J. Byrne
The University of Queensland

Nancy A. Pachana
The University of Queensland

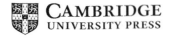
CAMBRIDGE
UNIVERSITY PRESS

CAMBRIDGE
UNIVERSITY PRESS

University Printing House, Cambridge CB2 8BS, United Kingdom

One Liberty Plaza, 20th Floor, New York, NY 10006, USA

477 Williamstown Road, Port Melbourne, VIC 3207, Australia

314–321, 3rd Floor, Plot 3, Splendor Forum, Jasola District Centre, New Delhi – 110025, India

79 Anson Road, #06–04/06, Singapore 079906

Cambridge University Press is part of the University of Cambridge.

It furthers the University's mission by disseminating knowledge in the pursuit of education, learning, and research at the highest international levels of excellence.

www.cambridge.org
Information on this title: www.cambridge.org/9781107018181
DOI: 10.1017/9781139087469

First published 2021

Printed in the United Kingdom by TJ Books Limited, Padstow Cornwall

A catalogue record for this publication is available from the British Library.

ISBN 978-1-108-82636-5 Paperback

Cambridge University Press has no responsibility for the persistence or accuracy of URLs for external or third-party internet websites referred to in this publication and does not guarantee that any content on such websites is, or will remain, accurate or appropriate.

Every effort has been made in preparing this book to provide accurate and up-to-date information that is in accord with accepted standards and practice at the time of publication. Although case histories are drawn from actual cases, every effort has been made to disguise the identities of the individuals involved. Nevertheless, the authors, editors, and publishers can make no warranties that the information contained herein is totally free from error, not least because clinical standards are constantly changing through research and regulation. The authors, editors, and publishers therefore disclaim all liability for direct or consequential damages resulting from the use of material contained in this book. Readers are strongly advised to pay careful attention to information provided by the manufacturer of any drugs or equipment that they plan to use.

Contents

List of Contributors   vi

1   **Introduction and Conceptual Overview**   1
Gerard J. Byrne and Nancy A. Pachana

2   **Epidemiology, Risk and Protective Factors**   10
Gerard J. Byrne and Nancy A. Pachana

3   **Diagnosis of Anxiety Disorders in Older Adults**   20
Christina Bryant

4   **Subthreshold Anxiety in Later Life: Epidemiology and Treatment Strategies**   33
Sébastien Grenier and Marie-Josée Richer

5   **Cross-cultural Issues in Late-Life Anxiety**   63
Xiaoping Lin and Charissa Hosseini

6   **Clinical Assessment of Late-Life Anxiety**   79
Christine E. Gould, Brian C. Kok, Vanessa K. Ma, and Barry A. Edelstein

7   **Late-Life Anxiety and Comorbid Depression: The Role of Attentional Bias**   97
Emily S. Bower and Julie Loebach Wetherell

8   **Anxiety and Cognitive Functioning**   117
Sherry A. Beaudreau, Andrew J. Petkus, Nathan C. Hantke, and Christine E. Gould

9   **Anxiety in Parkinson's Disease**   139
Nadeeka N. W. Dissanayaka

10   **Anxiety in Older Adults across Care Settings**   157
Veronica L. Shead, Rachel L. Rodriguez, Samuel J. Dreeben, and Shalagh A. McBride

11   **Psychosocial Treatment of Anxiety in Later Life**   173
Katherine Ramos and Melinda A. Stanley

12   **Pharmacological Treatment of Anxiety in Later Life**   189
Gerard J. Byrne

13   **Animal Models in Anxiety Research**   205
Madhusoothanan Bhagavathi Perumal and Pankaj Sah

14   **Late-Life Anxiety: Where to from Here?**   226
Nancy A. Pachana and Gerard J. Byrne

Index   241

Contributors

Sherry A. Beaudreau
Stanford University

Madhusoothanan Bhagavathi Perumal
The University of Queensland

Emily S. Bower
Pacific University

Christina Bryant
University of Melbourne

Gerard J. Byrne
The University of Queensland

Nadeeka N. W. Dissanayaka
The University of Queensland

Samuel J. Dreeben
Schreiner University

Barry A. Edelstein
West Virginia University

Christine E. Gould
VA Palo Alto Health Care System

Sébastien Grenier
University of Montreal

Nathan C. Hantke
Oregon Health and Science University

Charissa Hosseini
Palo Alto University

Brian C. Kok
Palo Alto University

Xiaoping Lin
Monash University

Vanessa K. Ma
Palo Alto University

Shalagh A. McBride
Chillicothe VA Medical Center

Nancy A. Pachana
The University of Queensland

Andrew J. Petkus
University of Southern California

Katherine Ramos
Duke University

Marie-Josée Richer
University of Montreal

Rachel L. Rodriguez
Durham Veterans Affairs Health Care System

Pankaj Sah
The University of Queensland

Veronica L. Shead
VA St. Louis Health Care System

Melinda A. Stanley
Baylor College of Medicine

Julie Loebach Wetherell
VA San Diego Healthcare System

Introduction and Conceptual Overview

Gerard J. Byrne and Nancy A. Pachana

Introduction

Historically, clinicians and researchers interested in the mental health of older people have focused on depression and dementia and have given little attention to anxiety except as a complication of depression or dementia. Over recent years, however, research into anxiety in older people has increased substantially, leading to both a burgeoning scientific literature and increasing clinical interest in the field.

In this book, expert clinicians and researchers combine to provide readers with a detailed and scholarly overview of current knowledge in relation to anxiety in older people. They also highlight gaps in both theory and practice, pointing the way forward. Before introducing each chapter, we will provide a brief conceptual overview of anxiety in older people to set the scene for the rest of the book.

Conceptual Overview

Naturalist Charles Darwin noted that fear and anxiety are phylogenetically ancient emotions that confer a survival advantage across species (Darwin, 1872). These emotions facilitate escape from immediate danger and prepare the individual to respond to future threat. Although a moderate level of anxiety may be adaptive and may even improve performance (Yerkes & Dodson, 1908), high and prolonged levels of anxiety are maladaptive and may represent a mental disorder.

Complex brain mechanisms underpin both adaptive and maladaptive responses to threat in humans and other animals. While the prefrontal cortex is involved in social cognition and threat appraisal, the limbic system is most involved in generating fear and anxiety responses. Neuroimaging studies with both functional magnetic resonance imaging (fMRI) and positron emission tomography (PET) have confirmed the existence of fear-related circuits involving the amygdala, insula, and anterior cingulate (Sehlmeyer et al., 2009). Studies in rodents have shown that the amygdala is critical to the generation of panic, and fear responses in the amygdala are difficult to extinguish (Sah & Westbrook, 2008). The hippocampus modulates stress responses through the hypothalamic–pituitary–adrenal (HPA) axis, and there is evidence that individuals with greater hippocampal volume and neurogenesis have greater resilience to stress (Martin et al., 2009).

Although no genes of large effect have been discovered in this area, studies in twins indicate that about 30–40% of the variation in risk of anxiety disorder is of genetic origin (Norrholm & Ressler, 2009) and that genetic mechanisms may play a larger role in panic disorder than in generalized anxiety disorder (GAD). Genetic factors continue to play an important role in late-life anxiety (Gillespie et al., 2004), and epigenetic mechanisms may also play a part (Gottschalk & Domschke, 2016).

Early-life experiences appear to be critical to the development of adult anxiety, and studies in rodents confirm this view. Rat pups separated from their mothers for relatively short periods of time during the early postnatal period demonstrate increased anxiety-related behaviours as adults (Kalinichev et al., 2002). In humans, childhood abuse has a persisting effect on the risk of late-life anxiety (Cougle et al., 2010), and this may be mediated through dysregulation of the negative feedback system of the HPA axis (Lähdepuro et al., 2019; Lupien et al., 2009). In adult life, adverse life events are also associated with new-onset anxiety disorders (Miloyan et al., 2018).

Until recently, the anxiety disorders were considered to include GAD, social anxiety disorder, panic disorder, agoraphobia, simple phobia, post-traumatic stress disorder (PTSD), obsessive–compulsive disorder (OCD), adjustment disorder with anxiety, and a group of organic and substance-related anxiety states. However, since the publication of the Diagnostic and Statistical Manual of Mental Disorders, 5th Edition (DSM-5) (American Psychiatric Association, 2013), the nosological status of PTSD and OCD has changed. These disorders have been assigned new categories separate from the anxiety disorders.

In DSM-5, PTSD is included in a chapter labelled 'Trauma- and Stressor-Related Disorders', and in the International Classification of Diseases, 10th Revision (ICD-10) (World Health Organization, 1992), it is included in a chapter labelled 'Reaction to Severe Stress, and Adjustment Disorders'. In both taxonomies, acute stress reactions and adjustment disorders are now in the same section as PTSD. ICD-10 includes this section under the broader rubric of 'Neurotic, Stress-Related and Somatoform Disorders' with the codes F40–F48.

The splitting off of stress-related disorders, including PTSD, from the anxiety disorders in contemporary nosologies may provide a measure of conceptual clarity for some clinicians and insurers, but this makes less sense from an aetiological perspective. It is clear that adverse life events, whether experienced in childhood or adulthood, are associated with the onset of many different psychiatric disorders, including anxiety disorders.

Placement of OCD in its own chapter in DSM-5 brings the American nosology in line with ICD-10. OCD shares a chapter on 'Obsessive-Compulsive and Related Disorders' with 'Body Dysmorphic Disorder', 'Hoarding Disorder', and a variety of other conditions, as recommended by commentators (e.g., Stein et al., 2010)

Certain personality traits, especially neuroticism and conscientiousness, predispose individuals to the development of anxiety symptoms and anxiety disorders (Rosellini & Brown, 2011), and about one-third of the genetic influence on GAD is shared with neuroticism (Mackintosh et al., 2006). In people with dementia due to probable Alzheimer's disease, informant-rated premorbid neuroticism is associated with current anxiety measured on the Neuropsychiatric Inventory (Archer et al., 2007). Neuroticism has been found to increase with age in cognitively normal older people who have a positive amyloid PET scan and are at increased risk of future dementia due to Alzheimer's disease (Fredericks et al., 2018).

Anxiety, at least when it is experienced as fear or worry, is scalable and lends itself to dimensional thinking. This is helpful for researchers, but it is of less utility when clinicians are dealing with third-party payers, who generally require a categorical diagnosis rather than a scale score. As a consequence, there is tension between dimensional measurement and categorical assignment when thinking about anxiety symptoms and anxiety disorders.

DSM-5 has attempted to deal with this by requiring a certain number of symptoms over a certain period of time, together with impairment of social or occupational function, before a categorical diagnosis can be made. The construction of syndromes in this way aids clinical case formulation, communication with patients and between clinicians, and planning of therapeutic interventions, but it does little to assist scientific enquiry into causal mechanisms.

Existing diagnostic criteria for anxiety disorders do not provide for age-related variations in aetiology, clinical presentation, or course. This leaves open the possibility that the epidemiology of anxiety disorders in older adults has been biased by the use of criteria better suited to use in younger people or in early-onset cases rather than in older people or in late-onset cases. In keeping with this concern, there is evidence that sub-threshold cases of anxiety make up a larger proportion of clinically significant cases in older people (Grenier et al., 2011; Miloyan et al., 2015).

It is instructive to consider the burden of disease due to anxiety disorders. Burden is measured using estimates of years lived with disability (YLDs) and years of life lost (YLLs) due to premature mortality. Disability-adjusted life years (DALYs) represent the sum of YLDs and YLLs. Mental disorders are responsible for 22.9% of global YLDs and 7.4% of global YLLs (Whiteford et al., 2015). Among mental disorders, anxiety disorders are second only to major depressive disorder in terms of global DALYs. There is a greater global burden due to anxiety disorders than due to schizophrenia and bipolar disorder. In 2010, anxiety disorders accounted for 10.4% of the global burden due to mental, neurological, and substance use disorders when measured in DALYs (Whiteford et al., 2015). The burden associated with anxiety disorders differs markedly between individuals; it is higher among women and young people than among men and older people (Baxter et al., 2014). Burden associated with anxiety disorders also varies considerably between countries or regions. Burden due to anxiety disorders is highest in North Africa/the Middle East and North America and lowest in East Asia and Eastern Europe (Baxter et al., 2014). Burden also varies by age. Among adult men and women, the global burden associated with anxiety disorders is highest among those aged 20–34 years and lowest among those aged 75 years and over (Baxter et al., 2014).

The available epidemiological data, albeit mostly from developed countries, indicate that anxiety symptoms and anxiety disorders decline in prevalence after the age of about 50 years (Byrne, 2020). This decline in prevalence occurs in parallel with a decline in trait neuroticism. However, most of the available evidence also suggests that the prevalence of anxiety increases in people with mild cognitive impairment and dementia. Anxiety has conventionally been considered to be a reaction to cognitive impairment, but anxiety has also been postulated as a potential cause of dementia (Gulpers et al., 2016).

Anxiety disorders as they are currently understood exhibit considerable co-morbidity with other anxiety disorders. This means that individuals often meet diagnostic criteria for more than one anxiety disorder at the same time. For example, in the National Epidemiologic Survey on Alcohol and Related Conditions – III (NESARC-III) population survey of the USA (Grant et al., 2014), in which 5,806 individuals aged 65 years and over were sampled, 658 (11.3%) older people met draft DSM-5 diagnostic criteria for an anxiety disorder in the past year. Of these, 126 met criteria for more than one anxiety disorder in the past year. Thus, 19.1% of older people with an anxiety disorder (or 2.2% of the general US population of older people) met criteria for more than one current anxiety disorder.

Anxiety disorders also exhibit co-morbidity with other mental disorders. In the NESARC-III survey, 387 (6.7%) older people met diagnostic criteria for major depression in the past year. Of these, 141 (36.4%) also met diagnostic criteria for one or more anxiety disorders in the past year. Conversely, 21.4% of those with a past-year anxiety disorder met criteria for a past-year major depressive episode. The anxiety disorders most often associated with major depression were GAD, PTSD, specific phobia, and social anxiety disorder.

In the NESARC-III survey, 139 (2.4%) older people met criteria for past-year alcohol use disorder. Of these, 26 (18.7%) also met criteria for one or more past-year anxiety disorders. Conversely, of 658 older people with past-year anxiety disorder, 4% had a co-morbid past-year history of alcohol use disorder. The anxiety disorders most often associated with alcohol use disorder were GAD, PTSD, social anxiety disorder, and specific phobia.

Anxiety disorders generally have their onset in young and middle-aged people. In the Australian National Survey of Mental Health and Wellbeing 2007, the median age of onset for GAD was 26 years. Only 10% of cases of GAD had their onset after the age of 60 years (Gonçalves & Byrne, 2012). However, when anxiety disorders have their onset in later life, they may be markers for undiagnosed cognitive impairment or incipient dementia.

The search for risk factors for incident anxiety disorders in later life requires adequately powered prospective studies. Such studies are uncommon due to their high cost and the natural attrition of older people. Findings from the small number of available prospective studies are conflicting (e.g., see Chou et al., 2011; Zhang et al., 2015). More work is needed.

There has been considerable recent activity in the development of anxiety rating scales for use in older people. This has been important because the Hamilton Anxiety Rating Scale (HAM-A; Hamilton, 1959) and the Beck Anxiety Inventory (BAI; Beck et al., 1988) have generally been considered inappropriate for use in older people because they are both dominated by somatic items, assessment of which can be confounded by the symptoms of general medical conditions that become more prevalent with advancing age. More recently, several scales have been developed specifically for use in older people. These include the 10-item Self-rated Anxiety Screening Test (SAST; Sinoff et al., 1999) designed for use in geriatric medicine settings, the 20-item self-rated Geriatric Anxiety Inventory (GAI; Pachana et al., 2007) designed for the self-assessment of generalized anxiety, the 30-item self-rated Geriatric Anxiety Scale (GAS; Segal et al., 2010), and the 18-item clinician-rated Rating Anxiety in Dementia instrument (RAID; Shankar et al., 1999). The GAI is available in a 5-item short form (GAI-SF; Byrne & Pachana, 2011) and the GAS is available in a 10-item form (GAS-10; Mueller et al., 2015). Several of these scales are available in multiple languages. Further work is needed in examining the performance of anxiety rating scales in the context of disabling physical illness and cognitive impairment.

The study of treatment interventions for anxiety disorders in older people is a relatively underdeveloped field. Conventional interventions for anxiety disorders in older people include the development of a therapeutic alliance, psychoeducation about the nature of anxiety and its treatment, lifestyle modification including stimulant reduction, sleep hygiene, physical exercise, relaxation training, behavioural activation, non-specific and specific exposure, formal psychotherapy including cognitive behaviour therapy (CBT), and antidepressant medication. Whilst conventional treatments delivered by trained clinicians are moderately effective (e.g., Gonçalves & Byrne, 2012), there are major problems with treatment accessibility for many older people. To date, most treatment outcome data in older people have been for GAD in cognitively intact individuals. There is a need for clinical trials in other anxiety disorders in later life and for clinical trials for anxiety disorders in the context of cognitive impairment and dementia. It is encouraging to see that work is being done to adapt psychotherapy for older people with Parkinson's disease, a neurodegenerative disorder commonly associated with anxiety (Dissanayaka et al., 2016; Knight et al., 2016).

The development of new and more effective biological treatments is likely to be predicated upon advances in the basic neuroscience of anxiety. In the absence of such advances, clinical trial work is likely to be limited to currently available psychotropic medications and the repurposing of drugs used for other disorders. Sophisticated laboratory techniques, including the use of optogenetics in living mice, have demonstrated the ability to turn anxiety circuits on and off (Tye et al., 2011). The search for molecular mechanisms underpinning anxiety and stress-related disorders is in its infancy, but one possibility is cAMP-specific 3′,5′-cyclic phosphodiesterase 4B, an enzyme that in humans is encoded by the *PDE4B* gene (Meier et al., 2019). *PDE4B* is also involved in memory and long-term plasticity in rodents, providing a potential mechanism by which anxiety and memory are linked. It is thus likely that our knowledge of the basic biological mechanisms underpinning anxiety will advance rapidly. We look forward to the translation of these laboratory findings into treatments for humans.

Research into psychosocial treatments for late-life anxiety has both a shorter history and arguably a lower success rate than research targeting depression in later life. For example, for GAD in later life, a meta-analysis of studies demonstrated CBT to be superior to wait-list or 'treatment-as-usual' conditions, but not to active controls such as supportive counselling (Hall et al., 2016). Other interventions, such as those using mindfulness, have received mixed support and require further studies with better control conditions (Geiger et al., 2016). Translations of findings from clinical trials of psychosocial as well as combination therapy using psychosocial interventions with pharmacotherapy have suffered from the inclusion of participants under age 65, a lack of data on the growing demographic segment of those over age 75, and a paucity of studies targeting co-morbid depression and anxiety in older persons – a relatively common clinical presentation (Moller et al., 2016). Technological innovations have opened up the possibility of anxiety treatments within a 'virtual reality' setting (e.g., Meyerbröker & Emmelkamp, 2014); these are a promising new approach for specific phobias.

Chapter Summary

The first chapters of the text deal with broader aspects of anxiety disorders. In Chapter 2, Byrne and Pachana address the epidemiology of anxiety disorders in older people. They discuss likely sources of variation in population estimates and consider both prevalent and incident anxiety disorders. They highlight conflicting findings in relation to risk factors for anxiety disorders in older people. In Chapter 3, Bryant discusses diagnostic issues in late-life anxiety. She considers the value of diagnosis as well as its limitations. In Chapter 4, Grenier and Richer deal with sub-threshold anxiety in later life. They note its high prevalence and association with insomnia, impaired daily functioning, suicidality, and increased use of health services. They highlight inconsistent findings in the scientific literature about the temporal stability of sub-threshold anxiety. They discuss the relationship of anxiety to depression and to several important physical disorders, as well as treatment implications.

Cultural issues are not raised often enough in discussions of anxiety. In Chapter 5, Lin and Hosseini address cross-cultural issues in late-life anxiety. They note conceptual differences between Western and non-Western cultures in the perception of anxiety, including non-Western holistic models in which the distinction between physical and mental health is not as strongly demarcated. They caution that much cross-cultural research into anxiety has been undertaken in immigrants and may not generalize well to their countries of origin. They note that, in some cultures, the notion of mental illness refers to serious but low-prevalence mental disorders such as schizophrenia and bipolar disorder, rather than to high-prevalence disorders such as anxiety and depression.

The following chapters address assessment as well as the cognitive sequelae of anxiety. In Chapter 6, Gould, Kok, Ma, and Edelstein discuss the clinical assessment of late-life anxiety. They note common differences between the clinical presentation of anxiety in older and younger people. They provide useful overviews of the properties of the diagnostic interviews and rating scales that might be used in the assessment of older people with anxiety problems. They deal with specific issues including the assessment of anxiety in the presence of physical illness. In Chapter 7, Bower and Wetherell address attention bias in older people with anxiety and co-morbid depression. They indicate that biased attention to negative information is a core component of cognitive models of anxiety and depression. They discuss the interference effect of negative information for anxious older people and report evidence from fMRI studies of failure of the dorsolateral prefrontal cortex to dampen down the amygdala in older people with GAD. In Chapter 8, Beaudreau, Petkus, Hantke, and Gould address anxiety and cognitive function. They note that older adults with anxiety symptoms exhibit poorer performance on global measures of cognitive functioning. They also note that anxiety in older people is a predictor of future cognitive decline and dementia. They discuss cognitive and biological models that may account for the link between anxiety and cognitive function.

Therapeutic interventions across a variety of settings and specific disorders is the focus of the following chapters. In Chapter 9, Dissanayaka addresses anxiety in Parkinson's disease. She emphasizes the specific nature of anxiety in this progressive neurodegenerative disorder, which often has its onset in later life. She deals in detail with putative biological underpinnings and therapeutic interventions. In Chapter 10, Shead, Rodriguez, Dreeben, and McBride deal with anxiety in older adults across various care settings, including home care, long-term care, and palliative care. They discuss the challenges of assessment and management in these diverse settings. In Chapter 11, Ramos and Stanley detail the role of psychosocial interventions in the treatment of anxiety in later life. They note that CBT is effective for late-life GAD when compared with wait-list controls, minimal contact, or treatment as usual, but not when compared with other active interventions. However, they indicate that CBT has efficacy as an augmentation strategy in older people with GAD treated with antidepressant medication. They suggest that relaxation training and other behavioural approaches may be preferable to cognitive skills acquisition, particularly in the context of memory impairment. They discuss modification to standard techniques for use with older people with cognitive or sensory changes. They discuss psychosocial interventions in several specific situations, including hoarding and fear of falling. They also discuss novel modes of delivery of psychosocial interventions. In Chapter 12, Byrne addresses the role of psychotropic medication in the management of anxiety disorders. He notes that if medication is to be used, antidepressants are preferred. He summarizes the evidence from clinical trials for the use of antidepressants and several other classes of psychotropic medication. He notes that most of the clinical trial evidence in older people has been obtained from studies of short duration and relates to the treatment of GAD. There is scant evidence for the pharmacological treatment of anxiety disorders other than GAD in older people.

Potential avenues meriting further research are the focus of the final chapters of this text. In Chapter 13, Perumal and Sah discuss the findings from recent animal models in anxiety research. They emphasize the role of the amygdala and its connections with the medial prefrontal cortex and the hippocampus. They show there are different circuits mediating fear learning and extinction. They outline how these findings in laboratory animals could be translated into humans. And finally, in Chapter 14, Pachana and Byrne summarize the field of anxiety disorders in older people, highlight important clinical issues, and make suggestions for future research.

References

American Psychiatric Association (2013). *Diagnostic and Statistical Manual of Mental Disorders*, 5th ed. Washington, DC: American Psychiatric Association.

Archer, N., Brown, R. G., Reeves, S. J., et al. (2007). Premorbid personality and behavioural and psychological symptoms in probable Alzheimer disease. *American Journal of Geriatric Psychiatry*, 15, 202–213.

Baxter, A. J., Vos, T., Scott, K. M., Ferrari, A. J. and Whiteford, H. A. (2014). The global burden of anxiety disorders in 2010. *Psychological Medicine*, 44, 2363–2374.

Beck, A. T., Epstein, N., Brown, G. and Steer, R. A. (1988). An inventory for measuring clinical anxiety: psychometric properties. *Journal of Consulting and Clinical Psychology*, 56, 893–897.

Byrne, G. J. (2020). Anxiety disorders in older people. In T. Dening, A. Thomas, J.-P. Taylor and R. Stewart, eds., *The Oxford Textbook of Old Age Psychiatry*, 3rd ed. Oxford: Oxford University Press, pp. 655–670.

Byrne, G. J. and Pachana, N. A. (2011). Development and validation of a short form of the Geriatric Anxiety Inventory – the GAI-SF. *International Psychogeriatrics*, 23(1), 125–131.

Chou, K. L., Mackenzie, C. S., Liang, K. and Sareen, J. (2011). Three-year incidence and predictors of first-onset of DSM-IV mood, anxiety, and substance use disorders in older adults: results from Wave 2 of the National Epidemiologic Survey on Alcohol and Related Conditions. *Journal of Clinical Psychiatry*, 72(2), 144–155.

Cougle, J. R., Timpano, K. R., Sachs-Ericsson, N., Keough, M. E. and Riccardi, C. J. (2010). Examining the unique relationships between anxiety disorders and childhood physical and sexual abuse in the National Comorbidity Survey – Replication. *Psychiatry Research*, 177(1–2), 150–155.

Darwin, C. (1872). *The Expression of the Emotions in Man and Animals*. London: John Murray.

Dissanayaka, N. N., O'Sullivan, J. D., Pachana, N. A., et al. (2016). Disease-specific anxiety symptomatology in Parkinson's disease. *International Psychogeriatrics*, 28(7), 1153–1163.

Fredericks, C. A., Sturm, V. E., Brown, J. A., et al. (2018). Early affective changes and increased connectivity in preclinical Alzheimer's disease. *Alzheimer's & Dementia*, 10, 471–479.

Geiger, P. J., Boggero, I. A., Brake, C. A., et al. (2016). Mindfulness-based interventions for older adults: a review of the effects on physical and emotional well-being. *Mindfulness*, 7(2), 296–307.

Gillespie, N. A., Kirk, K. M., Evans, D. M., et al. (2004). Do the genetic or environmental determinants of anxiety and depression change with age? A longitudinal study of Australian twins. *Twin Research*, 7, 39–53.

Gonçalves, D. C. and Byrne, G. J. (2012). Sooner or later: age at onset of generalized anxiety disorder in older adults. *Depression & Anxiety*, 29(1), 39–46.

Gottschalk, M. G. and Domschke, K. (2016). Novel developments in genetic and epigenetic mechanisms of anxiety. *Current Opinion in Psychiatry*, 29(1), 32–38.

Grant, B. F., Amsbary, M., Chu, A., et al. (2014). *Source and Accuracy Statement: National Epidemiologic Survey on Alcohol and Related Conditions-III (NESARC-III)*. Rockville, MD: National Institute on Alcohol Abuse and Alcoholism.

Grenier, S., Préville, M., Boyer, R., et al. (2011). The impact of DSM-IV symptom and clinical significance criteria of the prevalence estimates of subthreshold and threshold anxiety in the older adult population. *American Journal of Geriatric Psychiatry*, **19** (4), 316–326.

Gulpers, B., Ramakers, I., Hamel, R., et al. (2016). Anxiety as a predictor for cognitive decline and dementia: a systematic review and meta-analysis. *American Journal of Geriatric Psychiatry*, **24**(10), 823–842.

Hall, J., Kellett, S., Berrios, R., Bains, M. K. and Scott S. (2016). Efficacy of cognitive behavioral therapy for generalized anxiety disorder in older adults: systematic review, meta-analysis, and meta-regression. *American Journal of Geriatric Psychiatry*, **24** (11), 1063–1073.

Hamilton, M. (1959). The assessment of anxiety states by rating. *British Journal of Medical Psychology*, **32**, 50–55.

Kalinichev, M., Easterling, K. W., Plotsky, P. M. and Holtzman, S. G. (2002). Long-lasting changes in stress-induced corticosterone response and anxiety-like behaviors as a consequence of neonatal maternal separation in Long-Evans rats. *Pharmacology Biochemistry and Behavior*, **73**, 131–140.

Knight, B., Dissanayaka, N. N. and Pachana, N. A. (2016). Adapting psychotherapy for older patients with Parkinson's disease. *International Psychogeriatrics*, **28**(10), 1631–1636.

Lähdepuro, A., Savolainen, K., Lahti-Pulkkinen, M., et al. (2019). The impact of early life stress on anxiety symptoms in late adulthood. *Scientific Reports*, **9**, 4395.

Lupien, S. J., McEwen, B. S., Gunnar, M. R. and Heim, C. (2009). Effects of stress throughout the lifespan on the brain, behaviour and cognition. *Nature Reviews Neuroscience*, **10**, 434–445.

Mackintosh, M. A., Gatz, M., Wetherell, J. L. and Pedersen, N. L. (2006). A twin study of lifetime generalized anxiety disorder (GAD) in older adults: genetic and environmental influences shared by neuroticism and GAD. *Twin Research in Human Genetics*, **9**, 30–37.

Martin, E. I., Ressler, K. J., Binder, E. and Nemeroff, C. B., (2009). The neurobiology of anxiety disorders: brain imaging, genetics, and psychoneuroendocrinology. *Psychiatric Clinics of North America*, **32**, 549–575.

Meier, S. M., Trontti, K., Purves, K. L. et al. (2019). Genetic variants associated with anxiety and stress-related disorders: a genome-wide association study and mouse-model study. *JAMA Psychiatry*, **76**(9), 924–932.

Meyerbröker, K. and Emmelkamp, P. M. G. (2014). Virtual reality techniques in older adults: exposure therapy, memory training, and training of motor balance. In N. A. Pachana and K. Laidlaw, eds., *The Oxford Handbook of Clinical Geropsychology*, Oxford: Oxford University Press, pp. 1011–1024.

Miloyan, B., Byrne, G. J. and Pachana, N. A. (2015). Threshold and subthreshold generalized anxiety disorder in later life. *American Journal of Geriatric Psychiatry*, **23** (6), 633–641.

Miloyan, B., Joseph Bienvenu, O., Brilot, B. and Eaton, W. W. (2018). Adverse life events and the onset of anxiety disorders. *Psychiatry Research*, **259**, 488–492.

Moller, H. J., Bandelow, B., Volz, H. P., Barnikol, U. B., Seifritz, E. and Kasper, S. (2016). The relevance of 'mixed anxiety and depression' as a diagnostic category in clinical practice. *European Archives of Psychiatry and Clinical Neuroscience*, **266**(8), 725–736.

Mueller, A. E., Segal, D. L., Gavett, B., et al. (2015). Geriatric Anxiety Scale: item response theory analysis, differential item functioning, and creation of a ten-item short form (GAS-10). *International Psychogeriatrics*, **27**(7), 1099–1111.

Norrholm, S. D. and Ressler, K. J. (2009). Genetics of anxiety and trauma-related disorders. *Neuroscience*, **164**, 272–287.

Pachana, N. A., Byrne, G. J., Siddle, H., Koloski, N., Harley, E. and Arnold, E. (2007). Development and validation of the Geriatric Anxiety Inventory. *International Psychogeriatrics*, **19**(1), 103–114.

Reynolds, C., Richmond, B. and Lowe, P. (2003). *The Adult Manifest Anxiety Scale – Elderly Version (AMAS-E)*. Los Angeles, CA: Western Psychological Services.

Rosellini, A. J. and Brown, T. A. (2011). The NEO Five-Factor Inventory: latent structure and relationships with dimensions of anxiety and depressive disorders in a large clinical sample. *Assessment*, 18(1), 27–38.

Sah, P. and Westbrook, R. F. (2008). Behavioural neuroscience: the circuit of fear. *Nature*, 454, 589–590.

Segal, D. L., June, A., Payne, M., Coolidge, F. L., Yochim, B. (2010). Development and initial validation of a self-report assessment tool for anxiety among older adults: the Geriatric Anxiety Scale. *Journal of Anxiety Disorders*, 24(7), 709–714.

Sehlmeyer, C., Schöning, S., Zwitserlood, P., et al. (2009). Human fear conditioning and extinction in neuroimaging: a systematic review. *PLoS ONE*, 4, e5865.

Shankar, K. K., Walker, M., Frost, D. and Orrell, M. W. (1999). The development of a valid and reliable scale for rating anxiety in dementia (RAID). *Aging & Mental Health*, 3(1), 39–49.

Sinoff, G., Ore, L., Zlogtogorsky, D. and Tamir, A. (1999). Short Anxiety Screening Test – a brief instrument for detecting anxiety in the elderly. *International Journal of Geriatric Psychiatry*, 14(12), 1062–1071.

Stein, D. J., Fineberg, N. A., Bienvenu, O. J., et al. (2010). Should OCD be classified as an anxiety disorder in DSM-V? *Depression & Anxiety*, 27(6), 495–506.

Tye, K. M., Prakash, R., Kim, S.-Y., et al. (2011). Amygdala circuitry mediating reversible and bidirectional control of anxiety. *Nature*, 471, 358–362.

Whiteford, H. A., Ferrari, A. J., Degenhardt, F. V. and Vos, T. (2015). The global burden of mental, neurological and substance use disorders: An analysis from the Global Burden of Disease Study 2010. *PLoS ONE*, 10(2), e0116820.

World Health Organization (1992). *The ICD-10 Classification of Mental and Behavioural Disorders: Clinical Descriptions and Diagnostic Guidelines*. Geneva: World Health Organization.

Yerkes, R. M. and Dodson, J. D. (1908). The relation of strength of stimulus to rapidity of habit-formation. *Journal of Comparative Neurology and Psychology*, 18, 459–82.

Zhang, X., Norton, J., Carriere, I., Ritchie, K., Chaudieu, I. and Ancelin, M. L. (2015). Risk factors for late-onset generalized anxiety disorder: results from a 12-year prospective cohort (the ESPIRT study). *Translational Psychiatry*, 5, e536.

Epidemiology, Risk and Protective Factors

Gerard J. Byrne and Nancy A. Pachana

Introduction

Anxiety disorders in later life have historically been overshadowed by strong clinical and epidemiological interest in mood disorders and cognitive disorders. This chapter reviews the key scientific literature on the epidemiology of anxiety disorders in older people and putative risk and protective factors.

Methodological Issues

Although a number of important population-based epidemiological studies have yielded data on anxiety symptoms and anxiety disorders in older people, there remain substantial methodological challenges to the interpretation of their findings. The first challenge is that many studies have been underpowered, leading to point estimates with wide confidence intervals (CIs). In most studies, a single diagnostic instrument has been used to generate anxiety diagnoses across a wide age range with little consideration as to whether the instrument is as valid and reliable in advanced old age as it is in young and middle-aged persons.

Additional challenges arise from the use of differing age ranges to represent older people. Some studies have increased their sample sizes and improved the precision of their estimates by including people as young as 50 or 55 years in their cohorts. While this may improve measurement precision, it does so at a cost to the applicability of the findings to genuinely older people. Epidemiological studies that include middle-aged persons are not very useful for clinical or service planning purposes when the focus is on later life. It is not appropriate to compare later-life epidemiological data coming from samples with differing age ranges because there is evidence of age-related differences in anxiety symptoms and in the prevalence and incidence of anxiety disorders (Gonçalves & Byrne, 2012, 2013; Miloyan, Byrne, & Pachana, 2014; Miloyan et al., 2014).

Another source of variation arises from the use of differing sets of diagnostic criteria. Although the Diagnostic and Statistical Manual of Mental Disorders (DSM) (American Psychiatric Association, 2013) is now the most commonly used diagnostic system in research publications, late-life anxiety data have also been collected using International Classification of Diseases (ICD) (World Health Organization, 2018) criteria and using the older Geriatric Mental State/Automatic Geriatric Examination for Computer-Assisted Taxonomy (GMS/AGECAT) system (Copeland & Dewey, 1999). The latter system generates the broad diagnostic category of anxiety neurosis rather than the individual anxiety diagnosis favoured by the DSM and ICD. Even when the same underlying diagnostic system is employed, investigators may choose from a range of diagnostic interviews. Contemporary research relies mainly upon fully structured interviews administered by trained laypersons. Examples include the Comprehensive International Diagnostic Interview (CIDI), the Mini International Neuropsychiatric Interview (MINI), and the Alcohol Use Disorder and Associated Disabilities Interview (AUDADIS). Each of these structured diagnostic interviews uses slightly different approaches to eliciting the symptoms required to meet the criteria for DSM or ICD diagnoses. In addition, each of these instruments has multiple versions.

The main implication of these methodological differences is that estimates of the prevalence and incidence of anxiety disorders among older people are difficult to compare across studies.

Burden of Disease

In both high-income countries and low- and middle-income countries, anxiety disorders ranked sixth among the ten leading causes of years of life lived with disability in 2010 (Baxter et al., 2014). There were substantial variations in rank according to age. Among persons aged 15–49 years anxiety disorders were ranked fourth, whereas among persons aged 50–69 years anxiety disorders were ranked tenth, and among persons aged 70 years and over anxiety disorders were ranked twentieth. Thus, the relative burden of disease associated with anxiety disorders falls with advancing age as the prevalence of other disabling conditions increases.

Overview of Epidemiology

In the Guy's/Age Concern survey conducted in the Lewisham and North Southwark health districts in London (Lindesay, Briggs, & Murphy, 1989), 890 people aged 65 years and over were interviewed with a structured schedule. The prevalence of generalized anxiety was 3.7% and phobic anxiety was 10.0%.

The Longitudinal Aging Study Amsterdam (LASA) investigated the prevalence of anxiety disorders in a random community sample of 3,107 people aged 55–85 years in the Netherlands (Beekman et al., 1998). The overall prevalence of anxiety disorders was estimated at 10.2%. At six-year follow-up, just under one in four of those with an anxiety disorder at baseline still met the diagnostic criteria, although almost half had subclinical anxiety symptoms. In those with persistent anxiety disorder, benzodiazepine use was high, but use of mental healthcare and antidepressants was low (Schuurmans et al., 2005).

Bryant, Jackson, and Ames (2008) reviewed the prevalence of anxiety disorders in older people in studies published between 1980 and 2007 and found that prevalence estimates varied between 1.2% and 15.0% in community samples of adults aged 60 years and over.

Using data from the Burden of Disease study, Baxter et al. (2013) reported that the global current prevalence of anxiety disorders was 7.3% (95% CI: 4.8–10.9%). To obtain this estimate, they combined estimates of point prevalence, one-month prevalence, and three-month prevalence from 87 studies conducted in 44 countries. They found a higher prevalence estimate in Euro/Anglo cultures (10.4%; 95% CI: 7.0–15.5%) than in African cultures (5.3%; 95% CI: 3.5–8.1%). In a multivariate model, the adjusted odds ratio (OR) for persons aged 55 years and over was 0.8 (95% CI: 0.7–0.9%), with a predicted current prevalence of 6.7% (95% CI: 4.4–10.1%). The authors did not provide estimates for any other older age categories.

Population-Based Prevalence Estimates

We found eight population studies that reported prevalence estimates for any anxiety disorder in older people (Andreas et al., 2017; Byers et al., 2010; Byrne, 2013; Fung et al., 2017; Grenier et al., 2011; Kang et al., 2016; Prina et al., 2011; Reynolds et al., 2015).

As noted above, it is difficult to compare prevalence estimates from different studies due to the use of differing diagnostic instruments, differing diagnostic systems, and differing age ranges. In addition, the inclusion of differing sets of anxiety disorders within the rubric of 'any anxiety disorder' further complicates comparisons between studies.

In high-income regions, including the United States, Canada, Europe, Australia, and the Republic of Korea, 12-month prevalence estimates for any anxiety disorder in older people, based mainly on DSM-IV criteria, varied from 4.3% to 11.4%. These estimates come from studies that varied in the age ranges covered and the conditions included in estimates of any anxiety disorder.

Andreas et al. (2017) studied a random sample of 3,142 people aged 65–84 years from Italy, Spain, England, Germany, Israel, and Switzerland using the fully structured Composite International Diagnostic Interview 65+ (CIDI65+) diagnostic interview. They reported 12-month and lifetime prevalence estimates for agoraphobia, panic disorder, post-traumatic stress disorder, simple phobia, and any anxiety disorder. They did not report prevalence estimates for generalized anxiety disorder or social phobia, and it is not clear from their paper whether these conditions were included in their estimate of the prevalence of any anxiety disorder.

In a subsequent report based on the same study, a more complete set of prevalence data was provided (Canuto et al., 2018). After adjustment for site, age, and sex, the overall 12-month prevalence of any anxiety disorder was 17.3% (95% CI: 14.0–20.4%), with the prevalence being significantly greater in females than males (23.5% vs 9.5%; $F_{1,20} = 143.2$, $p < 0.001$). The adjusted prevalence estimates for individual anxiety disorders were as follows: agoraphobia 4.9% (95% CI: 3.3–6.6%), panic disorder 3.8% (95% CI: 2.6–5.0%), generalized anxiety disorder 3.1% (95% CI: 1.9–4.3%), post-traumatic stress disorder 1.4% (95% CI: 0.4–2.4%), social phobia 1.3% (95% CI: 0.6–2.1%), and obsessive-compulsive disorder 0.8% (95% CI: 0.3–1.4%). Prevalence estimates for simple phobia were provided by type: animal phobia 3.5% (95% CI: 2.5–4.6%), environmental phobia 3.3% (95% CI: 2.1–4.4%), blood injection phobia 1.7% (95% CI: 1.1–2.4%), and situation phobia 3.0% (95% CI: 2.0–4.0%). Canuto et al. (2018) also reported a linear trend for decreased prevalence of any anxiety disorder with age: 65–69 years 20.6%, 70–74 years 19.3%, 75–79 years 13.7%, and 80+ years 12.4% ($F_{1,20} = 20.9$, $p < 0.001$).

In the United States, Byers et al. (2010), using data from the National Comorbidity Survey – Replication (NCS-R) study, found that the 12-month prevalence estimates for any DSM-IV anxiety disorder in persons aged 55 years and over were 7.6% in males and 14.7% in females.

In another report from the United States, Reynolds et al. (2015), using data from 12,312 persons aged 55 years and over participating in the National Epidemiologic Survey on Alcohol and Related Disorders – II (NESARC-II) study, found a 12-month weighted prevalence estimate for any DSM-IV anxiety disorder of 11.4%. In this analysis, prevalence estimates for individual anxiety disorders were as follows: panic disorder 1.4%, social phobia 1.5%, specific phobia 5.8%, generalized anxiety disorder 2.8%, and post-traumatic stress disorder 3.5%. Among this nationally representative sample of community-residing individuals, the likelihood of having a diagnosis of an anxiety disorder in the past year varied with age. Compared to the oldest-old (85+ years) reference group, those aged 55–64 years had an OR for any anxiety disorder of 2.26, those aged 65–74 years had an OR of 1.3, and those aged 75–84 years had an OR of 1.19. Only the CI for the OR for the young-old (those aged 55–64 years) did not overlap with unity and was statistically significant.

The prevalence of anxiety symptoms and disorders among older people in nursing homes and other residential aged care facilities has been reviewed by Creighton, Davison, and Kissane (2016). They found nine studies that estimated the prevalence of anxiety *symptoms* in people living in residential aged care facilities. These prevalence estimates varied between 6.5% and 58.4%, although the prevalence of clinically significant anxiety varied between 6.5% and 29.7%. Studies with larger sample sizes tended to give higher prevalence estimates. These investigators also found nine studies that estimated the overall prevalence of anxiety *disorders* in residential aged care facilities. Prevalence estimates varied between 3.2% and 20.0% (Creighton et al., 2016). Studies with better methodologies and larger sample sizes tended to give lower prevalence estimates.

Population-Based Incidence Estimates

The incidence of anxiety disorders in older people has not often been estimated in population-based surveys, although incidence studies provide a more robust basis for risk factor identification than prevalence studies.

The Enquête sur la Santé des Aînés (ESA) study was conducted in 2,784 community-dwelling persons aged 65 years and over living in Quebec, Canada (Préville et al., 2010). Diagnostic interviews employed the ESA-Q, a computer-assisted instrument similar to the Diagnostic Interview Schedule (DIS) and the Composite International Diagnostic Interview (CIDI). The overall one-year incidence of any DSM-IV anxiety disorder was found to be 2.3% (standard error (SE) 0.38). The one-year incidence rates for individual anxiety disorders were as follows: generalized anxiety disorder 0.8% (SE 0.20), panic disorder 0.1% (SE 0.07), specific phobia 1.1% (SE 0.21), social phobia 0.3% (SE 0.12), agoraphobia without panic disorder 0.4% (SE 0.13), and obsessive-compulsive disorder 0.3% (SE 0.12).

Using data from the United States, Chou et al. (2011) reported three-year weighted incidence estimates among 8,012 persons aged 60 years and over for selected DSM-IV anxiety disorders based on NESARC-II interviews employing the Alcohol Use Disorder and Associated Disabilities Interview Schedule – DSM-IV (AUDADIS-IV). The weighted incidence estimates were as follows: panic disorder 0.76% (SE 0.13), specific phobia 1.35% (SE 0.17), social phobia 0.58% (SE 0.10), and generalized anxiety disorder 1.63% (SE 0.18). These authors did not provide estimates of the incidence of agoraphobia, obsessive-compulsive disorder, or post-traumatic stress disorder, or an overall estimate of the incidence of anxiety disorders as a group.

In the Kwangju study from the Republic of Korea, Kang et al. (2016) found a two-year incidence of anxiety neurosis in 909 persons aged 65 years and over of 6.7% using the GMS/AGECAT diagnostic system. These authors did not report the incidence of individual anxiety disorders.

Cultural Differences

Cultural differences are another source of epidemiological variation. As Hofmann and Hinton (2014) have noted, cross-cultural comparisons of the prevalence of anxiety disorders are challenging because of differences in language and assessment instruments and differences in culturally specific political, geographical, and socio-demographic contexts. There may also be differences in the constructs underlying particular anxiety disorders or particular anxiety symptoms.

In an attempt to overcome some of these challenges, Asnaani et al. (2010) examined cross-ethnic lifetime prevalence rates for anxiety disorders among English-speaking adults from different ethnic backgrounds residing in the United States. They used data from the Collaborative Psychiatric Epidemiology Survey (CPES), which amalgamated data from three separate epidemiologic surveys with similar methodologies. Findings from older adults were not reported separately. The CPES sampled the following groups, oversampling ethnic minorities (count, mean age, percentage female): White Americans (6,870, 46.5 years, 54.3%), African Americans (4,598, 42.7 years, 63.9%), Hispanic Americans (3,615, 39.7 years, 55.8%), and Asian Americans (1,628, 42.2 years, 53.2%). There were lower rates of social anxiety disorder, generalized anxiety disorder, panic disorder, and post-traumatic stress disorder among Asian Americans than among any other ethnic group. White Americans had higher rates of social anxiety disorder, generalized anxiety disorder, and panic disorder than African Americans, Hispanic Americans, and Asian Americans. African Americans had higher rates of post-traumatic stress disorder than Asian Americans or Hispanic Americans.

It is unclear from these findings whether degree of acculturation is a risk factor for anxiety disorder across ethnic groups. Work by Breslau et al. (2007) in immigrants and their US-born descendants based on the NCS-R suggests that risk of psychiatric disorder rises shortly after migration. The authors posit that this might be due to post-migration experiences or to early socialization effects.

One study that did report transcultural prevalence estimates for anxiety disorder in older people used data from the 10/66 survey (Prina et al., 2011). This ambitious study investigated the one-month prevalence of anxiety neurosis using the GMS/AGECAT diagnostic system in persons aged 65 years and over at 11 sites in 7 low- and middle-income countries. Prevalence estimates in China, Cuba, Dominican Republic, India, Mexico, Peru, and Venezuela varied between 0.1% and 9.6%. In China, India, Mexico, and Peru, rural areas had lower prevalence estimates than urban areas. The prevalence estimates in older people in China (urban 0.2%; rural 0.1%) are so low as to raise questions about the cultural validity of the Western concept of anxiety disorder there.

The MentDis_ICF65+ study reported findings from five European countries and Israel (Canuto et al., 2018). After Bonferroni correction (critical value of $\alpha = 0.007$), there was no significant difference in the 12-month prevalence of any anxiety disorder across the six centres ($F_{5,16} = 3.4$, $p = 0.028$). However, agoraphobia, panic disorder, and social phobia were more prevalent in London (England) and post-traumatic stress disorder was more prevalent in Jerusalem (Israel).

Overall, these transcultural findings are fascinating and certainly suggest the presence of substantial differences in the prevalence of anxiety disorders across cultures, including in older people. In Chapter 5, Xiaoping Lin and Charissa Hosseini deal in more detail with cross-cultural dimensions of anxiety in later life.

Risk and Protective Factors

Most of the population-based epidemiological surveys of anxiety disorders in older people have generated prevalence estimates rather than incidence estimates and have reported only a limited range of variables that might permit consideration of risk and protective factors.

Clinical studies of anxiety symptoms and anxiety disorders in older people allow consideration of risk and protective factors, but limit generalizability to the setting in which the data have been collected.

Using data from the Kwangju study in the Republic of Korea, Kang et al. (2016) investigated factors associated with the prevalence, incidence, and persistence of anxiety disorders in people aged 65 years and over using a multivariate model. Prevalent anxiety disorders were associated with rented housing, physical inactivity, depression, insomnia, and cognitive impairment. Incident anxiety disorders were associated with physical inactivity and insomnia. Persistent anxiety disorders (present at both baseline and follow-up) were associated with rented housing, stressful life events, and depression. These authors noted that anxiety *symptoms* were associated with different sets of factors from anxiety *disorders*.

Using data from the NESARC-II study in the United States, Chou et al. (2011) investigated whether certain health indicators (obesity, pain, self-rated health, number of medical conditions, presence of psychosis) or stressful life events were associated with *incident* anxiety disorders in 8,012 persons aged 60 years and over using a multivariate model. They found no such associations.

Using data from the same study, Mackenzie et al. (2014) investigated the prevalence and predictors of persistent and remitting anxiety disorders. These investigators used data from 1,994 persons aged 55 years and over who had a 12-month mental disorder at Wave 1 of NESARC and who participated in Wave 2 of NESARC. The presence of any persistent anxiety disorder was predicted by the mental component score of the 12-item Short Form Health Survey (SF-12; Ware et al., 1996), by the presence of any personality disorder, and by any past-year mood disorder. Persistent panic disorder was predicted by the physical component score of the SF-12 and by a lifetime history of suicide attempts. Social phobia was predicted by lifetime anxiety treatment.

Using data from the Enquête de Santé Psychologique – Risques, Incidence et Traitement (ESPRIT) study, a prospective cohort study in France, Zhang et al. (2015) investigated risk factors for *incident* generalized anxiety disorder in 1,711 participants aged 65 years and over who were free of generalized anxiety disorder at baseline. Participants were randomly recruited from electoral rolls and examined at baseline and on five subsequent occasions over 12 years. The investigators generated DSM-IV diagnoses using the MINI, which were validated by a clinical panel. Over the follow-up period, 8.4% of the participants developed incident generalized anxiety disorder, 80% of which were first episodes. Independent risk factors for incident generalized anxiety disorder derived from a multivariate Cox model were as follows: female gender, recent adverse life events, chronic physical and mental disorders, poverty, parental loss or separation, low affective support during childhood, and parental mental illness. It is unclear why the findings from this French study differed substantially from those of the US study of Chou et al. (2011).

Almeida et al. (2012) investigated associations of persisting anxiety *symptoms* over two years in 20,036 people aged 60 years and over attending Australian primary care physicians. The large sample size gave sufficient statistical power to examine a wide range of associations. Clinically significant anxiety was defined as a self-rated score of 11 or more on the anxiety subscale of the Hospital Anxiety and Depression Scale (HADS-A) and persistent anxiety was defined as a HADS-A score of 11 or more at baseline and at 24 months. Clinically significant anxiety at baseline was associated with a number of socio-demographic and lifestyle factors: younger age, female gender, migrant status, no post-school education, physical inactivity, risky alcohol consumption, poor social support, financial strain, and childhood physical abuse. It was also associated with several clinical factors: past anxiety disorder, past depressive disorder, pain, poor perceived health, and use of antidepressants or benzodiazepines. Being overweight or obese was protective. Persistent anxiety was associated with younger age, female gender, being married, no post-school education, poor social support, financial strain, past depressive disorder, past anxiety disorder, pain, and poor perceived health.

Co-morbidity among Anxiety Disorders

Co-morbidity among DSM-IV anxiety disorders in 8,012 people aged 60 years and over was examined by Chou et al. (2011) using data from NESARC-II. Baseline panic disorder was associated with incident social phobia at three years post-baseline (OR: 9.6; 95% CI: 2.7–33.9). Baseline post-traumatic stress disorder was associated with incident panic disorder (OR: 7.7; 95% CI: 1.8–32.5), incident specific phobia (OR: 3.1; 95% CI: 1.1–9.2), and incident generalized anxiety disorder (OR: 3.4; 95% CI: 1.4–8.2) at three years post-baseline.

Co-morbidity with Depression

In the multisite MentDis_ICF65+ study, Canuto et al. (2018) found that panic disorder (OR: 2.54; 95% CI: 1.71–3.76) and specific phobia (OR: 2.37; 95% CI: 1.31–4.27) but not the other anxiety disorders predicted cross-sectional major depressive disorder.

Anxiety Associated with Other Conditions

Anxiety symptoms and anxiety disorders are associated with a range of general medical conditions (Gonçalves, Pachana, & Byrne, 2011; Vancampfort et al., 2017). For example, there appears to be a strong association between idiopathic Parkinson's disease and anxiety, with 25% of a clinical sample of people with Parkinson's disease meeting DSM-IV criteria for an anxiety disorder (Dissanayaka et al., 2010). In the LASA, older people with intellectual disability (IQ < 70) reported more anxiety symptoms on the HADS than older people with normal intelligence (Hermans et al., 2014). Anxiety in older people is also associated with an increased risk for subsequent dementia. The pattern of the association suggests that anxiety is a prodromal symptom of dementia rather than a cause of dementia (Gulpers et al., 2016) and that it is associated with conversion from mild cognitive impairment to dementia (Li & Li, 2017).

Summary

Anxiety symptoms and anxiety disorders are highly prevalent in later life, although they are less prevalent than in middle age. There is a relative paucity of epidemiological data on anxiety in people aged 80 years and over, so it is not entirely clear whether rates of anxiety rise after this age. Although most anxiety disorders in older people appear to have their onset earlier in life, there is evidence that most incident anxiety disorders in later life represent new-onset cases rather than the re-emergence of early-onset cases. Anxiety disorders predict the future development of other anxiety disorders. There is divided opinion about risk and protective factors for late-life anxiety disorders, but stressful life events both recent and remote appear relevant, as do indicators of socio-economic status and general physical health.

References

Almeida, O. P., Draper, B., Pirkis, J., et al. (2012). Anxiety, depression, and comorbid anxiety and depression: risk factors and outcome over two years. *International Psychogeriatrics*, **24**(10), 1622–1632.

American Psychiatric Association (2013). *Diagnostic and Statistical Manual of Mental Disorders*, 5th ed. Washington, DC: American Psychiatric Association.

Andreas, S., Schulz, H., Volkert, J., et al. (2017). Prevalence of mental disorders in elderly people: the European MentDis_ICF65+ study. *British Journal of Psychiatry*, **210**(2), 125–131.

Asnaani, A., Richey, J. A., Dimaite, R., Hinton, D. E. and Hofmann, S. G. (2010). A cross-ethnic comparison of lifetime prevalence rates of anxiety disorders. *Journal of Nervous and Mental Disorders*, **198**, 551–555.

Baxter, A. J., Scott, K. M., Vos, T. and Whiteford, H. A. (2013). Global prevalence of anxiety disorders: a systematic review and meta-regression. *Psychological Medicine*, **43**(5), 897–910.

Baxter, A. J., Vos, T., Scott, K. M., Ferrari, A. J. and Whiteford, H. A. (2014). The global burden of anxiety disorders in 2010. *Psychological Medicine*, **44**, 2363–2374.

Beekman, A. T., Bremmer, M. A., Deeg, D. J., et al. (1998). Anxiety disorders in later life: a report from the Longitudinal Aging Study Amsterdam. *International Journal of Geriatric Psychiatry*, **13**(1), 717–726.

Breslau, J., Aguilar-Gaxiola, S., Borges, G., Kendler, K. S., Su, M. and Kessler, R. C. (2007). Risk for psychiatric disorder among immigrants and their US-born descendants: evidence from the National Comorbidity Survey – Replication. *Journal of Nervous and Mental Disorders*, **195**, 189–195.

Bryant, C., Jackson, H. and Ames, D. (2008). The prevalence of anxiety in older adults: methodological issues and a review of the literature. *Journal of Affective Disorders*, **109**, 233–250.

Byers, A. L., Yaffe, K., Covinsky, K. E., Friedman, B. M. and Bruce, M. L. (2010). High occurrence of mood and anxiety disorders among older adults: the National Comorbidity Survey Replication. *Archives of General Psychiatry*, **67**(5), 489–496.

Byrne, G. J. (2013). Anxiety disorders in older people. In T. Denning and A. Thomas, eds., *The Oxford Textbook of Old Age Psychiatry*, 2nd ed. Oxford: Oxford University Press, pp. 589–602.

Canuto, A., Weber, K., Bartschi, M., et al. (2018). Anxiety disorders in old age: psychiatric comorbidities, quality of life, and prevalence according to age, gender, and country. *American Journal of Geriatric Psychiatry*, **26**(2), 174–185.

Chou, K. L., Mackenzie, C. S., Liang, K. and Sareen, J. (2011). Three-year incidence and predictors of first-onset of DSM-IV mood, anxiety, and substance use disorders in older adults: results from Wave 2 of the National Epidemiologic Survey on Alcohol and Related Conditions. *Journal of Clinical Psychiatry*, **72**(2), 144–155.

Copeland, J. and Dewey, M. (1999). The AGECAT system. www.researchgate.net/publication/2512924_The_AGECAT_system (last accessed 24 July 2018).

Creighton, A. S., Davison, T. E. and Kissane, D. W. (2016). The prevalence of anxiety among older adults in nursing homes and other residential aged care facilities: a systematic review. *International Journal of Geriatric Psychiatry*, **31**(6), 555–566.

Dissanayaka, N. N., Sellbach, A., Matheson, S., et al. (2010). Anxiety disorders in Parkinson's disease: prevalence and risk factors. *Movement Disorders*, **25**(7), 838–845.

Fung, A. W., Chan, W. C., Wong, C. S., et al. (2017). Prevalence of anxiety disorders in community dwelling older adults in Hong Kong. *International Psychogeriatrics*, **29**(2), 259–267.

Gonçalves, D. C. and Byrne, G. J. (2012). Sooner or later: age at onset of generalized anxiety disorder in older adults. *Depression & Anxiety*, **29**(1), 39–46.

Gonçalves, D. C. and Byrne, G. J. (2013). Who worries most? Worry prevalence and patterns across the lifespan. *International Journal of Geriatric Psychiatry*, 28(1), 41–49.

Gonçalves, D. C., Pachana, N. P. and Byrne, G. J. (2011). Prevalence and correlates of generalized anxiety disorder among older adults in the Australian National Survey of Mental Health and Well-Being. *Journal of Affective Disorders*, 132, 223–230.

Grenier, S., Préville, M., Boyer, R., et al. (2011). The impact of DSM-IV symptom and clinical significance criteria on the prevalence estimates of subthreshold and threshold anxiety in the older adult population. *American Journal of Psychiatry*, 19(4), 316–326.

Gulpers, B., Ramakers, I., Hamel, R., Kohler, S., Oude Voshaar, R. and Verhey, F. (2016). Anxiety as a predictor for cognitive decline and dementia: a systematic review and meta-analysis. *American Journal of Geriatric Psychiatry*, 24(10), 823–842.

Hermans, H., Beekman, A. T. and Evenhuis, H. M. (2014). Comparison of anxiety as reported by older people with intellectual disabilities and by older people with normal intelligence. *American Journal of Geriatric Psychiatry*, 22(12), 1391–1398.

Hofmann, S. G. and Hinton, D. E. (2014). Cross-cultural aspects of anxiety disorders. *Current Psychiatry Reports*, 16(6), 450.

Kang, H. J., Bae, K. Y., Kim, S. W., Shin, I. S., Yoon, J. S. and Kim, J. M. (2016). Anxiety symptoms in Korean elderly individuals: a two-year longitudinal community study. *International Psychogeriatrics*, 28(3), 423–433.

Li, X. X. and Li, Z. (2017). The impact of anxiety on the progression of mild cognitive impairment to dementia in Chinese and English databases: a systematic review and meta-analysis. *International Journal of Geriatric Psychiatry*, 33(1), 131–140.

Lindesay, J., Briggs, K. and Murphy, E. (1989). The Guy's/Age Concern survey. Prevalence rates of cognitive impairment, depression and anxiety in an urban elderly community. *British Journal of Psychiatry*, 155, 317–329.

Mackenzie, C. S., El-Gabalawy, R., Chou, K. L. and Sareen, J. (2014). Prevalence and predictors of persistent versus remitting mood, anxiety, and substance disorders in a national sample of older adults. *American Journal of Psychiatry*, 22(9), 854–865.

Miloyan, B., Byrne, G. J. and Pachana, N. A. (2014). Age-related changes in generalized anxiety disorder symptoms. *International Psychogeriatrics*, 26(4), 565–572.

Miloyan, B., Bulley, A., Pachana, N. A. and Byrne, G. J. (2014). Social phobia symptoms across the adult lifespan. *Journal of Affective Disorders*, 16, 86–90.

Préville, M., Boyer, R., Vasiliadis, H. M., et al. (2010). Scientific Committee of the ESA Study. One-year incidence of psychiatric disorders in Quebec's older adult population. *Canadian Journal of Psychiatry*, 55(7), 449–457.

Prina, A. M., Ferri, C. P., Guerra, M., Brayne, C. and Prince, M. (2011). Prevalence of anxiety and its correlates among older adults in Latin America, India and China: cross-cultural study. *British Journal of Psychiatry*, 199(6), 485–491.

Reynolds, K., Pietrzak, R. H., El-Gabalawy, R., Mackenzie, C. S. and Sareen, J. (2015). Prevalence of psychiatric disorders in U.S. older adults: findings from a nationally representative survey. *World Psychiatry*, 14(1), 74–81.

Schuurmans, J., Comijs, H. C., Beekman, A. T., et al. (2005). The outcomes of anxiety disorders in older people at 6-year follow-up: results from the Longitudinal Aging Study Amsterdam. *Acta Psychiatrica Scandinavica*, 111(6), 420–428.

Vancampfort, D., Koyanagi, A., Hallgren, M., Probst, M. and Stubbs, B. (2017). The relationship between chronic physical conditions, multimorbidity and anxiety in the general population: a global perspective across 42 countries. *General Hospital Psychiatry*, 45, 1–6.

Ware, J. E. J., Kosinski, M. and Keller, S. D. (1996). A 12-item Short-Form Health Survey:

construction of scales and preliminary tests of reliability and validity. *Medical Care*, **34**, 220–233.

World Health Organization (2018). *International Classification of Diseases*, 11th revision. Geneva: World Health Organization Press.

Zhang, X., Norton, J., Carriere, I., Ritchie, K., Chaudieu, I. and Ancelin, M. L. (2015). Risk factors for late-onset generalized anxiety disorder: results from a 12-year prospective cohort (the ESPIRT study). *Translational Psychiatry*, **5**, e536.

Diagnosis of Anxiety Disorders in Older Adults

Christina Bryant

Debates about diagnosis in psychiatry and clinical psychology are both ever-present and controversial. They have gained greater prominence in the context of the publication of the fifth edition of the Diagnostic and Statistical Manual (DSM-5) of the American Psychiatric Association (2013). On the one hand, some authors are concerned that diagnostic processes impose unhelpful labels on human experience and lead to an over-reliance on their imperfect categories (Healy, 2011), while others suggest that the importance of diagnosis is growing rather than diminishing (Craddock & Mynors-Wallis, 2014). It is well documented that there are a number of features of anxiety disorders in older adults that pose specific challenges to both recognition and diagnosis (Bryant, 2010). This chapter considers some of the factors that make the diagnosis of anxiety disorders particularly complex in older adults. It proposes that a therapeutically useful approach to diagnosis in this context must go beyond mere consideration of diagnostic criteria to an attempt at a much broader formulation. This formulation needs to take into account the cultural, cohort-specific, and developmental challenges of ageing. It is suggested that one helpful perspective in this context is the Contextual Adult Lifespan Theory for Adapting Psychotherapy (CALTAP) model, developed as a way of conceptualizing psychological work with older clients (Knight & Pachana, 2015). First, however, we return to the broad question of the nature and importance of diagnosis.

The Importance of Diagnosis

The publication in 2013 of the DSM-5 (American Psychiatric Association, 2013) both reflected old controversies about diagnosis and triggered new debates about the place of diagnosis in psychiatry and psychology. The DSM-5 itself has been roundly criticized for medicalizing normal experience (Gornall, 2013) and for the apparently inflated role of the pharmaceutical industry and specialized interest groups in the 'creation' of new diagnostic entities, such as premenstrual dysphoric disorder (Frances & Widiger, 2012). Moreover, attempts to move away from purely categorical ways of defining personality disorders to a more dimensional system were a very public failure (Shedler et al., 2010). The upshot appears to be something of a crisis of confidence in relation to psychiatric diagnosis (Craddock & Mynors-Wallis, 2014), which has perhaps also created an opportunity to arrive at a more balanced perspective on the utility of psychiatric diagnosis. Craddock and Mynors-Wallis (2014) proposed that psychiatric diagnosis is both impersonal and imperfect, but also important.

One of the fundamental problems with psychiatric diagnosis – in contrast to the diagnosis of physical ailments – is that it is based on the observation of behaviours and self-reported symptoms. Currently, there are few direct measures of brain functioning that aid the diagnosis of psychological symptoms such as depression and anxiety. This gives rise to one of the difficulties at the heart of the DSM: namely, whether an observed cluster of symptoms (or syndrome) maps sufficiently well onto the 'diagnostic criteria' for a particular disorder to justify regarding it as a case, say, of social anxiety disorder, a problem that is particularly common in older adults. For example, Flint has argued that a common constellation of anxious symptoms in older adults is the experience of anxious mood, being unable to relax, and the presence of somatic complaints such as dizziness and feeling shaky or nauseous (Flint, 2005). Yet, this combination of symptoms does not map onto any single anxiety disorder in the DSM-5.

Nevertheless, diagnosis is indisputably important. As Craddock and Mynors-Wallis (2014) argue, it is important for communication between clinicians and for treatment planning. It is also increasingly important to clients themselves, serving purposes as diverse as providing reassurance that their situation is not unique, providing hope that a condition is treatable, and perhaps allaying fears or shame that their symptoms are a result of a moral failing or weakness. Having a shared diagnosis may also encourage support amongst people with similar symptoms and enable clients to seek out appropriate information and education (Craddock & Mynors-Wallis, 2014).

It is clear that psychiatric diagnosis is far from perfect and that it behoves all clinicians to take a critical perspective with regard to their approach to this core clinical activity. Used carefully, diagnosis can open the way to effective treatments and de-stigmatization. We need to be aware of its limitations, however, and not be afraid to enhance its utility by assessing not just symptoms, but also their context, their specific features, and how they affect day-to-day functioning. This poses particular challenges in the older adult.

Challenges in Diagnosing Anxiety Disorders in Older Adults

At the outset, it is important to note that when we talk about 'older adults' or 'old age', we are referring to a period of enormous heterogeneity (Zarit & Zarit, 2012). Potentially encompassing a period of 40 years or more from the age of 60 upwards, there are likely to be significant differences in the health and well-being of the typical 65-year-old and that of their 85-year-old counterpart. This degree of heterogeneity makes the experience of anxiety across older individuals more variable and idiosyncratic. Moreover, there are also significant variations between older individuals of the same chronological age, such that some 75-year-olds have few age-related impairments and remain physically and socially active, while other 75-year-olds have experienced significant physical and/or cognitive declines with associated loss of role functioning and quality of life. This may be one of the many reasons that anxiety disorders tend to be under-diagnosed in older adults (Bryant, 2010).

Before a diagnosis can be made, however, detection and recognition of symptoms has to take place, but this, too, is less likely to occur in older adults. The reasons for this are varied, but they include a lower likelihood that general practitioners (GPs; primary care physicians) will enquire about anxiety symptoms (perhaps through having a greater focus on dementia and depression) and the fact that older people themselves are less likely to volunteer information about anxiety symptoms. One factor may be their greater ease of avoidance of situations that could provoke anxiety (Mohlman et al., 2012a). For example, an older person may find that impaired hearing leads to anxiety in social situations, which are then avoided; age-related stereotyping may lead well-meaning friends and relatives to explain this as expected behaviour for somebody of their age. In this way, a cycle of anxiety, avoidance and decline in social participation can quickly set in and remain unchallenged unless detailed enquiry is made about the underlying reasons for the activity avoidance.

There is no doubt that stigma remains a major barrier to the diagnosis of anxiety disorders in older adults. Although the baby boomers are now reaching old age with higher awareness of mental illness and its treatment (Karel et al., 2012), older adults in the 70-plus age group may be less aware of these issues and may see them as a moral failing rather than as treatable conditions (Knight & Pachana, 2015). The tendency to stoicism sometimes seen in older people (Bei et al., 2013) may also hold back help-seeking and lead to symptoms not being regarded as 'excessive' – a key criterion for the diagnosis of most anxiety disorders. Finally, different use of language to describe symptoms of anxiety creates a further barrier to the detection of anxiety in older adults. It may be, then, that before the question of diagnosis even arises, older adults have fallen at the first hurdle: namely, detection and recognition of symptoms.

The second broad challenge in relation to the diagnosis of anxiety is that its presentation may be different in older adults at a both a quantitative and qualitative level. With regard to the former, older adults are more likely than younger adults to experience anxiety disorders at a sub-threshold level because they do not meet certain diagnostic criteria (Jeste et al., 2005; see also Chapter 4 in this volume). This can be illustrated by a study by Karlsson et al. (2009), who compared the prevalence of social anxiety depending on the application or suspension of DSM-IV criteria in a sample of 914 community-dwelling older adults. The full criteria for social anxiety include (1) a fear of social situations, which (2) needs to be experienced as excessive or unreasonable, (3) avoidance of those situations or tolerance of them with great difficulty or distress, and (4) social consequences of this distress. When these criteria were strictly applied, the prevalence of DSM-IV social anxiety was 1.86%, but this increased substantially when the criteria were relaxed. 'Broadly defined social anxiety', which meant the lifting of the 'excessiveness' criterion, and the presence of symptoms (1), (3) and (4), had a prevalence of around 4%, while fear of social situations only had a prevalence of around 9%. In a similar vein, a study by Creamer and Parslow (2008) based on data from the Australian National Survey of Mental Health on a sample of 1,792 community-residing individuals aged 65–85 years showed that 11.7% of men and 8.6% of women reported re-experiencing symptoms associated with past events, yet only 0.4% met criteria for post-traumatic stress disorder (PTSD). Without further assessment, it is not possible to evaluate the functional impact of these symptom levels, but both of these studies illustrate the high prevalence of symptoms that do not meet diagnostic criteria, but could arguably restrict functioning.

A further challenge to the diagnosis of anxiety in older adults is that of co-morbidity with physical illness, an important issue given the potential consequences of anxiety on the outcomes of medical illnesses and the benefits of addressing both physical and mental health concerns (Bryant et al., 2013). While it may appear an obvious statement, it should be noted that the presence of a medical illness does not preclude the existence of co-morbid anxiety that can exacerbate functional decline and increase the use of health services (Yohannes et al., 2000). Many older adults experience physical health problems and/or take medications that may mimic, mask, or exacerbate anxiety symptoms. The medical and anxiety symptoms can be hard to distinguish, however, such as in the case of diabetes and thyroid disease and the use of corticosteroids. Even if certain somatic symptoms, like shortness of breath, are directly attributable to a medical condition, pathological behaviours in response to those symptoms may not be. For example, a patient with chronic obstructive pulmonary disease may develop agoraphobic avoidance of situations that physiologically do not cause panic, such as wearing certain clothing or spending time in smaller rooms within the home (Bryant et al., 2013).

These complex relationships between physical and psychological symptoms can make it hard to disentangle physical from psychological distress. The first step in overcoming this is to be aware of the potential relationships between physical and psychological symptoms. The next step is to pursue lines of enquiry that can help to distinguish symptoms of anxiety from physiological manifestations of illnesses or their treatment. Useful questions may include whether the anxiety predates or follows the onset of the medical condition, whether there are other life events that could account for increased anxiety, and whether recently started medications are known to have side effects that mimic anxiety symptoms.

A further issue with regard to the diagnosis of anxiety in older adults is the co-morbidity of anxiety with dementia. Research in this area is sparse, possibly because of the lack of valid criteria and measures for diagnosing anxiety in people with dementia (Shankar et al., 1999). The course of anxiety in dementia appears to be complex, and some studies suggest that anxiety is more common in people with vascular dementia than those with an Alzheimer's pathology (Seignourel et al., 2008). Assessment of anxiety in dementia will require careful questioning of the relative chronologies of the cognitive and anxiety symptoms, as well as seeking corroboration from somebody who knows the patient well. The individual's own understanding and insight into their cognitive impairment may also be informative, as it is likely that anxious worry decreases as insight declines, when behavioural manifestations of anxiety such as agitation become more common (Bierman et al., 2007).

A final issue with regard to the diagnosis of anxiety in older adults is that of commonly occurring anxieties that do not map well onto existing DSM-5 criteria. Perhaps the most important example of this is the anxiety commonly known as fear of falling. Said to be the most commonly occurring fear of older adults, with a prevalence of up to 54% in community-dwelling older adults (Lachman et al., 1998), this fear is characterized by physiological arousal when confronted by the feared situation and marked avoidance of such situations. Despite the obvious similarities with phobic disorders, few older people would be classified as having a phobia in the DSM-5. One reason for this is that most older adults would not describe their fear as being out of proportion to the situation. Gagnon et al. (2005) found that among a sample of 48 people with fear of falling, most of whom manifested moderate avoidance, only one deemed their anxiety to be excessive. Thus, the remaining 47 failed to meet criteria for a phobic disorder. This is an example of an age-specific fear that 'falls through the cracks' of the DSM classification system (Bryant et al., 2013).

Finally, it should be noted that a number of changes were made to the DSM-5 criteria (American Psychiatric Association, 2013). First, there were some conceptual changes resulting in obsessive–compulsive disorder (OCD) being removed from the section on anxiety disorders and placed in a new section for obsessive–compulsive and related disorders. These share difficulties with impulse control and include conditions such as trichotillomania and hoarding disorder. Similarly, PTSD was removed from the chapter on anxiety disorders and is now part of a chapter for trauma- and stressor-related disorders. These have in common that exposure to an identified traumatic event is an explicit and necessary diagnostic criterion. Other changes to the DSM criteria that may prove beneficial for older adults include removal of the 'excessiveness' criterion for specific phobias and social anxiety disorder and the replacement of this with the term 'out of proportion to'.

A further potentially important change is that the text of the DSM-5 now includes guidance as to the recognition of these disorders in older adults, stating, for example, that co-morbid illness and changes to the social environment constitute challenges to the detection of social anxiety in older adults. Until now, the text has included guidance on diagnostic challenges in relation to children and adolescents, but no supplementary information on issues of relevance to older adults. These changes may help to increase awareness of these conditions as experienced by older adults, thereby increasing their detection.

Screening for Anxiety: Which Instruments Are Most Helpful?

Given the complexities in diagnosing anxiety just outlined, we now turn to a discussion of the clinical processes involved. We start by considering the role of screening instruments, considering their strengths and shortcomings, then we discuss approaches to clinical interviewing with older adults, and we conclude by proposing that formulation using the CALTAP model is a useful adjunct to diagnosis.

In clinical settings, the first step towards making a diagnosis is likely to involve a clinical interview: a client has been referred, and the clinician seeks to engage that individual and build rapport in an effort to understand the clinical picture. This process is likely to include taking a personal history, including important life events that could contribute towards the current symptoms, and making enquiries about how these symptoms affect the ability to carry out valued activities (Mohlman et al., 2012b). Screening tools may be useful at this point, although they do not, in themselves, enable a diagnosis to be made. However, they may help clinicians to gather initial information about the mental state of their patient or client. This may then prompt more extensive clinical examination, perhaps leading to a formal diagnosis. In research settings, screening instruments may be used alone or, if resources permit, before formal assessment using a structured diagnostic interview schedule, such as the Composite International Diagnostic Interview (CIDI) (Wittchen et al., 1993).

A number of screening instruments are widely used with older adults, including the Hospital Anxiety and Depression Scale (HADS) (Zigmond & Snaith, 1983), the Short Anxiety Screening Test (SAST) (Sinoff et al., 1999), the Hamilton Anxiety Scale (HAMA) (Hamilton et al., 1976), the Beck Anxiety Inventory (BAI) (Beck et al., 1988), the Rating Scale for Anxiety in Dementia (RAID) (Shankar et al., 1999), and the Geriatric Anxiety Inventory (GAI) (Pachana et al., 2007). Of these, only the GAI, SAST, and RAID were designed specifically for older people.

The GAI uses a yes–no/agree–disagree response format with no reverse-scored items, an approach modelled on that of the Geriatric Depression Scale (GDS) (Yesavage et al., 1983), thus making the reporting of symptoms easier for older adults, especially for those with cognitive impairment, physical disability, and/or sensory impairment (Byrne & Pachana, 2011). The HADS, for example, has been criticized for having reversals of wording and varying response keys in an attempt to avoid the effects of response bias, but these reversals can be disorientating, and some users may miss the changes in direction of the items (Coyne & van Sonderen, 2012). The GAI avoids somatic items, with a view to limiting the impact of physical illnesses. This is said to confer an advantage over other scales, especially the BAI, which includes items measuring feeling 'unsteady', 'lightheaded', and 'wobbliness in the legs', all symptoms that could easily have physical causes in an older person. The GAI is reported to have sound psychometric properties among community-dwelling older people (Pachana et al., 2007), and it is one of the four tools (together with the SAST, the HADS, and the RAID) recommended by the US National Guideline Clearinghouse for the assessment of late-life anxiety (Lin et al., 2016).

The HADS (Zigmond & Snaith, 1983) has been very widely used in research with older adults: its supposed strength is that it was developed for use in the outpatient physical health setting, and therefore it includes few items that can confuse physical and psychological symptoms. Some have suggested that this is misguided, as somatic symptoms may actually reflect anxiety states (Coyne & van Sonderen, 2012). The HADS also has the advantage of brevity, with seven items each in two subscales that assess both anxiety and depression – useful because of the high co-morbidity between anxiety and depression. Studies have shown that the two subscales do work as intended as a two-factor measure of anxiety and depression in older adults (Flint & Rifat, 2002), but concerns have been raised about the functioning of this measure in certain populations. For example, in a geriatric inpatient population, Davies et al. (1993) compared the HADS and the Geriatric Mental State/ Automatic Geriatric Examination for Computer-Assisted Taxonomy (GMS-AGECAT), a semi-structured diagnostic instrument that produces computerized diagnoses using a hierarchical diagnostic algorithm (Copeland et al., 1986), and they reported poor correspondence between the two instruments. Davies et al. found that the HADS failed to detect cases of depression identified by the GMS-AGECAT, and that 16 of the 26 people identified by the HADS as clinically anxious were GMS-AGECAT cases of depression. A somewhat similar study by Bryant et al. (2009) examined the prevalence and course of anxiety in medically unwell older adults using both the HADS as a symptom measure and the GMS-AGECAT (Copeland et al., 1986). This, too, showed a low correspondence between symptom scores on the HADS and the GMS-AGECAT, especially in relation to depression, but also with regard to anxiety. The HADS identified clinically significant anxiety in 17% of the sample, whereas the GMS-AGECAT identified only 8% of the sample as cases of anxiety. In the absence of a third, gold-standard measure of psychopathology, such as a clinical interview conducted by an experienced clinician, it is difficult to say whether the HADS was over-diagnosing or the GMS-AGECAT underdiagnosing anxiety.

More recently, a study by Campbell et al. (2015) highlighted weaknesses of the measure in people with cognitive impairment, although these were more marked for the depression subscale, where there was poor correspondence between the depression subscale of the HADS and scores on the GDS. It is not surprising, then, that the HADS has its critics, with some going so far as to say that it should no longer be used (Coyne & van Sonderen, 2012). In summary, it is probably fair to say that that the HADS has definite limitations, and its results should be interpreted carefully and corroborated by further enquiry.

The SAST (Sinoff et al., 1999) was developed in part to overcome some of the difficulties identified in the HADS. It was validated against psychiatric evaluation in a sample of 150 geriatric inpatients and outpatients in Israel, and with only 10 items, it has the advantage of brevity, while also explicitly including a number of somatic symptoms that some have argued are associated with anxiety in older adults, such as back and neck pain and poor sleep (Flint, 2005). The authors argued that the omission of somatic items from measures of psychopathology in older adults is a mistake, since those somatic symptoms are themselves manifestations of anxiety and should therefore be measured (Sinoff et al., 1999). Sinoff et al. reported good internal reliability for the scale, together with good reliability in distinguishing anxiety from depression.

While the SAST was developed in part to address concerns about the co-morbidity between anxiety and physical health, the RAID was developed to provide a measure of anxiety in people with dementia (Shankar et al., 1999). There are particular challenges in diagnosing anxiety in people with dementia, including a lack of consensus about how to define and conceptualize anxiety in this population. Several other issues complicate this challenge, including how to distinguish between symptoms of anxiety and symptoms of dementia, as well as the overlap between anxiety, depression, and agitation (Seignourel et al., 2008; Selwood et al., 2005). Unlike all of the scales previously discussed, the RAID is not based on self-report, but rather on the combination of carer and clinician observations over the past two weeks across six domains, namely worry, apprehension and vigilance, motor tension, autonomic hyperactivity, and panic attacks and phobias. Although originally tested on only a sample of 33 patients, thorough psychometric evaluation confirmed the reliability, validity, and clinical utility of the scale and its factor structure (Seignourel et al., 2008). The authors reported that it was easy to use and acceptable to both patients and carers, a finding confirmed in a number of subsequent studies (e.g., Selwood et al., 2005).

Cross-Cultural Issues in Anxiety Diagnosis

While the instruments described above have been developed and been validated in a range of samples in order to address the challenges of physical and neurodegenerative co-morbidities, a further challenge arises as to their cultural appropriateness. Most of the measures described were originally developed in the English language and in Western cultures, apart from the SAST, which was developed in Israel. Concerns have been raised about their adequacy for people from different language and cultural backgrounds. For example, the majority of outlying (both low and high prevalence) findings with regard to the prevalence of anxiety and depression are found to originate in non-English-speaking countries (Lin et al., 2016). On the one hand, this finding might suggest that there are true differences in the prevalence of psychological disorders in older people from different cultural backgrounds, but there are other possible explanations. Taking another perspective, this disparity might reflect cultural differences in how mental disorders are defined, conceptualized, and experienced. This view would be supported by a review by Parker et al. (2001) on the presentation of depression among Chinese participants, which found evidence that Chinese people tend to deny depression or express it somatically. The reasons for this are complex, and they include the stigma associated with mental illness, as well as a tendency to stoicism. Finally, and of particular relevance to the use of screening instruments to identify and diagnose anxiety, this finding might be related to differences across languages in vocabulary and grammar and systematic bias due to the translation of screening instruments (Lin et al., 2016). This therefore raises the question of how to assess and diagnose anxiety in individuals from non-Western backgrounds. Some of the measures described above have been translated into languages other than English – the HADS, for example, has been translated into all of the major European languages, in addition to Arabic, Hebrew, Chinese (both Mandarin and Cantonese), Japanese, Farsi, Malayalam, and Urdu. Such translations are not without their difficulties, as highlighted by Coyne and van Sonderen (2012), who point out that the original wording of the HADS is strongly based on British English colloquialisms, such as 'I get a sort of frightened feeling like butterflies in the stomach', which is very difficult to translate into other languages.

Indeed, the question of translation of instruments is itself complex, potentially time-consuming, and expensive. While translation and back-translation can go some way to ensuring the appropriateness of measures, this may not be sufficient (Eremenco et al., 2005).

Eremenco et al. authors suggest an approach that includes review in several countries, the use of qualitative and quantitative methods in testing, and the use of more sophisticated methods derived from item response theory to evaluate item equivalence through differential item functioning analysis. Once again, the clinician may not be able to work in an ideal situation with perfectly designed measures, but they will need to use even apparently carefully translated measures with a degree of critical evaluation and caution.

Best Practice in the Diagnosis of Anxiety

The above discussion has illustrated the challenges of diagnosis in older adults and highlighted key questions, some of which remain unresolved. Should screening instruments explicitly exclude somatic items because these confuse physical and psychological symptoms (the approach taken by the HADS)? Should they include some somatic items because these reflect the concerns of older adults (the approach taken by the SAST)? How can diagnoses be made when the client themselves has limited ability to articulate their distress when they have a co-morbid neurodegenerative disorder? How can clinicians and researchers best take into account the effects of culture on the conceptualization and subsequent measurement of anxiety? And what of the manifestations of anxiety commonly seen in older adults that only map imperfectly onto the existing DSM-5 criteria for anxiety, such as fear of falling? It is clear that screening instruments may have a place in assisting with this process, and in the research environment, the use of diagnostic interviews such as the GMS-AGECAT (Copeland et al., 1986), the Structured Diagnostic Interview (SCID) (First, 2002), or the CIDI (Wittchen et al., 1993) may be needed to supplement prior screening in order to arrive at a definitive diagnosis. Of these, only the GMS-AGECAT was developed for use with older adults, and it may not be the best instrument for the diagnosis of anxiety. This is because of its hierarchical algorithm, in which depression is a higher-order diagnosis than anxiety, resulting in very low prevalence rates of anxiety, as only symptoms of anxiety that present in the absence of significant symptoms of depression will result in an anxiety diagnosis (Copeland et al., 1987). Some would argue that this merely highlights the high co-morbidity of anxiety and depression, but it is a significant limitation for those researchers with an *a priori* focus on anxiety. Finally, it should be mentioned that the anxiety diagnostic categories of the GMS-AGECAT are now quite dated and do not reflect current nosology.

In the clinical arena, however, the approach is more likely to involve detailed interviews and evaluations of symptoms. This process, also known as case formulation, is regarded as a fundamental skill of the mental health clinician (Johnstone & Dallos, 2013). I would suggest that careful case formulation provides the best chance of making an accurate assessment and diagnosis of anxiety in older adults, and that this is the foundation for subsequent therapeutic work. The essential feature of case formulation is its focus on integrating information gathered about a client and their symptoms and functioning. Multiple aspects of the client's background – development, biological, medical, psychiatric, and psychological – are brought together by clinician and client to produce a shared and nuanced understanding of the client's current situation, with a view to generating working hypotheses as to its origins and meaning and developing a treatment plan (Johnstone & Dallos, 2013). In the area of psychotherapy with older adults, one of the most useful frameworks for doing this is the CALTAP model (Knight & Pachana, 2015; Knight & Poon, 2008).

The CALTAP model is conceived of as a trans-diagnostic as well as trans-theoretical perspective that takes into account important features of late life to assist the clinician in thinking sensitively about their client (Knight & Pachana, 2015). The CALTAP model contains a number of elements, which are represented in Figure 3.1.

At the centre of the diagram, the clinician is alerted to the specific challenges and positive and negative aspects of maturation as they relate to the presenting problem. Here, the model is reminding us that we need an accurate understanding of how factors that may be unique to or more common in old age can affect a presentation. These factors include the greater likelihood of experiencing losses ranging from bereavements to loss of physical functioning, medication side effects, or cognitive decline. Negative aspects of ageing refer to normal age-related developmental changes, such as reduced speed of processing and working memory capacity. On the other hand, there may be some aspects of development that are positive and favour the client's capacity to understand their situation. For example, most older adults have developed a repertoire of coping mechanisms and experience of the world that may contribute to 'wisdom' or affective complexity. These changes are important because they may affect the way in which an assessment is conducted and, ultimately, have a bearing on the quality of the formulation. These challenges sit alongside the social context in which they present: an older person living in supported and age-segregated accommodation may have quite different anxieties from an older person living alone. These changes are also contrasted with so-called cohort effects, which are those effects attributable to being part of a particular generation; these often interact with culture. Examples include the likelihood that a woman born in rural Italy 80 years ago will have had fewer years of education than

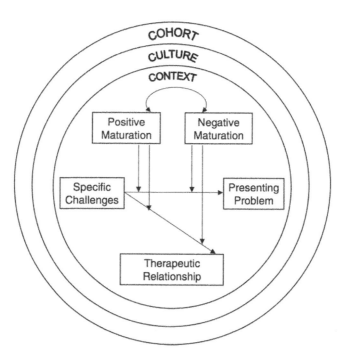

Figure 3.1 CALTAP: Contextual Adult Lifespan Theory for Adapting Psychotherapy.

a 65-year-old woman born in the USA. The implications of this for the diagnostic process are that the clinician needs to be alert to the possibility that the language used to describe psychological experiences may be quite different in these two instances, which could potentially lead to symptoms of anxiety being completely missed. Moreover, personal and social values may also be very different: for example, urbanization has had a profound effect on the structure of families in East Asian societies over the last 20 years (Lin et al., 2015), leading to marked changes in traditional attitudes towards intergenerational relationships and filial piety.

Future Directions

The prevalence and significance of anxiety disorders in older adults are increasingly well recognized, but there is still some way to go in terms of their optimal recognition and diagnosis (Mohlman et al., 2012a). How might we further improve on their diagnosis? First, clinicians and researchers need to challenge stereotypical assumptions about older people, including the idea that that avoidance of activities is normative. Moreover, there is still room for the DSM-5 (American Psychiatric Association, 2013) to be more attuned to the needs of older adults by providing more clinically relevant material in the text accompanying the diagnostic criteria. For example, in relation to impairment and avoidance, there is scope for examples that show greater sensitivity to the social worlds of older people, where caring duties or club participation may be more pertinent than job or school participation (Bryant et al., 2013). The text could also include age-specific examples of avoidance (e.g., avoiding purchasing needed items because of financial fears or avoiding asking for help for fear of being a burden), which could help clinicians ask the right questions.

The diagnosis of anxiety in older adults may also benefit from a dimensional rather than categorical approach to diagnosis. This can be illustrated by reference to generalized anxiety disorder (GAD) – probably the most prevalent anxiety disorder among older people (Beekman et al., 1998). GAD is a controversial diagnosis, partly because of its strong co-morbidity with depression: up to 40% of people who are initially diagnosed with GAD subsequently develop depression or mixed anxiety–depression (Lenze et al., 2001, 2005). A more dimensional approach may benefit older adults by reducing the reliance on the distinction between depression and anxiety, while also helping to address the issue that older adults may experience psychiatric symptoms at a level that is clinically significant while not meeting current DSM diagnostic criteria (Jeste et al., 2005).

Conclusion

In summary, I would suggest that the use of a trans-theoretical framework such as the CALTAP model offers the clinician a way forward out of what can, at times, seem a challenging problem: how to make meaningful diagnoses of anxiety in older adults when there are so many unique aspects of their presentation and the diagnostic system does not always work well for these disorders in this population. To return to where we started: diagnosis is indeed important (Craddock & Mynors-Wallis, 2014). In the research context, it can help to ensure that the needs of older adults are recognized, better understood, and provided for, while in the clinical context, it can open the door to appropriate treatments. Given the complexities of the issues and the shortcomings of many of the extant screening instruments and diagnostic tools, the clinician must use their therapeutic rapport-building, assessment, and formulation skills to ensure that the diagnoses they make are relevant and appropriate.

References

American Psychiatric Association (2013). *Diagnostic and Statistical Manual of Mental Disorders*, 5th ed. Washington, DC: American Psychiatric Association.

Beck, A. T., Epstein, N., Brown, G. and Steer, R. A. (1988). An inventory for measuring clinical anxiety: psychometric properties. *Journal of Consulting and Clinical Psychology*, 56(6), 893–897.

Beekman, A. T., Bremmer, M. A., Deeg, D. J., et al. (1998). Anxiety disorders in later life: a report from the Longitudinal Aging Study Amsterdam. *International Journal of Geriatric Psychiatry*, 13(10), 717–726.

Bei, B., Bryant, C., Gilson, K.-M., et al. (2013). A prospective study of the impact of floods on the mental and physical health of older adults. *Aging and Mental Health*, 17(8), 992–1002.

Bierman, E., Comijs, H., Jonker, C. and Beekman, A. (2007). Symptoms of anxiety and depression in the course of cognitive decline. *Dementia and Geriatric Cognitive Disorders*, 24(3), 213–219.

Bryant, C. (2010). Anxiety and depression in old age: challenges in recognition and diagnosis. *International Psychogeriatrics*, 22(4), 511–513.

Bryant, C., Jackson, H. and Ames, D. (2009). Depression and anxiety in medically unwell older adults: prevalence and short-term course. *International Psychogeriatrics*, 21(4), 754–763.

Bryant, C., Mohlman, J., Gum, A., et al. (2013). Anxiety disorders in older adults: Looking to DSM5 and beyond. . . *American Journal of Geriatric Psychiatry*, 21(9), 872–876.

Byrne, G. J. and Pachana, N. A. (2011). Development and validation of a short form of the Geriatric Anxiety Inventory – the GAI-SF. *International Psychogeriatrics*, 23(1), 125–131.

Campbell, G., Bryant, C., Ellis, K. A., Buckley, R. and Ames, D. (2015). Comparing the Performance of the HADS and the GDS-15 in the AIBL study. *International Psychogeriatrics*, 27(9), 1577–1578.

Copeland, J., Dewey, M. E. and Griffiths-Jones, H. (1986). A computerized psychiatric diagnostic system and case nomenclature for elderly subjects: GMS and AGECAT. *Psychological Medicine*, 16(1), 89–99.

Copeland, J. R., Dewey, M. E., Wood, N., Searle, R., Davidson, I. and McWilliam, C. (1987). Range of mental illness among the elderly in the community. Prevalence in Liverpool using the GMS-AGECAT package. *British Journal of Psychiatry*, 150(6), 815–823.

Coyne, J. C. and van Sonderen, E. (2012). No further research needed: abandoning the Hospital and Anxiety Depression Scale (HADS). *Journal of Psychosomatic Research*, 72(3), 173–174.

Craddock, N. and Mynors-Wallis, L. (2014). Psychiatric diagnosis: impersonal, imperfect and important. *British Journal of Psychiatry*, 204(2), 93–95.

Creamer, M. and Parslow, R. (2008). Trauma exposure and posttraumatic stress disorder in the elderly: a community prevalence study. *American Journal of Geriatric Psychiatry*, 16 (10), 853–856.

Davies, K. N., Burn, W. K., McKenzie, F. R., Brothwell, J. A. and Wattis, J. P. (1993). Evaluation of the hospital anxiety and depression scale as a screening instrument in geriatric medical inpatients. *International Journal of Geriatric Psychiatry*, 8(2), 165–169.

Eremenco, S. L., Cella, D. and Arnold, B. J. (2005). A comprehensive method for the translation and cross-cultural validation of health status questionnaires. *Evaluation & the health professions*, 28(2), 212–232.

First, M. B. (2002). *User's Guide for the Structured Clinical Interview for DSM-IV-TR Axis I Disorders: SCID-I*. New York: Biometrics Research Department, New York State Psychiatric Institute.

Flint, A. J. (2005). Generalised anxiety disorder in elderly patients. *Drugs and Aging*, 22(2), 101–114.

Flint, A. J. and Rifat, S. L. (2002). Factor structure of the hospital anxiety and depression scale in older patients with major depression. *International Journal of Geriatric Psychiatry*, **17**(2), 117–123.

Frances, A. J. and Widiger, T. (2012). Psychiatric diagnosis: lessons from the DSM-IV past and cautions for the DSM-5 future. *Annual Review of Clinical Psychology*, **8**, 109–130.

Gagnon, N., Flint, A. J., Naglie, G. and Devins, G. M. (2005). Affective correlates of fear of falling in elderly persons. *American Journal of Geriatric Psychiatry*, **13**(1), 7–14.

Gornall, J. (2013). DSM-5: a fatal diagnosis? *BMJ*, **346**, f3256.

Hamilton, M., Schutte, N. and Malouff, J. (1976). Hamilton anxiety scale (HAMA). In N. S. Schutte and J. M. Malouff, eds., *Sourcebook of Adult Assessment: Applied Clinical Psychology*. New York: Plenum Press, pp. 154–157.

Healy, P. (2011). DSM diagnosis and beyond: on the need for a hermeneutically-informed biopsychosocial framework. *Medicine, Health Care and Philosophy*, **14**(2), 163–175.

Jeste, D. V., Blazer, D. G. and First, M. (2005). Aging-related diagnostic variations: need for diagnostic criteria appropriate for elderly psychiatric patients. *Biological Psychiatry*, **58**(4), 265–271.

Johnstone, L. and Dallos, R. (2013). *Formulation in Psychology and Psychotherapy: Making Sense of People's Problems*. Abingdon: Routledge.

Karel, M. J., Gatz, M. and Smyer, M. A. (2012). Aging and mental health in the decade ahead: what psychologists need to know. *American Psychologist*, **67**(3), 184–198.

Karlsson, B., Klenfeldt, I. F., Sigström, R., et al. (2009). Prevalence of social phobia in non-demented elderly from a Swedish population study. *American Journal of Geriatric Psychiatry*, **17**(2), 127–135.

Knight, B. G. and Pachana, N. A. (2015). *Psychological Assessment and Therapy with Older People*. Oxford: Oxford University Press.

Knight, B. G. and Poon, C. (2008). The socio-cultural context in understanding older adults: contextual adult life span theory for adapting psychotherapy. In B. Woods and L. Clare, eds., *The Handbook of the Clinical Psychology of Ageing*. Hoboken, NJ: John Wiley & Sons, pp. 439–456.

Lachman, M. E., Howland, J., Tennstedt, S., et al. (1998). Fear of falling and activity restriction: the survey of activities and fear of falling in the elderly (SAFE). *Journals of Gerontology Series B: Psychological Sciences and Social Sciences*, **53**(1), P43–P50.

Lenze, E. J., Mulsant, B. H., Mohlman, J., et al. (2005). Generalized anxiety disorder in late life: lifetime course and comorbidity with major depressive disorder. *American Journal of Geriatric Psychiatry*, **13**(1), 77–80.

Lenze, E. J., Mulsant, B. H., Shear, M. K., Alexopoulos, G. S., Frank, E. and Reynolds, C. F. (2001). Comorbidity of depression and anxiety disorders in later life. *Depression and Anxiety*, **14**(2), 86–93.

Lin, X., Bryant, C., Boldero, J. and Dow, B. (2015). Older Chinese immigrants' relationships with their children: a literature review from a solidarity–conflict perspective. *The Gerontologist*, **55**(6), 990–1005.

Lin, X., Haralambous, B., Pachana, N. A., et al. (2016). Screening for depression and anxiety among older Chinese immigrants living in Western countries: the use of the Geriatric Depression Scale (GDS) and the Geriatric Anxiety Inventory (GAI). *Asia-Pacific Psychiatry*, **8**(1), 32–43.

Mohlman, J., Bryant, C., Lenze, E. J., et al. (2012a). Improving recognition of late life anxiety disorders in Diagnostic and Statistical Manual of Mental Disorders: observations and recommendations of the Advisory Committee to the Lifespan Disorders Work Group. *International Journal of Geriatric Psychiatry*, **27**(6), 549–556.

Mohlman, J., Sirota, K. G., Papp, L. A., Staples, A. M., King, A. and Gorenstein, E. E. (2012b). Clinical interviewing with older adults. *Cognitive and Behavioral Practice*, **19**(1), 89–100.

Pachana, N. A., Byrne, G. J., Siddle, H., Koloski, N., Harley, E. and Arnold, E. (2007). Development and validation of the Geriatric Anxiety Inventory. *International Psychogeriatrics*, **19**(1), 103–114.

Parker, G., Gladstone, G. and Chee, K. T. (2001). Depression in the planet's largest ethnic group: the Chinese. *American Journal of Psychiatry*, **158**(6), 857–864.

Seignourel, P. J., Kunik, M. E., Snow, L., Wilson, N. and Stanley, M. (2008). Anxiety in dementia: a critical review. *Clinical Psychology Review*, **28**(7), 1071–1082.

Selwood, A., Thorgrimsen, L. and Orrell, M. (2005). Quality of life in dementia – a one-year follow-up study. *International Journal of Geriatric Psychiatry*, **20**(3), 232–237.

Shankar, K. K., Walker, M., Frost, D. and Orrell, M. W. (1999). The development of a valid and reliable scale for rating anxiety in dementia (RAID). *Aging and Mental Health*, **3**(1), 39–49.

Shedler, J., Beck, A., Fonagy, P., et al. (2010). Personality disorders in DSM-5. *American Journal of Psychiatry*, **167**(9), 1026–1028.

Sinoff, G., Ore, L., Zlotogorsky, D. and Tamir, A. (1999). Short anxiety screening test – a brief instrument for detecting anxiety in the elderly. *International Journal of Geriatric Psychiatry*, **14**(12), 1062–1071.

Wittchen, H.-U., Robins, L. N., Semler, W. J., Cottler, L. and World Health Organization (1993). *Composite International Diagnostic Interview (CIDI): Interviewer's Manual.* Geneva: World Health Organization.

Yesavage, J. A., Brink, T., Rose, T. L., et al. (1983). Development and validation of a geriatric depression screening scale: a preliminary report. *Journal of Psychiatric Research*, **17**(1), 37–49.

Yohannes, A. M., Baldwin, R. C. and Connolly, M. J. (2000). Depression and anxiety in elderly outpatients with chronic obstructive pulmonary disease: prevalence, and validation of the BASDEC screening questionnaire. *International Journal of Geriatric Psychiatry*, **15**(12), 1090–1096.

Zarit, S. H. and Zarit, J. M. (2012). *Mental Disorders in Older Adults: Fundamentals of Assessment and Treatment.* New York: Guilford Press.

Zigmond, A. S. and Snaith, R. P. (1983). The hospital anxiety and depression scale. *Acta Psychiatrica Scandinavica*, **67**(6), 361–370.

Subthreshold Anxiety in Later Life
Epidemiology and Treatment Strategies

Sébastien Grenier and Marie-Josée Richer

Introduction

Subthreshold anxiety is defined as a condition in which anxiety symptoms, although present, do not meet all of the diagnostic criteria for anxiety disorder as specified in the international classification systems for mental disorders (i.e., the Diagnostic and Statistical Manual of Mental Disorders, 5th Edition (DSM-5) or the International Classification of Diseases, 10th Revision (ICD-10)). Over time, several terms have been used interchangeably to characterize anxiety symptoms in older adults, the most common being subthreshold anxiety, subclinical anxiety, subsyndromal anxiety disorders, and anxiety disorder not otherwise specified (ADNOS). In this chapter, we review epidemiological data and treatment strategies for subthreshold anxiety in later life. The term "subthreshold anxiety" will include all of the aforementioned conditions.

Prevalence and Associated Factors

According to epidemiological studies, between 0.1% and 32.3% of community-dwelling individuals aged 60 years and over have subthreshold anxiety varying in intensity and severity (Almeida et al., 2012; Blyth et al., 2011; Braam et al., 2014; Forlani et al., 2014; Forsell & Winblad, 1998; Grenier et al., 2011a; Heun et al., 2000; Mehta et al., 2003; Papassotiropoulos & Heun, 1999; Prina et al., 2011a). In clinical settings (e.g., nursing homes, geriatric hospitals), between 3.2% and 47.0% of older patients have subthreshold anxiety (Ames et al., 1994; Drageset et al., 2013; Kvaal et al., 2001; Simning et al., 2012; Smalbrugge et al., 2005; Yohannes et al., 2008). Prevalence rates for subthreshold anxiety vary depending on the reporting period (e.g., current vs. lifetime prevalence), the study population (community vs. clinical samples), and the definition used to identify subthreshold anxiety cases (see Table 4.1). Indeed, some authors identify subthreshold anxiety cases based on the sole presence of a few anxiety symptoms (which inflates the prevalence), while others use a stricter definition that includes other DSM diagnostic criteria (e.g., anxiety symptoms need to be present for at least 1 month). Epidemiological studies show that the prevalence of anxiety disorders tends to diminish with age (Flint, 2005; Kessler et al., 2005), yet it is not clear whether this also applies to subthreshold anxiety. In fact, results of a recent Italian study (366 individuals aged 74 and over without cognitive impairment randomly selected from the Faenza Community Aging Study: $n = 7,930$ participants) showed that 21.0% of participants were affected by subthreshold anxiety (Forlani et al., 2014), a proportion similar to that found (18.5%) in a previous study (Heun et al., 2000; seniors aged 60 and over, mean age: 77.7 years). In a larger study of general practice patients (20,036 persons aged 60 years and over; Almeida et al., 2012), it was shown that the

Table 4.1 Description of studies reporting prevalence data on subthreshold anxiety among community-dwelling older adults and older patients.

Authors (in alphabetical order) and name of the study	Country	Definition of subthreshold anxiety	Measure used to assess subthreshold anxiety	Study design and description of the sample	Prevalence of late-life subthreshold anxiety
Studies conducted with older adults living in the community					
Almeida et al. (2012) Depression and Early Prevention of Suicide in General Practice (DEPS-GP)	Australia	A score ≥11 on the HADS-A was used to identify the presence of clinically significant anxiety.	Anxiety subscale of the Hospital Anxiety and Depression Scale (HADS-A)	- Data came from a clustered randomized trial (DEPS-GP) originally designed to investigate how a GP-centred intervention changed the prevalence of depression among their patients. Participants were assessed twice (baseline and 24 months later) - n = 20,036 adults aged 60 years or over	- At baseline: 4.7% (presence of anxiety without depression) - After 24 months: 31% of older adults with anxiety at baseline were also anxious at follow-up
Blyth et al. (2011) The Concord Health and Ageing in Men Project (CHAMP)	Australia	Respondents who answered positively to at least 2 of the first 4 items of the Goldberg Anxiety Subscale and scored 5 or more overall were classified as having clinically significant anxiety	Goldberg Anxiety Subscale of the Goldberg Anxiety and Depression Scale (GADS)	- Population-based epidemiological cohort study - n = 1511 men aged 70 years and older - Recruited men came from three geographical regions: Local Government Areas of Burwood, Canada Bay and Strathfield	- At baseline of the CHAMP: 6.3% (respondents having clinically significant anxiety; last 4 weeks) - Worry about health: 22.4% - The prevalence of other anxiety symptoms varied from 15.4% to 29.2%

Study	Country	Instrument	Definition	Method/Sample	Results
Braam et al. (2014) EURODEP concerted action	The Netherlands, Germany, Iceland, Ireland, England, Spain and Albania	Geriatric Mental State Examination (GMS-AGECAT package)	Respondents having a diagnostic confidence of 0 or 1 estimated by the GMS-AGECAT (within six levels of diagnostic confidence ranging from no symptoms (0) to very severely affected (5)) were classified as subthreshold cases	- Population-based multicentre study including 15 research groups from 12 European countries - n = 14,200 adults aged between 65 and 104 years old (mean age: 76 years) - The sampling frames were based either on municipality registers or on GP registers. Except for Dublin, London and Iceland, where the complete registers were used, the samples were drawn randomly	- Among respondents without depression: 32.3% - Among respondents having a subthreshold depression: 67.3% - Among respondents having a threshold depression: 86.2%
Grenier et al. (2011a) ESA study	Canada	Étude sur la Santé des Aînés diagnostic Questionnaire (ESA-Q). This questionnaire is similar to the Diagnostic Interview Schedule and the Composite International Diagnostic Interview.	Symptoms of anxiety meeting symptom criteria without significant disabilities or symptoms of anxiety not meeting symptom criteria	- Cross-sectional survey - n = 2,784 adults aged 65 years and older (mean age: 73.8 years) - Households within each of the 16 administrative regions of Quebec were selected according to a random sampling method. A random process was also used to select only one older adult within the household	- Symptoms of anxiety not meeting symptom criteria: 15.9% (12 months) - Symptoms of anxiety meeting symptom criteria without significant disabilities: 4.6% (12 months) - Total prevalence of cases with subthreshold anxiety: 20.5% (12-months)
Forlani et al. (2014) Faenza Project	Italy	Geriatric Anxiety Inventory short form (GAI-sf)	A score ≥3 on the GAI-sf was used to detect the	- Cross-sectional population-based study	- Anxiety symptoms occurred in 77 participants (21.04%)

Table 4.1 (cont.)

Authors (in alphabetical order) and name of the study	Country	Definition of subthreshold anxiety	Measure used to assess subthreshold anxiety	Study design and description of the sample	Prevalence of late-life subthreshold anxiety
		presence of anxiety symptoms		- n = 366 non-demented older adults (mean age: 83.7 years). - Participants came from Faenza, a city located in northern Italy	- The proportion of individuals with anxiety symptoms decreased with increasing age: after 90 years (7.8%)
Forsell and Winblad (1998)	Sweden	Respondents were categorized into three groups according to the frequency of their anxiety feelings: (1) those who felt calm most of the time; (2) those who felt anxious now and then; and (3) those who had anxiety most of the time with or without panic attacks	The Comprehensive Psychopathological Rating Scale (CPRS)	- The present study utilized data from the follow-up phase of a longitudinal investigation of adults registered in the district of Kungsholmen in Stockholm. - n = 966 persons aged 78 years and over (mean age: 84.2 years)	- Feeling anxious now and then: 19.4% - Feeling anxious most of the time with or without panic attacks: 5.0% - Total prevalence of people reporting feelings of anxiety: 24.4%
Heun et al. (2000)	Germany	Subthreshold generalized anxiety disorder: unrealistic anxiety or worry about two or more life situations, anxious for at least 6 months without fulfilling full diagnostic criteria, at least one physical or vegetative symptom of anxiety	Composite International Diagnostic Interview (CIDI)	- Cross-sectional study - n = 286 elderly subjects aged above 60 years (mean age: 77.7 years) - Participants came from the general population and were selected with the support of the city census office in Mainz, Germany	- Participants reported at least one subthreshold anxiety disorder: 18.5% - Subthreshold generalized anxiety disorder: 0% (current); 5.2% (lifetime)

Study	Country	Definition	Measure	Sample	Prevalence
		Subthreshold panic disorder: presence of acute unexpected anxiety attacks (criterion A) and one to four physical symptoms Subthreshold agoraphobia: unreasonable fear in places or situations from which it is difficult to leave; lack of avoidance or of symptoms of anxiety Subthreshold social phobia: persistent fear of situations in which the person is exposed to social interactions (criterion A is fulfilled), but lack of avoidance or social consequences Subthreshold simple phobia: persistent fear of circumscribed stimulus (criterion A is fulfilled), but lack of avoidance or consequences			- Subthreshold panic disorder: 1.7% (current); 8.4% (lifetime) - Subthreshold agoraphobia: 0.7% (current); 2.1% (lifetime). - Subthreshold social phobia: 1.4% (current); 2.1% (lifetime) - Subthreshold simple phobia: 8.4% (current); 15.0% (lifetime)
Mehta et al. (2003) Health, Aging and Body Composition Study (Heath ABC)	USA	Participants were defined as having anxiety symptoms if they experienced during the last week any two of these	Anxiety subscale of the Hopkins Symptom Checklist	- Prospective cohort study - n = 3,041 adults aged 70–79 years (mean age: 74 years) - The cohort was uniquely constructed with balanced	- Approximately 19% of all participants reported one or more anxiety

Table 4.1 (cont.)

Authors (in alphabetical order) and name of the study	Country	Definition of subthreshold anxiety	Measure used to assess subthreshold anxiety	Study design and description of the sample	Prevalence of late-life subthreshold anxiety
		three symptoms (feeling fearful, nervous/shaky or tense/keyed up) at least "a little" or any one symptom at least "quite a bit"		participation of Blacks and Whites and men and women who were recruited from Medicare beneficiary lists at two field centres in Pittsburgh, Pennsylvania, and Memphis, Tennessee	symptom(s) in the past week - Anxiety symptoms occurred in 15% of older people without depression and in 43% of those with depression
Miloyan et al. (2015) The National Epidemiological Survey of Alcohol and Related Conditions (NESARC)	USA	Participants were categorized as having a subthreshold generalized anxiety disorder (GAD) if they met the following diagnostic criteria: reporting 6 months or more of worry, tension or nervousness and not meeting all diagnostic criteria for a threshold GAD	Non-hierarchical GAD diagnostic procedure based on DSM-IV criteria	- National survey including 43,093 non-institutionalized adults (18–98 years old) from all 50 US states and the District of Columbia. Wave 1 of the NESARC was conducted in 2001–2002. Three years later, wave 2 follow-up re-interviews were conducted with 34,653 of the original participants. - Wave 1: *n* = 13,420 participants aged 55 years or over (mean age: 68.88 years) - Wave 2: *n* = 10,409 participants aged 55 years or over (mean age: 70.67 years)	- 12-month prevalence of subthreshold GAD (wave 1): 7.1% - 12-month prevalence of subthreshold GAD (wave 2): 3.26%
Papassotiropoulos and Heun (1999)	Germany	Subthreshold panic disorder: presence of acute unexpected anxiety	CIDI/DSM-III-R and ICD-10 diagnostic criteria	- Community-based study - *n* = 274 participants aged above 60 years	- Prevalence of subthreshold anxiety (including

	Country	Definition of subthreshold anxiety	Instrument	Sample	Results
		attacks (criterion A); one to four physical symptoms Subthreshold agoraphobia: unreasonable fear in places or situations from which it is difficult to flee; lack of avoidance or of symptoms of anxiety Subthreshold social phobia: persistent fear of situations in which the subject is exposed to social interactions (criterion A); lack of avoidance or of social consequences Subthreshold simple phobia: persistent fear of a circumscribed stimulus (criterion A); lack of avoidance or of social consequences		- With the support of the local Census Bureau and the regional Board of Data Protection (Rheinland-Pfalz, Germany), a stratified random sample aged over 60 years was selected from the general population	subthreshold panic disorder, agoraphobia, social phobia and simple phobia): 9.5% or 26 participants out of 274 (last 4 weeks) - Prevalence rates were not reported for each subthreshold anxiety disorder
Prina et al. (2011a)	China, India, Cuba, Dominican Republic, Venezuela, Mexico and Peru	Participants who obtained a score under 3 in the GMS/AGECAT Stage I anxiety cluster were classified as subthreshold cases	Geriatric Mental State Examination (GMS-AGECAT package)	- Cross-sectional surveys of all residents aged 65 or over (n = 15,021) recruited in 11 catchment sites (low-socioeconomic status districts) from seven countries	Prevalence rates of subthreshold anxiety according to countries: - China (0.1–0.2%) - India (0.8–3.0%) - Cuba (6.3%) - Dominican Republic (8.5%) - Venezuela (8.1%)

Table 4.1 (cont.)

Authors (in alphabetical order) and name of the study	Country	Definition of subthreshold anxiety	Measure used to assess subthreshold anxiety	Study design and description of the sample	Prevalence of late-life subthreshold anxiety
					- Mexico (4.9–5.7%) - Peru (2.2–9.6%)
Studies conducted with older patients					
Ames et al. (1994)	Australia	Respondents having a diagnostic confidence of 0 or 1 estimated by the GMS-AGECAT (within six levels of diagnostic confidence ranging from no symptoms (0) to very severely affected (5)) were classified as subthreshold cases	Geriatric Mental State Examination (GMS-AGECAT package)	- Cross-sectional study - n = 81 patients aged 60 years or more (mean age: 81.8 years) recruited in a geriatric hospital located in the north-west of Melbourne. The study was confined to the acute wards, to which patients were admitted directly from the community for management of complex medical problems. Wards were visited in turn at the same time each week. At each visit, ten beds were enumerated in numerical sequence (starting with Bed 1 on the uppermost floor) and the occupants of those beds were approached for an interview	- 1-month prevalence of subthreshold anxiety: 15%
Drageset et al. (2013)	Norway	A score ≥8 on the HADS-A was used to identify the	HADS-A	- Cross-sectional observation study	

Study	Country	Definition	Instrument	Sample/Design	Results
		presence of probable anxiety (cases that should undergo further clinical examination)		- Convenience sample of 227 residents aged 65 years or more (mean age: 85.4 years) without cognitive impairment living for more than 6 months in 30 nursing homes (Bergen, Norway)	- Prevalence of probable cases of anxiety: 14%
Kvaal et al. (2001)	Norway	A threshold value for the sumscore of 39/40 on the STAI was used to identify the presence of clinically significant anxiety	Spielberger's State–Trait Anxiety Inventory (STAI)	- Controlled cross-sectional study - $n = 98$ geriatric inpatients aged 70 years and over (mean age: 81.8 years) without cognitive impairment and 68 healthy home-dwelling controls (mean age: 80.5 years) recruited from three senior citizen centres in Oslo	- Prevalence of significant anxiety in female patients: 41%. - In male patients: 47% - In healthy female controls: 2% - In healthy male controls: 0%
Simning et al. (2012)	USA	Residents who obtained a score ≥10 on the GAD-7 with the absence of a current (syndromal) anxiety disorder (according to the SCID) were classified as subsyndromal cases	Structured Clinical Interview for the DSM-IV (SCID) and the Generalized Anxiety Disorder – 7 item (GAD-7)	- Two-stage cross-sectional study within four public housing high-rises reserved for older adults in Rochester, New York - $n = 190$ residents aged 60 years and older (mean age: 66 years) - 80% of the sample were Black	- 1-month prevalence of subsyndromal anxiety: 3.2%
Smalbrugge et al. (2005)	The Netherlands	Subthreshold panic disorder: a subthreshold	Schedules for Clinical Assessment in	- Cross-sectional study	- Prevalence of subthreshold

Table 4.1 (cont.)

Authors (in alphabetical order) and name of the study	Country	Definition of subthreshold anxiety	Measure used to assess subthreshold anxiety	Study design and description of the sample	Prevalence of late-life subthreshold anxiety
Amsterdam Groningen Elderly Depression (AGED) study		panic attack (a panic attack with one or more physical symptoms) during the last 4 weeks Subthreshold agoraphobia: unreasonable fear in places or situations from which it is difficult to leave during the last 4 weeks and at least some avoidance or symptoms of anxiety Subthreshold specific phobia: persistent fear of circumscribed stimulus during the last 4 weeks and at least some avoidance or consequences Subthreshold social phobia: persistent fear of situations in which a person is exposed to social interactions during	Neuropsychiatry (SCAN)	- n = 333 nursing home patients over 55 years old (mean age: 79.3 years) without severe cognitive impairment - Fourteen nursing homes in the north-west of the Netherlands were selected to participate	anxiety disorders: 4.2%

		the last 4 weeks and at least some avoidance or consequences Subthreshold generalized anxiety disorder: unrealistic anxiety or worry about two or more life situations during the last 4 weeks and at least one physical or vegetative symptom			
Yohannes et al. (2008)	UK	Participants who obtained a score ≥8 on the HADS-A were categorized as having anxiety symptoms	HADS-A	- Observational cohort study - $n = 173$ patients aged 60 years and more (mean age: 80 years) referred from a acute hospital setting or from GPs to a post-acute 36-bedded intermediate-care unit (north-west of England)	- Prevalence of anxiety symptoms: 43%

prevalence of anxiety symptoms (deemed clinically significant) decreased from 31.7% in the 60–64 age group to 3.3% in those aged 85 and over. These findings are supported by Prina et al. (2011a) (n = 15,021 participants representing all residents aged 65 and over of 11 low- and middle-income catchment areas in China, India, Cuba, the Dominican Republic, Venezuela, Mexico, and Peru), who showed that higher anxiety prevalence was related to younger age. In contrast, a study by Braam et al. (2014; involving 14,200 community-dwelling individuals aged 65 and over living in 7 European countries) suggested that subthreshold anxiety remains frequent in the oldest seniors. The discrepancy between these results indicates that more studies are needed to understand how age and other factors impact subthreshold anxiety rates. In particular, late-life subthreshold anxiety seems more frequent in women, people with lower education levels, people with poor social support, as well as in those affected by multiple physical illnesses, sleep disorders, or depression (Almeida et al., 2012; Forlani et al., 2014; Grenier et al., 2011a; Heun et al., 2000; Mehta et al., 2003). Depression can be viewed as a factor increasing the risk of developing subthreshold anxiety, but it may also be a consequence of subthreshold anxiety (see "Psychiatric Comorbidities" section).

Subthreshold anxiety is expressed in older individuals through diverse symptoms, among which the most frequent are specific phobias and generalized anxiety. The prevalence of subthreshold specific phobias varies between 8.7% (12-month prevalence; Grenier et al., 2011b) and 15% (lifetime prevalence; Heun et al., 2000). The prevalence of subthreshold generalized anxiety disorder (GAD) varies between 3.0% (12-month prevalence; Grenier et al., 2011a) and 7.1% (12-month prevalence; Miloyan et al., 2015) in older community-dwelling people. Some seniors therefore live with subthreshold worries that may affect them in different domains, including their family lives and health. Moreover, an Australian epidemiological study of normal aging (Blyth et al., 2011; 1,217 men aged 70 years or older) found that 22.4% of participants answered affirmatively to the question: Have you been worried about your health? Notably, the men concerned about their health were 2.8 times more at risk of suffering from chronic and intrusive pain compared to the other participants.

In addition, some studies have suggested that worry content evolves across the lifespan. Older individuals tend to worry more about their health (Hunt et al., 2003), welfare of loved ones (Gonçalves & Byrne, 2013), and interpersonal/family relationships (Diefenbach et al., 2001) than their younger counterparts. However, the frequency of these subthreshold worries did not differ between younger and older adults in another study (Gould & Edelstein, 2010). These inconsistent findings suggest that more studies are needed in order to better understand how the different worry themes vary across the lifespan. It is worth noting that worry themes do not significantly differ between older adults suffering from subthreshold and threshold GAD (Diefenbach et al., 2001).

Analogous results were found in another study investigating phobias: the subtypes of fear for older individuals with subthreshold specific phobias did not differ significantly from those with a full DSM diagnosis of specific phobia (Grenier et al., 2011b). The situational phobia subtype (e.g., bridges, elevators, etc.) was the most prevalent, being reported by more than 50% of participants, followed by the natural environment subtype (e.g., storms, lightning) and the animal subtype (e.g., dogs, insects). A previous population study (Fredrikson et al., 1996) also demonstrated that older participants (mean age: 53.3 years) without specific phobias were less afraid of animals, insects, and injections than younger participants (mean age: 29.0 years). However, the former were more afraid of heights, airplanes, and lightning than the latter. This study is the only one comparing subthreshold fear subtypes between age groups. More studies should thus be conducted to understand the fear subtypes that specifically affect older adults with subthreshold specific phobia.

The fear of falling is a fear subtype that particularly affects older individuals (Bryant et al., 2008). Currently, there is no psychiatric diagnosis associated with this fear, sometimes called ptophobia (Bhala et al., 1982) or post-fall syndrome (Murphy & Isaacs, 1982); it is found in 21–85% of adults over 65 years of age (see the systematic review of the literature conducted by Scheffer et al., 2008). Results from a recent meta-analysis (including 20 studies; $n = 4,738$) demonstrate that anxiety is moderately and significantly associated with fear of falling (Payette et al., 2016). When this fear reaches the threshold for a DSM specific phobia, it may be classified in the "other subtype" category. Fear of falling may also be diagnosed in older people with GAD or agoraphobia (Gagnon et al., 2005). However, some seniors report a fear of falling without necessarily suffering from a specific anxiety disorder (Gagnon et al., 2005). Previous studies have shown that the risk of developing a fear of falling is higher in women, older and physically frail people, and in those with cognitive deficits, anxiety, or depression (Drozdick & Edelstein, 2001; Murphy et al., 2002; Nagamatsu et al., 2011; van Haastregt et al., 2008).

Impact on Sleep, Well-Being, and Health Behaviors

Research evidence shows that anxious older adults report many sleep problems that cannot be explained by depressive symptoms (e.g., difficulty in falling asleep, frequent awakenings, daytime sleepiness, etc.; Mallon et al., 2000; Spira et al., 2009). Rumination (i.e., imagining catastrophic scenarios), which characterizes anxiety, could be the source of these sleep problems. In other words, sleep problems are often a consequence of subthreshold anxiety; the anxious person imagines catastrophic scenarios (e.g., son dying in a car accident), sleeps badly, wakes up tired, feels more anxious, which in turn increases sleep problems, thus continuing the cycle (Magee & Carmin, 2010). Apart from sleep disturbances, subthreshold anxiety may cause psychological distress and significantly disrupt the daily functioning of seniors, as is the case for threshold anxiety (Grenier et al., 2011a; Haller et al., 2014; Prina et al., 2011a; van Zelst et al., 2006; Wetherell et al., 2003). It is therefore questionable to suggest that anxiety symptoms not meeting all diagnostic criteria for a specific anxiety disorder are automatically less severe than for those who fulfill all criteria. In fact, in a population study, 15% of subjects with subthreshold specific phobia reported that their symptoms prevented them from functioning normally (Grenier et al., 2011b). The remaining 85% with subthreshold fears were not significantly affected in their day-to-day functioning. Nonetheless, about 40% of the latter reported the use of avoidance strategies, which tends to question the reported negligible impact on daily functioning. It is thus possible that anxious seniors may underestimate the impact of their symptoms on daily life. They may also consider that their reduced productivity is a normal consequence of aging, instead of attributing it to anxiety symptoms (Kelley-Moore et al., 2006). These findings suggest that a meaningful evaluation of anxiety symptom severity should not be limited to reports by anxious seniors exclusively, but should also include those of friends or close relatives. In addition, the impact of anxiety symptoms on daily living should be assessed not only through one general question (e.g., "Are your symptoms interfering with your daily functioning?") – specific questions related to behaviors affecting daily activities also need to be asked (e.g., "Are you avoiding some situations because of fear?"). For example, avoidance is a major behavioral component of the fear of falling. Indeed, an older person afraid of falling will, as a first reaction to fear, limit his/her movements and activities. The resulting inactivity can lead to serious consequences including decreased functional abilities and quality of life (QoL), increased frailty, social isolation, and depressive symptoms (Bertera & Bertera, 2008). Moreover, QoL is affected not only by the fear of falling, but also by other subthreshold anxiety types (e.g., subthreshold post-traumatic stress disorder; van Zelst et al., 2006).

Older individuals with subthreshold anxiety and avoidance behaviors are also more prone to take several medications (e.g., benzodiazepines (BZDs); Almeida et al., 2012; Grenier et al., 2011a; Wetherell et al., 2003). For instance, it was shown in Wetherell et al. (2003) that 54.5% of older people with subthreshold GAD used psychotropic medication compared to 30.6% of those with threshold GAD and 6.3% of seniors without anxiety. The authors considered that these results indicated that seniors with subthreshold GAD may benefit from the medication. However, it is also possible that this medication was inappropriately prescribed and triggered subthreshold anxiety symptoms. Indeed, it has been recognized that prolonged BZD use may cause many paradoxical effects, including an increase of anxiety symptoms (Lader, 2014). Given this finding, alternative non-pharmacological approaches should be considered first (see "Treatment Strategies" section). Furthermore, it was shown in an Italian study (Forlani et al., 2014; 366 seniors aged 74 years and over) that anxiety symptoms were associated with alcohol consumption, with alcohol intake being higher in more anxious subjects. Alcohol use may be seen by anxious seniors (especially men) as a self-medication. Moderate alcohol consumption may indeed help seniors to feel better (somehow helping them to cope with stress), and it is even associated with prevention of cognitive decline (Kim et al., 2012). Excessive drinking, however, may intensify and prolong anxiety symptoms (Almeida et al., 2012; Sorocco & Ferrell, 2006). Finally, it was shown in another study (Garrido et al., 2009; $n = 2,626$ community-dwelling adults aged 65 and over) that 23.2% of those with subthreshold GAD perceived a need for treatment to address their mental health problems compared to 48.1% of participants with full GAD. Garrido et al. (2009) concluded by saying that subthreshold anxiety expressed by seniors should not be overlooked when assessing the need for mental health services.

Expressing a need to consult for mental health problems is a phase that usually precedes the consultation (Andersen, 2008). Only a few studies have examined the use of health services by older patients reporting subthreshold anxiety. One of these studies showed that during the preceding year, 26.2% of older people with subthreshold anxiety consulted a health professional to relieve their anxiety symptoms (Grenier et al., 2011a). This consultation rate even exceeded that reported (i.e., 20.6%) by older participants with GAD. Another study has shown that seniors with subthreshold GAD and threshold GAD had received psychotherapy services at similar rates (72.7% vs. 77.8%; Wetherell et al., 2003). Lastly, results from a Canadian study ($n = 12,792$) showed that 21.7% of older persons with clinically significant anxiety symptoms sought consultation during the preceding year compared to 34.2% of seniors with an anxiety disorder (Scott et al., 2010). Of these, 21.7% went to the general medical sector, 31.0% went to the mental health sector, and 34.9% went to both sectors.

Given these findings, we can say that late-life subthreshold anxiety is a serious condition that can cause sleep problems, affect daily functioning, and increase the use of healthcare services and the propensity to consume psychotropic drugs. Subthreshold anxiety has also been associated with suicidal feelings. Indeed, a Swedish study ($n = 560$ participants aged 70 years and over without dementia living in private households or institutions) showed that the presence of anxiety symptoms was significantly related to suicidal feelings after controlling for depression (Jonson et al., 2012). This study reiterates the need to seriously address the manifestations of subthreshold anxiety in older people, regardless of the presence of depressive symptoms.

Psychiatric Comorbidities

Depressive Symptoms and Disorder

A large number of studies have shown that subthreshold anxiety is frequently associated with depression in older people (Beekman et al., 2000; Braam et al., 2014; Lenze, 2003; Lenze et al., 2000; Mackenzie et al., 2011; Mehta et al., 2003; Prina et al., 2011b; Schoevers et al., 2005). In particular, 33–63% of older patients suffering from a major depressive disorder also display anxiety symptoms that vary in intensity and severity (Kirby et al., 1999; Mehta et al., 2003; Mulsant et al., 1996). For depressed seniors living in the community, the comorbidity rate falls to 20% (Forlani et al., 2014; Heun et al., 2000). In fact, the study by Forlani et al. (2014) suggests that a higher intensity of depressive symptoms is associated with a lower comorbidity rate; while 32.9% of seniors suffering from mild depression (according to the ICD-10) also experience anxiety symptoms, comorbid anxiety is reported by 21.1% of participants with moderate to severe levels of depression. In contrast, Braam et al. (2014) found that the prevalence of anxiety symptoms increased with depression severity (according to Geriatric Mental State/Automatic Geriatric Examination for Computer-Assisted Taxonomy (GMS/AGECAT)), from 63.7% in patients with subthreshold depression to 86.2% in those with case-level depression. The discrepancy between these two findings might be due to the instruments used to assess anxiety and depression and to differences between definitions of subthreshold cases. Moreover, another study showed that 15.4% of seniors suffering from subthreshold anxiety also had mild or severe depression, a comorbidity rate comparable (i.e., 16.8%) to that found among respondents with a full anxiety disorder (Grenier et al., 2011a). This result underlines that the clinical profile of older people suffering from subthreshold anxiety shows more similarities with anxiety disorder cases than with the profile of seniors without anxiety.

With respect to the comorbid symptoms occurring in depressive states, it was shown that 24% of seniors with depressive symptoms also had anxiety symptoms, and conversely, about 57% of participants aged 60 and over reporting anxiety symptoms also presented with depressive symptoms (Heun et al., 2000). Even if these comorbidity cases did not include full disorders, many studies have demonstrated that anxious and depressive symptomatology can significantly affect day-to-day functioning (Braam et al., 2014; Das-Munshi et al., 2008; Roy-Byrne et al., 1994). In order to better classify people presenting with subthreshold anxious and depressive symptoms, a new disorder was proposed in the 1990s: mixed anxiety–depression (Zinbarg et al., 1994). However, researchers did not unanimously support this new diagnostic category (Batelaan et al., 2012; Cassidy et al., 2005). The main arguments against it include its imprecision (for some authors, it includes the combination of subthreshold anxiety and depression meeting DSM criteria, while others limit it to the co-occurrence of subthreshold anxiety and subthreshold depression; Cassidy et al., 2005) and its lack of stability over time (Batelaan et al., 2012).

Evolution over Time of Late-Life Anxiety Symptoms and Related Conditions

The instability of late-life anxiety symptoms can be illustrated by the results of a recent population study (n = 20,036; Almeida et al., 2012): only 31.0% of participants aged 60 and over who had clinically significant anxiety symptoms at baseline (without depression) still showed anxiety symptoms at the 2-year follow-up, while 2.5% did not present these symptoms at follow-up, 10.7% had developed depression, and 25.5% had mixed anxiety–depression symptoms. Moreover, other studies have shown that late-life anxiety symptoms can later convert into a major depression with or without a comorbid GAD (Schoevers et al., 2005; Wetherell et al., 2001). A Dutch study that demonstrated that subthreshold anxiety increases the risk of developing a full anxiety disorder (Smit et al., 2007) also showed that treating subthreshold anxiety could prevent the conversion to a DSM-IV anxiety disorder in 55.9% of cases. Another Dutch study suggested that late-life anxiety disorders are unstable over time: 47% of participants presenting with an anxiety disorder at baseline converted to subthreshold anxiety 6 years later, while only 23% still met the criteria for a given anxiety disorder (Schuurmans et al., 2005). In addition, another study (Miloyan et al., 2015; 13,420 Americans aged 55–98 years old) showed that the presence of subthreshold GAD at baseline was not a good predictor of threshold GAD 3 years later. Therefore, the link between subthreshold and threshold anxiety was not consistently demonstrated in the existing research findings. Subthreshold late-life anxiety often (although not always) converts to threshold anxiety, but the inverse can also happen: threshold anxiety may also lead to subthreshold anxiety. Further longitudinal studies should thus be conducted in order to better understand how late-life anxious symptoms fluctuate over time and to identify conversion/preventive factors linking them to full anxiety disorder.

Neurologic Comorbidities

Cognitive Impairment and Dementia

More than 50% of patients with cognitive deficits (including Alzheimer's disease (AD)) suffer from a psychological distress characterized, in particular, by severe anxiety symptoms (Apostolova & Cummings, 2008; Beaudreau & O'Hara, 2008; Lyketsos et al., 2002; Seignourel et al., 2008). Psychological distress can disrupt daily functioning and worsen QoL for those patients (Hoe et al., 2006; Moyle & O'Dwyer, 2012). Moreover, many studies have demonstrated that anxiety, even at a subthreshold level, can contribute to cognitive decline in older people (Beaudreau & O'Hara, 2008; Gallacher et al., 2009; Palmer et al., 2007; Petkus et al., 2016; Potvin et al., 2011a). It has also been demonstrated that the association between anxiety and cognitive decline/dementia did not depend on the effects attributed to depressive symptoms (Petkus et al., 2016; Potvin et al., 2011a). In another cross-sectional study conducted by the same research group, results indicate that subthreshold GAD was significantly associated with the presence of cognitive impairment no dementia (CIND) in older men, after controlling for the statistical impacts of age, education, presence of depression, chronic diseases, and psychotropic drug use (Potvin et al., 2011b). In this study, subthreshold GAD was the only anxiety disorder significantly associated with CIND, irrespective of the presence or absence of depressive symptoms. These results also illustrate the need to account for gender in anxiety research in order to understand its impact on seniors' cognitive functioning.

Moreover, another study demonstrated that, in healthy older people without dementia, anxiety symptoms (measured by Symptom Checklist-90 – Revised (SCL-90-R)) were inversely related to cognitive functioning (based on the Repeatable Battery for the Assessment of Neuropsychological Status (RBANS) scores), independently of the depression level (Stillman et al., 2012). Although the study sample was small, the results underline that anxiety (and not solely depression) is an important variable influencing cognitive functioning in seniors. Various theories have been proposed to explain the effect of anxiety on the cognitive functioning of older adults. According to the Processing Efficiency Theory and Attentional Control Theory (the two most cited theories), worries overload the cognitive system (mainly working memory), which makes it more difficult for the brain to adequately process information (Eysenck & Calvo, 1992; Eysenck et al., 2007). When anxious people are performing a given task, they need to invest more effort than those not suffering from anxiety to reach the same level of cognitive performance. These findings suggest that subthreshold anxiety is significantly associated with cognitive deficits, regardless of the presence or absence of depression. However, more longitudinal studies are required in order to better understand how anxiety, depression, and cognitive functioning interact over time and, above all, to isolate the singular effects of subthreshold anxiety on cognitive performance in seniors.

Parkinson's Disease

According to clinical studies (Brown et al., 2011; Leentjens et al., 2011; Marinus et al., 2002; Pontone et al., 2009; Stefanova et al., 2013), the current prevalence rate of subthreshold anxiety in patients with Parkinson's disease (PD) is between 11% and 38%. A recent epidemiological study involving 450 PD patients even found that 51% of them presented possible/probable anxiety symptoms (according to Hospital Anxiety and Depression Rating Scale scores; Nègre-Pagès et al., 2010). In PD patients, anxiety can worsen motor symptoms and increase gait problems and dyskinesia, in addition to altering QoL (Marinus et al., 2002; Nègre-Pagès et al., 2010; Siemers et al., 1993; Vazquez et al., 1993). Furthermore, it has been shown that the prevalence of full anxiety disorder is higher (43%) than subthreshold anxiety (25%) in PD patients, in contrast to what has been observed for older people living at home (Pontone et al., 2009). Similar results were obtained in another study (Leentjens et al., 2011), in which 34% of PD patients were suffering from at least one anxiety disorder and 11.4% were suffering from subthreshold anxiety. The disparity between the results of PD patients and community-dwelling seniors could be explained by the impact of the disease on daily functioning (i.e., the probability of presenting all of the anxiety symptoms for anxiety diagnosis might be higher in people suffering from debilitating diseases such as PD). Nevertheless, this hypothesis is not supported by the results of Nègre-Pagès et al. (2010), whose study demonstrated that PD patients presented with more anxiety than non-PD patients with comparable disability levels. It is also noteworthy that even if the prevalence of anxiety disorders is different between these two groups (community-dwelling seniors vs. PD patients), their anxiety–depression comorbidity rates are similar. Indeed, subthreshold anxiety and depression are highly comorbid in PD patients (Nègre-Pagès et al., 2010; Martinez-Martin & Damian, 2010; Stefanova et al., 2013), as is the case for community-dwelling older adults. In light of these findings, further research is needed to better understand how anxiety symptoms affect the evolution and severity of Parkinsonian symptoms, regardless of depressive symptoms.

Other Medical Comorbidities

Cardiovascular Diseases and Related Conditions

There is now evidence that subthreshold anxiety is associated with cardiovascular diseases (CVDs) in older people (Grenier et al., 2012; Moser et al., 2010) and that anxious people with CVDs are at higher risk of mortality or morbidity (Frasure-Smith & Lesperance, 2008; Huffman et al., 2010). An epidemiological study conducted in Quebec (Canada) has shown that 14.8% of the study sample (613 individuals with CVDs aged ≥65 years) had subthreshold anxiety (Grenier et al., 2012). In these older participants with CVDs, the 12-month prevalence of subthreshold anxiety was approximately three times higher than that of anxiety disorders (5.1%). Other reported anxiety-related conditions in this study included subthreshold symptoms of social phobia (1.1%), obsessive–compulsive disorder (OCD; 1.3%), GAD (2.0%), panic disorder (3.1%), agoraphobia (7.5%), and specific phobia (8.0%). In addition, Grenier et al. (2012) showed that the presence of high blood pressure and depression in older people with CVDs increased the risk of suffering from subthreshold anxiety. It should also be noted that the risks of medical complications, CVDs, and mortality increase in people with anxiety and/or depression symptoms (Rutledge et al., 2009). Thus, it is important to evaluate and treat both symptom types in older cardiac patients. This conclusion is also supported by another study that demonstrated that anxiety and depression symptoms increase the risk of CVDs (Gallagher et al., 2012). However, a recent study concluded that anxiety (not depression) was the only predictor of CVD events in older primary care patients (Stewart et al., 2016). Finally, another study showed that diabetes, stroke, and hypertension were significantly related to anxious symptoms after adjusting for age, gender, race/ethnicity, marital status, and education (Jones et al., 2016).

Chronic Obstructive Pulmonary Disease

Various studies suggest that between 10% and 60% of chronic obstructive pulmonary disease (COPD) patients (usually over 60 years old) present with subthreshold anxiety varying in intensity and severity (Brenes, 2003; Kunik et al., 2005; Yohannes et al., 2000). Patients with COPD are 10 times more likely to suffer from panic attacks or panic disorder compared to the general population (Livermore et al., 2010). This finding is not surprising given that the breathing difficulties in COPD resemble panic attacks. These patients also report more anxious symptoms than those with other medical conditions (e.g., heart diseases, cancer; Kvaal et al., 2001). Unlike the general older population, the prevalence rates of subthreshold anxiety and threshold anxiety are not different in patients with COPD. Indeed, between 10% and 55% of COPD inpatients present a full anxiety disorder, which is very similar to the prevalence mentioned above for subthreshold anxiety (Willgoss & Yohannes, 2013). In addition, if anxiety symptoms are not effectively treated, respiratory problems can worsen, thus reducing the QoL and even increasing the mortality risk of COPD patients (Panagioti et al., 2014). Anxious COPD patients are also frequently affected by comorbid depressive symptoms, as seen in other physical or neurodegenerative diseases associated with aging (e.g., heart disease, PD; Panagioti et al., 2014). In a study carried out with 1,334 patients with different chronic breathing disorders (including COPD), it was shown that 10% of them presented with only high-intensity anxiety symptoms, 20% with only high-intensity depression symptoms, and 70% with a combination thereof (Kunik et al., 2005).

Other Medical Comorbidities

Subthreshold anxiety is also found in other medical conditions associated with aging, such as chronic pain/headache (Feeney, 2004; Lucchetti et al., 2013; Rzewuska et al., 2015), psoriatic arthritis (McDonough et al., 2014; Ogdie et al., 2015), osteoporosis (Erez et al., 2012; Williams et al., 2011), and hearing/visual impairment (Contrera et al., 2017; van der Aa et al., 2015). Indeed, the higher the number of physical diseases, the greater the risk for an older person to suffer from anxiety (Jones et al., 2016). This was demonstrated by the fact that each additional comorbid physical disease increased anxiety symptoms by 0.257 standard deviations (vs. 0.276 standard deviations for depressive symptoms). Three mechanisms may explain the strong association between anxiety symptoms and physical diseases: (1) anxiety symptoms may increase a person's vulnerability to physical diseases; (2) physical diseases may cause anxiety symptoms; and (3) the side effects of medications taken for physical health problems may mimic anxiety symptoms (the reverse is also true). Further longitudinal studies should be undertaken to validate these mechanisms and to better understand how physical diseases and anxious and depressive symptoms interact over time.

Treatment Strategies

Pharmacological Treatments

Anxiolytic drugs (especially BZDs) are frequently prescribed to treat anxiety in older adults (Préville et al., 2011). However, the safety of these drugs has been questioned. For example, BZD use (even for some weeks) in older people may cause balance problems (increasing the risk of falls and hospitalization), affect memory and concentration, as well as worsen physical health and sleep quality (Béland et al., 2010, 2011; Bierman et al., 2007; Gleason et al., 1998; Gray et al., 2006; Lader, 2014; Landi et al., 2002; Quevillon & Bedard, 2003). Moreover, older BZD consumers may quickly become addicted to this medication (Ashton, 2005). For all of these reasons, if the costs outweigh the benefits, BZDs should not be routinely prescribed to anxious seniors. Antidepressants (mainly selective serotonin reuptake inhibitors) are deemed safer and more effective than BZDs to treat late-life anxiety in the long term, but their use is not without side effects (e.g., increased risk of falling, fractures, stroke, etc.), as suggested by an observational study including 60,746 older patients with depression (Coupland et al., 2011). See Chapter 12 for a further discussion of pharmacological approaches to anxiety in later life.

Psychosocial Interventions

In subthreshold anxiety cases, it is possible to reduce undesirable side effects by opting for non-pharmacological therapies. Four systematic reviews (with or without meta-analyses) evaluated the effectiveness of different psychological interventions (e.g., cognitive behavioral therapy (CBT), relaxation training, supportive therapy) in the treatment of late-life anxiety (Ayers et al., 2007; Gould et al., 2012; Hendriks et al., 2008; Thorp et al., 2009). These reviews concluded that CBT and relaxation training are effective treatments for full anxiety disorder in seniors (although the observed effects are generally smaller than in younger adults with anxiety). However, this conclusion cannot be generalized to subthreshold anxiety, since only seven studies (among the dozens considered) included patients with ADNOS or subthreshold anxiety (Barrowclough et al., 2001; DeBerry, 1982a, 1982b; DeBerry et al., 1989; Gorenstein et al., 2005; Scogin et al., 1992; Wetherell et al., 2009). It should also be noted that in the studies conducted by Barrowclough et al. (2001), Gorenstein et al. (2005), and Wetherell et al. (2009), the percentage of participants with ADNOS did not exceed 30% (the remaining participants had full anxiety disorder), thereby limiting the generalizability of results with regard to older adults suffering from subthreshold anxiety. Notably, a study including 55 subjects (mean age: 72 years; 28% with ADNOS) by Barrowclough et al. (2001) demonstrated that CBT reduced anxiety and depression more effectively than supportive counseling. The improvements noticed with CBT were maintained at the 3-, 6-, and 12-month follow-ups. Another study, involving participants wishing to reduce their use of anxiolytics (mean age: 68 years; 19% with ADNOS), also showed that CBT, in conjunction with a medical management (MM) approach, was a more effective way to wean patients off medication and reduce anxiety symptoms compared to the MM approach alone (Gorenstein et al., 2005). In particular, the CBT + MM treatment gains were maintained at the 6-month follow-up. Finally, a study by Wetherell et al. (2009), involving 31 primary care patients (mean age: 72.1 years; 13% with ADNOS), compared the effectiveness of two interventions for anxiety (CBT, usual care). The authors showed that both approaches were effective in reducing anxiety and depression symptoms. However, the protocol did not include a post-treatment follow-up.

Three other studies (DeBerry, 1982a, 1982b; DeBerry et al., 1989) have shown that relaxation training (often included in the CBT intervention strategy) was more effective in reducing anxiety than control treatment approaches (e.g., pseudo-relaxation) in recently widowed seniors. A later study involving 71 participants with subthreshold anxiety (mean age: 68 years; Scogin et al., 1992) has shown that progressive muscle relaxation and imaginal relaxation reduced anxiety more efficiently than a waiting list. The gains were maintained at the 1-month follow-up. Another study (Bains et al., 2014; not included in the meta-analysis done by Gould et al., 2012) suggests that CBT is an effective treatment for anxiety symptoms in older patients (mean age: 74.8 years) suffering from mixed anxiety–depression. A surprising result in this study was that CBT was not efficient in reducing depressive symptoms. It should be noted that methodological shortcomings (e.g., absence of comparison group) limit the conclusions that can be drawn from this study.

Other studies have shown that CBT was effective in reducing fear of falling (Dorresteijn et al., 2016; Huang et al., 2016; Tennstedt et al., 1998; Zijlstra et al., 2009, 2013) and subthreshold anxiety (with or without depression) in patients diagnosed with different diseases, such as COPD (de Godoy & de Godoy, 2003; Kunik et al., 2008), heart diseases (Yousefy et al., 2010), PD (Dobkin et al., 2011; Veazey et al., 2009), and AD (Kraus et al., 2008; Stanley et al., 2013). Finally, it has been demonstrated that mindfulness-based interventions (relying on relaxation strategies tested in the aforementioned studies; Foulk et al., 2013), life-review/reminiscence interventions (Haslam et al., 2010; Korte et al., 2012), spiritual/religious interventions (Elham et al., 2015), music interventions (Sung et al., 2012), and yoga (Bonura & Tenenbaum, 2014) could also effectively reduce anxiety symptoms in older adults with or without cognitive deficits. However, given the small number of studies with these methodologies and their uneven methodological controls, these results should be interpreted with caution.

In light of these findings, we consider that CBT and relaxation training are the two non-pharmacological interventions that should be prioritized to reduce subthreshold anxiety in later life. Currently, there is more empirical support for the effectiveness of CBT in the treatment of full anxiety disorders than for subthreshold anxiety. It should be kept in mind that an intervention that is effective at treating full anxiety disorder may not automatically alleviate subthreshold anxiety. Nonetheless, since subthreshold and threshold anxiety share many clinical similarities and few differences (Grenier et al., 2011a), both conditions may potentially be effectively addressed with CBT. We suggest that future studies include more seniors with subthreshold anxiety in their sample. Also, efficacy results for the different subtypes of anxiety disorders should be reported separately. Finally, the efficacy of CBT to relieve subthreshold anxiety in people suffering from physical or neurological diseases (e.g., COPD, PD, etc.), as well as the efficacy of new promising interventions (e.g., mindfulness, music, yoga), should be confirmed in additional studies.

Conclusion and Future Directions

There is ample research evidence indicating that the prevalence of subthreshold anxiety is high (even greater than full anxiety disorders) in older people with or without general medical comorbidities. Many studies have also shown that subthreshold anxiety (and not only anxiety disorders) can have an impact on the daily functioning of seniors and can compromise their well-being. Late-life anxiety symptoms may thus be severe or clinically significant even if all diagnostic criteria are not met. This implies that clinicians must remain vigilant and try to lower the anxiety symptoms reported by older patients. Indeed, some anxiety symptoms may indicate the presence of a previously unsuspected general medical condition or constitute warning signs of depression. Therefore, we recommend that screening of anxious and depressive symptoms be part of routine medical examinations, as is the case for blood pressure and body weight verification. In fact, the first challenge for clinicians is to recognize anxious and depressive symptoms that can either mimic symptoms that are seen in other physical illnesses or that are hidden behind somatic complaints. The second challenge is to respond quickly and effectively in order to minimize the deleterious effects of anxious and depressive symptoms on the old person's health. In this regard, the effectiveness of CBT and relaxation training appears to stand out among the different approaches. These interventions are not only effective at relieving late-life anxiety symptoms; they are also much less harmful to seniors' health than psychotropic drugs (e.g., BZDs). However, further studies are necessary to confirm their efficacy in samples comprising seniors with different subthreshold anxiety types or mixed anxious and depressive symptoms. Sometimes, researchers criticize their peers for not including older people with full anxiety disorder in their samples, implying that focusing on subthreshold anxiety cases decreases the quality or validity of a study. We argue that, on the contrary, choosing not to include subthreshold anxiety cases in samples decreases the generalizability of results. These results become less relevant to clinical settings, where subthreshold anxiety is more often the rule than the exception.

Therefore, it is important to better define subthreshold anxiety. For some researchers, subthreshold anxiety implies that some anxiety symptoms are present, while the definition is stricter for others. In all cases, however, anxiety is characterized as subthreshold when the threshold for a specific anxiety disorder is not met. One important question remains unresolved: At what point (moment) should the threshold be defined – when anxiety symptoms are severe enough to perturb daily functioning? Apparently not, since the severity/impact criteria based on functioning do not clearly differentiate people reporting subthreshold anxiety from those with full anxiety disorder. One way to overcome this threshold problem is to conceptualize late-life anxiety as a continuum extending from the absence of symptoms to full anxiety disorder. In older adults, anxiety may fluctuate throughout this continuum according to different biopsychological factors (biological vulnerability, diseases, life events, etc.). Additional studies are necessary to identify the strongest contributing factors for late-life anxiety fluctuations.

In addition, it would be worth investigating whether traditional CBT (including, among others, psychoeducation related to anxiety, relaxation training, and cognitive restructuration) is more effective than relaxation training only to reduce anxiety symptoms. If relaxation training alone provides comparable or better results than CBT, this would save time and money. Further studies should also be carried out to compare responses to treatment in older and middle-aged anxious adults. This would clarify the influence of aging on the effectiveness of interventions. These studies would finally provide the necessary evidence to better treat subthreshold anxiety in seniors and, possibly, add some years to their healthy life expectancy.

References

Almeida, O. P., Draper, B., Pirkis, J., et al. (2012). Anxiety, depression, and comorbid anxiety and depression: risk factors and outcome over two years. *International Psychogeriatrics*, 24, 1622–1632.

Ames, D., Flynn, E. and Harrigan, S. (1994). Prevalence of psychiatric disorders among inpatients of an acute geriatric hospital. *Australian Journal on Ageing*, 13, 8–11.

Andersen, R. M. (2008). National health surveys and the behavioral model of health services use. *Medical Care*, 46, 647–653.

Apostolova, L. G. and Cummings, J. L. (2008). Neuropsychiatric manifestations in mild cognitive impairment: a systematic review of the literature. *Dementia and Geriatric Cognitive Disorders*, 25, 115–126.

Ashton, H. (2005). The diagnosis and management of benzodiazepine dependence. *Current Opinion in Psychiatry*, 18, 249–255.

Ayers, C. R., Sorrell, J. T., Thorp, S. R. and Wetherell, J. L. (2007). Evidence-based psychological treatments for late-life anxiety. *Psychology and Aging*, 22, 8–17.

Bains, M. K., Scott, S., Kellett, S. and Saxon, D. (2014). Group psychoeducative cognitive–behaviour therapy for mixed anxiety and depression with older adults. *Aging and Mental Health*, 18, 1057–1065.

Barrowclough, C., King, P., Colville, J., Russell, E., Burns, A. and Tarrier, N. (2001). A randomized trial of the effectiveness of cognitive–behavioral therapy and supportive counseling for anxiety symptoms in older adults. *Journal of Consulting and Clinical Psychology*, 69, 756–762.

Batelaan, N. M., Spijker, J., De Graaf, R. and Cuijpers, P. (2012). Mixed anxiety depression should not be included in DSM-5. *Journal of Nervous and Mental Disease*, 200, 495–498.

Beaudreau, S. A. and O'Hara, R. (2008). Late-life anxiety and cognitive impairment: a review. *American Journal of Geriatric Psychiatry*, 16, 790–803.

Beekman, A. T., De Beurs, E., Van Balkom, A. J., Deeg, D. J., Van Dyck, R. and Van Tilburg, W. (2000). Anxiety and depression in later life: Co-occurrence and communality of risk factors. *American Journal of Psychiatry*, 157, 89–95.

Béland, S. G., Préville, M., Dubois, M.-F., et al. (2010). Benzodiazepine use and quality of sleep in the community-dwelling elderly population. *Aging and Mental Health*, 14, 843–850.

Béland, S. G., Préville, M., Dubois, M. F., et al. (2011). The association between length of benzodiazepine use and sleep quality in older population. *International Journal of Geriatric Psychiatry*, 26, 908–915.

Bertera, E. M. and Bertera, R. L. (2008). Fear of falling and activity avoidance in a national sample of older adults in the United States. *Health and Social Work*, 33, 54–62.

Bhala, R. P., O'donnell, J. and Thoppil, E. (1982). Ptophobia. Phobic fear of falling and its clinical management. *Physical Therapy*, 62, 187–190.

Bierman, E. J. M., Comijs, H. C., Gundy, C. M., Sonnenberg, C., Jonker, C. and Beekman, A. T. F. (2007). The effect of chronic benzodiazepine use on cognitive functioning in older persons: good, bad or indifferent? *International Journal of Geriatric Psychiatry*, **22**, 1194–1200.

Blyth, F. M., Cumming, R. G., Nicholas, M. K., et al. (2011). Intrusive pain and worry about health in older men: the CHAMP study. *Pain*, **152**, 447–452.

Bonura, K. B. and Tenenbaum, G. (2014). Effects of yoga on psychological health in older adults. *Journal of Physical Activity and Health*, **11**, 1334–1341.

Braam, A. W., Copeland, J. R. M., Delespaul, P. A. E. G., et al. (2014). Depression, subthreshold depression and comorbid anxiety symptoms in older Europeans: results from the EURODEP concerted action. *Journal of Affective Disorders*, **155**, 266–272.

Brenes, G. A. (2003). Anxiety and chronic obstructive pulmonary disease: prevalence, impact, and treatment. *Psychosomatic Medicine*, **65**, 963–970.

Brown, R. G., Landau, S., Hindle, J. V., et al. (2011). Depression and anxiety related subtypes in Parkinson's disease. *Journal of Neurology, Neurosurgery and Psychiatry*, **82**, 803–809.

Bryant, C., Jackson, H. and Ames, D. (2008). The prevalence of anxiety in older adults: Methodological issues and a review of the literature. *Journal of Affective Disorders*, **109**, 233–250.

Cassidy, E. L., Lauderdale, S. and Sheikh, J. I. (2005). Mixed anxiety and depression in older adults: clinical characteristics and management. *Journal of Geriatric Psychiatry and Neurology*, **18**, 83–88.

Contrera, K. J., Betz, J., Deal, J., et al. (2017). Association of hearing impairment and anxiety in older adults. *Journal of Aging and Health*, **29**, 172–184.

Coupland, C., Dhiman, P., Morriss, R., Arthur, A., Barton, G. and Hippisley-Cox, J. (2011). Antidepressant use and risk of adverse outcomes in older people: population based cohort study. *BMJ*, **343**, d4551.

Das-Munshi, J., Goldberg, D., Bebbington, P. E., et al. (2008). Public health significance of mixed anxiety and depression: beyond

current classification. *British Journal of Psychiatry*, **192**, 171–177.

de Godoy, D. V. and de Godoy, R. F. (2003). A randomized controlled trial of the effect of psychotherapy on anxiety and depression in chronic obstructive pulmonary disease1. *Archives of Physical Medicine and Rehabilitation*, **84**, 1154–1157.

DeBerry, S. (1982a). The effects of meditation-relaxation on anxiety and depression in a geriatric population. *Psychotherapy: Theory, Research and Practice*, **19**, 512–521.

DeBerry, S. (1982b). An evaluation of progressive muscle relaxation on stress related symptoms in a geriatric population. *International Journal of Aging and Human Development*, **14**, 255–269.

DeBerry, S., Davis, S. and Reinhard, K. E. (1989). A comparison of meditation-relaxation and cognitive/behavioral techniques for reducing anxiety and depression in a geriatric population. *Journal of Geriatric Psychiatry*, **22**, 231–247.

Diefenbach, G. J., Stanley, M. A. and Beck, J. G. (2001). Worry content reported by older adults with and without generalized anxiety disorder. *Aging and Mental Health*, **5**, 269–274.

Dobkin, R. D., Menza, M., Allen, L. A., et al. (2011). Cognitive–behavioral therapy for depression in Parkinson's disease: a randomized, controlled trial. *American Journal of Psychiatry*, **168**, 1066–1074.

Dorresteijn, T. A. C., Zijlstra, G. A. R., Ambergen, A. W., Delbaere, K., Vlaeyen, J. W. S. and Kempen, G. I. J. M. (2016). Effectiveness of a home-based cognitive behavioral program to manage concerns about falls in community-dwelling, frail older people: results of a randomized controlled trial. *BMC Geriatrics*, **16**, 1–11.

Drageset, J., Eide, G. E. and Ranhoff, A. H. (2013). Anxiety and depression among nursing home residents without cognitive impairment. *Scandinavian Journal of Caring Sciences*, **27**, 872–881.

Drozdick, L. and Edelstein, B. (2001). Correlates of fear of falling in older adults who have experienced a fall. *Journal of Clinical Geropsychology*, **7**, 1–13.

Elham, H., Hazrati, M., Momennasab, M. and Sareh, K. (2015). The effect of need-based spiritual/religious intervention on spiritual well-being and anxiety of elderly people. *Holistic Nursing Practice*, **29**, 136–143.

Erez, H., Weller, A., Vaisman, N. and Kreitler, S. (2012). The relationship of depression, anxiety and stress with low bone mineral density in post-menopausal women. *Archives of Osteoporosis*, **7**, 247–255.

Eysenck, M. W. and Calvo, M. G. (1992). Anxiety and performance: the Processing Efficiency Theory. *Cognition and Emotion*, **6**, 409–434.

Eysenck, M. W., Derakshan, N., Santos, R. and Calvo, M. G. (2007). Anxiety and cognitive performance: Attentional Control Theory. *Emotion*, **7**, 336–353.

Feeney, S. L. (2004). The relationship between pain and negative affect in older adults: anxiety as a predictor of pain. *Journal of Anxiety Disorders*, **18**, 733–744.

Flint, A. J. (2005). Generalised anxiety disorder in elderly patients: epidemiology, diagnosis and treatment options. *Drugs and Aging*, **22**, 101–114.

Forlani, M., Morri, M., Belvederi Murri, M., et al. (2014). Anxiety symptoms in 74+ community-dwelling elderly: associations with physical morbidity, depression and alcohol consumption. *PLoS ONE*, **9**, e89859.

Forsell, Y. and Winblad, B. (1998). Feelings of anxiety and associated variables in a very elderly population. *International Journal of Geriatric Psychiatry*, **13**, 454–458.

Foulk, M. A., Ingersoll-Dayton, B., Kavanagh, J., Robinson, E. and Kales, H. C. (2013). Mindfulness-based cognitive therapy with older adults: an exploratory study. *Journal of Gerontological Social Work*, **57**, 498–520.

Frasure-Smith, N. and Lesperance, F. (2008). Depression and anxiety as predictors of 2-year cardiac events in patients with stable coronary artery disease. *Archives of General Psychiatry*, **65**, 62–71.

Fredrikson, M., Annas, P., Fischer, H. and Wik, G. (1996). Gender and age differences in the prevalence of specific fears and phobias. *Behaviour Research and Therapy*, **34**, 33–39.

Gagnon, N., Flint, A. J., Naglie, G. and Devins, G. M. (2005). Affective correlates of fear of falling in elderly persons. *American Journal of Geriatric Psychiatry*, **13**, 7–14.

Gallacher, J., Bayer, A., Fish, M., et al. (2009). Does anxiety affect risk of dementia? Findings from the Caerphilly Prospective Study. *Psychosomatic Medicine*, **71**, 659–666.

Gallagher, D., O'regan, C., Savva, G. M., Cronin, H., Lawlor, B. A. and Kenny, R. A. (2012). Depression, anxiety and cardiovascular disease: which symptoms are associated with increased risk in community dwelling older adults? *Journal of Affective Disorders*, **142**, 132–138.

Garrido, M. M., Kane, R. L., Kaas, M. and Kane, R. A. (2009). Perceived need for mental health care among community-dwelling older adults. *Journals of Gerontology Series B: Psychological Sciences and Social Sciences*, **64B**, 704–712.

Gleason, P. P., Schulz, R., Smith, N. L., et al. (1998). Correlates and prevalence of benzodiazepine use in community-dwelling elderly. *Journal of General Internal Medicine*, **13**, 243–250.

Gonçalves, D. C. and Byrne, G. J. (2013). Who worries most? Worry prevalence and patterns across the lifespan. *International Journal of Geriatric Psychiatry*, **28**, 41–49.

Gorenstein, E. E., Kleber, M. S., Mohlman, J., Dejesus, M., Gorman, J. M. and Papp, L. A. (2005). Cognitive-behavioral therapy for management of anxiety and medication taper in older adults. *American Journal of Geriatric Psychiatry*, **13**, 901–909.

Gould, C. E. and Edelstein, B. A. (2010). Worry, emotion control, and anxiety control in older and young adults. *Journal of Anxiety Disorders*, **24**, 759–766.

Gould, R. L., Coulson, M. C. and Howard, R. J. (2012). Efficacy of cognitive behavioral therapy for anxiety disorders in older people: a meta-analysis and meta-regression of randomized controlled trials. *Journal of the American Geriatrics Society*, **60**, 218–229.

Gray, S. L., Lacroix, A. Z., Hanlon, J. T., et al. (2006). Benzodiazepine use and physical disability in community-dwelling older adults. *Journal of the American Geriatrics Society*, **54**, 224–230.

Grenier, S., Potvin, O., Hudon, C., et al. (2012). Twelve-month prevalence and correlates of subthreshold and threshold anxiety in community-dwelling older adults with cardiovascular diseases. *Journal of Affective Disorders*, **136**, 724–732.

Grenier, S., Préville, M., Boyer, R., et al. (2011a). The impact of DSM-IV symptom and clinical significance criteria on the prevalence estimates of subthreshold and threshold anxiety in the older adult population. *American Journal of Geriatric Psychiatry*, **19**, 316–326.

Grenier, S., Schuurmans, J., Goldfarb, M., et al. (2011b). The epidemiology of specific phobia and subthreshold fear subtypes in a community-based sample of older adults. *Depression and Anxiety*, **28**, 456–463.

Haller, H., Cramer, H., Lauche, R., Gass, F. and Dobos, G. (2014). The prevalence and burden of subthreshold generalized anxiety disorder: a systematic review. *BMC Psychiatry*, **14**, 128.

Haslam, C., Haslam, S. A., Jetten, J., Bevins, A., Ravenscroft, S. and Tonks, J. (2010). The social treatment: the benefits of group interventions in residential care settings. *Psychology and Aging*, **25**, 157–167.

Hendriks, G. J., Oude Voshaar, R. C., Keijsers, G. P. J., Hoogduin, C. A. L. and Van Balkom, A. J. L. M. (2008). Cognitive–behavioural therapy for late-life anxiety disorders: a systematic review and meta-analysis. *Acta Psychiatrica Scandinavica*, **117**, 403–411.

Heun, R., Papassotiropoulos, A. and Ptok, U. (2000). Subthreshold depressive and anxiety disorders in the elderly. *European Psychiatry*, **15**, 173–182.

Hoe, J., Hancock, G., Livingston, G. and Orrell, M. (2006). Quality of life of people with dementia in residential care homes. *British Journal of Psychiatry*, **188**, 460–464.

Huang, T.-T., Chung, M.-L., Chen, F.-R., Chin, Y.-F. and Wang, B.-H. (2016). Evaluation of a combined cognitive-behavioural and exercise intervention to manage fear of falling among elderly residents in nursing homes. *Aging and Mental Health*, **20**, 2–12.

Huffman, J. C., Celano, C. M. and Januzzi, J. L. (2010). The relationship between depression, anxiety, and cardiovascular outcomes in patients with acute coronary syndromes. *Neuropsychiatric Disease and Treatment*, **6**, 123–136.

Hunt, S., Wisocki, P. and Yanko, J. (2003). Worry and use of coping strategies among older and younger adults. *Journal of Anxiety Disorders*, **17**, 547–560.

Jones, S. M. W., Amtmann, D. and Gell, N. M. (2016). A psychometric examination of multimorbidity and mental health in older adults. *Aging and Mental Health*, **20**, 309–317.

Jonson, M., Skoog, I., Marlow, T., Mellqvist Fässberg, M. and Waern, M. (2012). Anxiety symptoms and suicidal feelings in a population sample of 70-year-olds without dementia. *International Psychogeriatrics*, **24**, 1865–1871.

Kelley-Moore, J. A., Schumacher, J. G., Kahana, E. and Kahana, B. (2006). When do older adults become "disabled"? Social and health antecedents of perceived disability in a panel study of the oldest old. *Journal of Health and Social Behavior*, **47**, 126–141.

Kessler, R. C., Berglund, P., Demler, O., Jin, R., Merikangas, K. R. and Walters, E. E. (2005). Lifetime prevalence and age-of-onset distributions of DSM-IV disorders in the National Comorbidity Survey Replication. *Archives of General Psychiatry*, **62**, 593–602.

Kim, J. W., Lee, D. Y., Lee, B. C., et al. (2012). Alcohol and cognition in the elderly: a review. *Psychiatry Investigation*, **9**, 8–16.

Kirby, M., Denihan, A., Bruce, I., Radic, A., Coakley, D. and Lawlor, B. A. (1999). Influence of symptoms of anxiety on treatment of depression in later life in primary care: questionnaire survey. *BMJ*, **318**, 579–580.

Korte, J., Bohlmeijer, E. T., Cappeliez, P., Smit, F. and Westerhof, G. J. (2012). Life review therapy for older adults with moderate depressive symptomatology:

a pragmatic randomized controlled trial. *Psychological Medicine*, **42**, 1163–1173.

Kraus, C. A., Seignourel, P., Balasubramanyam, V., et al. (2008). Cognitive-behavioral treatment for anxiety in patients with dementia: two case studies. *Journal of Psychiatric Practice*, **14**, 186–192.

Kunik, M. E., Roundy, K., Veazey, C., et al. (2005). Surprisingly high prevalence of anxiety and depression in chronic breathing disorders. *Chest*, **127**, 1205–1211.

Kunik, M. E., Veazey, C., Cully, J. A., et al. (2008). COPD education and cognitive behavioral therapy group treatment for clinically significant symptoms of depression and anxiety in COPD patients: a randomized controlled trial. *Psychological medicine*, **38**, 385–396.

Kvaal, K., Macijauskiene, J., Engedal, K. and Laake, K. (2001). High prevalence of anxiety symptoms in hospitalized geriatric patients. *International Journal of Geriatric Psychiatry*, **16**, 690–693.

Lader, M. (2014). Benzodiazepine Harm: How Can It Be Reduced? *British Journal of Clinical Pharmacology*, **77**, 295–301.

Landi, F., Cesari, M., Russo, A., Onder, G., Sgadari, A. and Bernabei, R. (2002). Benzodiazepines and the risk of urinary incontinence in frail older persons living in the community. *Clinical Pharmacology and Therapeutics*, **72**, 729–734.

Leentjens, A. F. G., Dujardin, K., Marsh, L., Martinez-Martin, P., Richard, I. H. and Starkstein, S. E. (2011). Symptomatology and markers of anxiety disorders in Parkinson's disease: a cross-sectional study. *Movement Disorders*, **26**, 484–492.

Lenze, E. (2003). Comorbidity of depression and anxiety in the elderly. *Current Psychiatry Reports*, **5**, 62–67.

Lenze, E. J., Mulsant, B. H., Shear, M. K., et al. (2000). Comorbid anxiety disorders in depressed elderly patients. *American Journal of Psychiatry*, **157**, 722–728.

Livermore, N., Sharpe, L. and McKenzie, D. (2010). Panic attacks and panic disorder in chronic obstructive pulmonary disease: a cognitive behavioral perspective. *Respiratory Medicine*, **104**, 1246–1253.

Lucchetti, G., Peres, M. F. P., Lucchetti, A. L. G., Mercante, J. P. P., Guendler, V. Z. and Zukerman, E. (2013). Generalized anxiety disorder, subthreshold anxiety and anxiety symptoms in primary headache. *Psychiatry and Clinical Neurosciences*, **67**, 41–49.

Lyketsos, C. G., Lopez, O., Jones, B., Fitzpatrick, A. L., Breitner, J. and Dekosky, S. (2002). Prevalence of neuropsychiatric symptoms in dementia and mild cognitive impairment: results from the cardiovascular health study. *JAMA*, **288**, 1475–1483.

Mackenzie, C. S., Reynolds, K., Chou, K. L., Pagura, J. and Sareen, J. (2011). Prevalence and correlates of generalized anxiety disorder in a national sample of older adults. *American Journal of Geriatric Psychiatry*, **19**, 305–315.

Magee, J. and Carmin, C. (2010). The relationship between sleep and anxiety in older adults. *Current Psychiatry Reports*, **12**, 13–19.

Mallon, L., Broman, J. E. and Jerker, H. (2000). Sleeping difficulties in relation to depression and anxiety in elderly adults. *Nordic Journal of Psychiatry*, **54**, 355–360.

Marinus, J., Leentjens, A. F., Visser, M., Stiggelbout, A. M. and Van Hilten, J. J. (2002). Evaluation of the hospital anxiety and depression scale in patients with Parkinson's disease. *Clinical Neuropharmacology*, **25**, 318–324.

Martinez-Martin, P. and Damian, J. (2010). Parkinson disease: Depression and anxiety in Parkinson disease. *Nature Reviews Neurology*, **6**, 243–245.

McDonough, E., Ayearst, R., Eder, L., et al. (2014). Depression and anxiety in psoriatic disease: prevalence and associated factors. *Journal of Rheumatology*, **41**, 887–896.

Mehta, K. M., Simonsick, E. M., Penninx, B. W., et al. (2003). Prevalence and correlates of anxiety symptoms in well-functioning older adults: findings from the health aging and body composition study. *Journal of the American Geriatrics Society*, **51**, 499–504.

Miloyan, B., Byrne, G. J. and Pachana, N. A. (2015). Threshold and subthreshold generalized anxiety disorder in later life. *American Journal of Geriatric Psychiatry*, 23, 633–641.

Moser, D. K., Dracup, K., Evangelista, L. S., et al. (2010). Comparison of prevalence of symptoms of depression, anxiety, and hostility in elderly patients with heart failure, myocardial infarction, and a coronary artery bypass graft. *Heart and Lung*, 39, 378–385.

Moyle, W. and O'Dwyer, S. (2012). Quality of life in people living with dementia in nursing homes. *Current Opinion in Psychiatry*, 25, 480–484.

Mulsant, B. H., Reynolds, C. F., Shear, M. K., Sweet, R. A. and Miller, M. (1996). Comorbid anxiety disorders in late-life depression. *Anxiety*, 2, 242–247.

Murphy, J. and Isaacs, B. (1982). The post-fall syndrome. A study of 36 elderly patients. *Gerontology*, 28, 265–270.

Murphy, S. L., Williams, C. S. and Gill, T. M. (2002). Characteristics associated with fear of falling and activity restriction in community-living older persons. *Journal of the American Geriatrics Society*, 50, 516–520.

Nagamatsu, L. S., Voss, M., Neider, M. B., et al. (2011). Increased cognitive load leads to impaired mobility decisions in seniors at risk for falls. *Psychology and Aging*, 26, 253–259.

Nègre-Pagès, L., Grandjean, H., Lapeyre-Mestre, M., et al. (2010). Anxious and depressive symptoms in Parkinson's disease: the French cross-sectional DoPaMiP study. *Movement Disorders*, 25, 157–166.

Ogdie, A., Schwartzman, S. and Husni, M. E. (2015). Recognizing and managing comorbidities in psoriatic arthritis. *Current Opinion in Rheumatology*, 27, 118–126.

Palmer, K., Berger, A. K., Monastero, R., et al. (2007). Predictors of progression from mild cognitive impairment to Alzheimer disease. *Neurology*, 68, 1596–1602.

Panagioti, M., Scott, C., Blakemore, A. and Coventry, P. A. (2014). Overview of the prevalence, impact, and management of depression and anxiety in chronic obstructive pulmonary disease. *International Journal of Chronic Obstructive Pulmonary Disease*, 9, 1289–1306.

Papassotiropoulos, A. and Heun, R. (1999). Detection of subthreshold depression and subthreshold anxiety in the elderly. *International Journal of Geriatric Psychiatry*, 14, 643–650.

Payette, M. C., Belanger, C., Leveille, V. and Grenier, S. (2016). Fall-related psychological concerns and anxiety among community-dwelling older adults: systematic review and meta-analysis. *PLoS ONE*, 11, e0152848.

Petkus, A. J., Reynolds, C. A., Wetherell, J. L., Kremen, W. S., Pedersen, N. L. and Gatz, M. (2016). Anxiety is associated with increased risk of dementia in older Swedish twins. *Alzheimer's and Dementia*, 12, 399–406.

Pontone, G. M., Williams, J. R., Anderson, K. E., et al. (2009). Prevalence of anxiety disorders and anxiety subtypes in patients with Parkinson's disease. *Movement Disorders*, 24, 1333–1338.

Potvin, O., Forget, H., Grenier, S., Préville, M. and Hudon, C. (2011a). Anxiety, depression, and 1-year incident cognitive impairment in community-dwelling older adults. *Journal of the American Geriatrics Society*, 59, 1421–1428.

Potvin, O., Hudon, C., Dion, M., Grenier, S. and Préville, M. (2011b). Anxiety disorders, depressive episodes and cognitive impairment no dementia in community-dwelling older men and women. *International Journal of Geriatric Psychiatry*, 26, 1080–1088.

Préville, M., Vasiliadis, H. M., Bosse, C., Dionne, P.-A., Voyer, P. and Brassard, J. (2011). Pattern of psychotropic drug use among older adults having a depression or an anxiety disorder: results from the longitudinal ESA study. *Canadian Journal of Psychiatry*, 56, 348–357.

Prina, A. M., Ferri, C. P., Guerra, M., Brayne, C. and Prince, M. (2011a). Prevalence of anxiety and its correlates among older adults in Latin America, India and China: cross-cultural study. *British Journal of Psychiatry*, 199, 485–491.

Prina, A. M., Ferri, C. P., Guerra, M., Brayne, C. and Prince, M. (2011b). Co-occurrence of anxiety and depression amongst older adults in low- and middle-income countries: findings from the 10/66 study. *Psychological Medicine*, **41**, 2047–2056.

Quevillon, F. and Bedard, M. A. (2003). [Benzodiazepines: consequences on memory in the elderly]. *Sante Mentale au Quebec*, **28**, 23–41.

Roy-Byrne, P., Katon, W., Broadhead, W. E., et al. (1994). Subsyndromal ("mixed") anxiety–depression in primary care. *Journal of General Internal Medicine*, **9**, 507–12.

Rutledge, T., Linke, S. E., Krantz, D. S., et al. (2009). Comorbid depression and anxiety symptoms as predictors of cardiovascular events: results from the NHLBI-sponsored Women's Ischemia Syndrome Evaluation (WISE) study. *Psychosomatic Medicine*, **71**, 958–964.

Rzewuska, M., Mallen, C. D., Strauss, V. Y., Belcher, J. and Peat, G. (2015). One-year trajectories of depression and anxiety symptoms in older patients presenting in general practice with musculoskeletal pain: a latent class growth analysis. *Journal of Psychosomatic Research*, **79**, 195–201.

Scheffer, A. C., Schuurmans, M. J., Dijk, N., Hooft, T. and Rooij, S. E. (2008). Fear of falling: measurement strategy, prevalence, risk factors and consequences among older persons. *Age and Ageing*, **37**, 19–24.

Schoevers, R. A., Deeg, D. J., Van Tilburg, W. and Beekman, A. T. (2005). Depression and generalized anxiety disorder: co-occurrence and longitudinal patterns in elderly patients. *American Journal of Geriatric Psychiatry*, **13**, 31–39.

Schuurmans, J., Comijs, H. C., Beekman, A. T. F., et al. (2005). The outcome of anxiety disorders in older people at 6-year follow-up: results from the Longitudinal Aging Study Amsterdam. *Acta Psychiatrica Scandinavica*, **111**, 420–428.

Scogin, F., Rickard, H. C., Keith, S., Wilson, J. and McElreath, L. (1992). Progressive and imaginal relaxation training for elderly persons with subjective anxiety. *Psychology and aging*, **7**, 419–424.

Scott, T., Mackenzie, C. S., Chipperfield, J. G. and Sareen, J. (2010). Mental health service use among Canadian older adults with anxiety disorders and clinically significant anxiety symptoms. *Aging and Mental Health*, **14**, 790–800.

Seignourel, P. J., Kunik, M. E., Snow, L., Wilson, N. and Stanley, M. (2008). Anxiety in dementia: A critical review. *Clinical Psychology Review*, **28**, 1071–1082.

Siemers, E. R., Shekhar, A., Quaid, K. and Dickson, H. (1993). Anxiety and motor performance in Parkinson's disease. *Movement Disorders*, **8**, 501–506.

Simning, A., Van Wijngaarden, E., Fisher, S. G., Richardson, T. M. and Conwell, Y. (2012). Mental health care need and service utilization in older adults living in public housing. *American Journal of Geriatric Psychiatry*, **20**, 441–451.

Smalbrugge, M., Pot, A. M., Jongenelis, K., Beekman, A. T. and Eefsting, J. A. (2005). Prevalence and correlates of anxiety among nursing home patients. *Journal of Affective Disorders*, **88**, 145–153.

Smit, F., Comijs, H., Schoevers, R., Cuijpers, P., Deeg, D. and Beekman, A. (2007). Target groups for the prevention of late-life anxiety. *British Journal of Psychiatry*, **190**, 428–434.

Sorocco, K. H. and Ferrell, S. W. (2006). Alcohol use among older adults. *Journal of General Psychology*, **133**, 453–467.

Spira, A. P., Stone, K., Beaudreau, S. A., Ancoli-Israel, S. and Yaffe, K. (2009). Anxiety symptoms and objectively measured sleep quality in older women. *American Journal of Geriatric Psychiatry*, **17**, 136–143.

Stanley, M. A., Calleo, J., Bush, A. L., et al. (2013). The peaceful mind program: a pilot test of a cognitive-behavioral therapy-based intervention for anxious patients with dementia. *American Journal of Geriatric Psychiatry*, **21**, 696–708.

Stefanova, E., Ziropadja, L., Petrović, M., Stojković, T. and Kostić, V. (2013). Screening for anxiety symptoms in parkinson disease: a cross-sectional study. *Journal of Geriatric Psychiatry and Neurology*, **26**, 34–40.

Stewart, J. C., Hawkins, M. A. W., Khambaty, T., Perkins, A. J. and Callahan, C. M. (2016). Depression and anxiety screens as predictors of 8-year incidence of myocardial infarction and stroke in primary care patients. *Psychosomatic Medicine*, **78**, 593–601.

Stillman, A. N., Rowe, K. C., Arndt, S. and Moser, D. J. (2012). Anxious symptoms and cognitive function in non-demented older adults: an inverse relationship. *International Journal of Geriatric Psychiatry*, **27**, 792–798.

Sung, H.-C., Lee, W.-L., Li, T.-L. and Watson, R. (2012). A group music intervention using percussion instruments with familiar music to reduce anxiety and agitation of institutionalized older adults with dementia. *International Journal of Geriatric Psychiatry*, **27**, 621–627.

Tennstedt, S., Howland, J., Lachman, M., Peterson, E., Kasten, L. and Jette, A. (1998). A randomized, controlled trial of a group intervention to reduce fear of falling and associated activity restriction in older adults. *Journals of Gerontology. Series B, Psychological Sciences and Social Sciences*, **53**, P384–P392.

Thorp, S. R., Ayers, C. R., Nuevo, R., Stoddard, J. A., Sorrell, J. T. and Wetherell, J. L. (2009). Meta-analysis comparing different behavioral treatments for late-life anxiety. *American Journal of Geriatric Psychiatry*, **17**, 105–115.

van der Aa, H. P. A., Comijs, H. C., Penninx, B. W. J. H., Van Rens, G. H. M. B. and Van Nispen, R. M. A. (2015). Major depressive and anxiety disorders in visually impaired older adults. *Investigative Ophthalmology and Visual Science*, **56**, 849–854.

van Haastregt, J. C., Zijlstra, G. A., Van Rossum, E., Van Eijk, J. T. and Kempen, G. I. (2008). Feelings of anxiety and symptoms of depression in community-living older persons who avoid activity for fear of falling. *American Journal of Geriatric Psychiatry*, **16**, 186-93.

van Zelst, W. H., De Beurs, E., Beekman, A. T., Van Dyck, R. and DeeG, D. D. (2006). Well-being, physical functioning, and use of health services in the elderly with PTSD and subthreshold PTSD. *International Journal of Geriatric Psychiatry*, **21**, 180–188.

Vazquez, A., Jimenez-Jimenez, F. J., Garcia-Ruiz, P. and Garcia-Urra, D. (1993). "Panic attacks" in Parkinson's disease. A long-term complication of levodopa therapy. *Acta Neurologica Scandinavica*, **87**, 14–18.

Veazey, C., Cook, K., Stanley, M., Lai, E. and Kunik, M. (2009). Telephone-administered cognitive behavioral therapy: a case study of anxiety and depression in Parkinson's disease. *Journal of Clinical Psychology in Medical Settings*, **16**, 243–253.

Wetherell, J. L., Gatz, M. and Pedersen, N. L. (2001). A longitudinal analysis of anxiety and depressive symptoms. *Psychology and Aging*, **16**, 187–195.

Wetherell, J. L., Le Roux, H. and Gatz, M. (2003). DSM-IV criteria for generalized anxiety disorder in older adults: distinguishing the worried from the well. *Psychology and Aging*, **18**, 622–627.

Wetherell, J. L. P., Ayers, C. R. P., Sorrell, J. T. P., et al. (2009). Modular psychotherapy for anxiety in older primary care patients. *American Journal of Geriatric Psychiatry*, **17**, 483–492.

Willgoss, T. G. and Yohannes, A. M. (2013). Anxiety disorders in patients with COPD: a systematic review. *Respiratory Care*, **58**, 858–866.

Williams, L. J., Bjerkeset, O., Langhammer, A., et al. (2011). The association between depressive and anxiety symptoms and bone mineral density in the general population: the HUNT study. *Journal of Affective Disorders*, **131**, 164–171.

Yohannes, A. M., Baldwin, R. C. and Connolly, M. J. (2000). Mood disorders in elderly patients with chronic obstructive pulmonary disease. *Reviews in Clinical Gerontology*, **10**, 193–202.

Yohannes, A. M., Baldwin, R. C. and Connolly, M. J. (2008). Prevalence of depression and anxiety symptoms in elderly patients admitted in post-acute intermediate care. *International Journal of Geriatric Psychiatry*, **23**, 1141–1147.

Yousefy, A., Khayyam-Nekouei, Z., Sadeghi, M., et al. (2010). The effect of cognitive–

behavioral therapy in reducing anxiety in heart disease patients. *ARYA Journal*, **2**, 84–88.

Zijlstra, G. A. R., van Haastregt, J. C. M., Ambergen, T., et al. (2009). Effects of a multicomponent cognitive behavioral group intervention on fear of falling and activity avoidance in community-dwelling older adults: results of a randomized controlled trial. *Journal of the American Geriatrics Society*, **57**, 2020–2028.

Zijlstra, G. A. R., van Haastregt, J. C. M., Du Moulin, M. F. M. T., de Jonge, M. C., van der Poel, A. and Kempen, G. I. J. M. (2013). Effects of the implementation of an evidence-based program to manage concerns about falls in older adults. *The Gerontologist*, **53**, 839–849.

Zinbarg, R. E., Barlow, D. H., Liebowitz, M., et al. (1994). The DSM-IV field trial for mixed anxiety–depression. *American Journal of Psychiatry*, **151**, 1153–1162.

Cross-cultural Issues in Late-Life Anxiety

Xiaoping Lin and Charissa Hosseini

This chapter discusses cross-cultural issues in late-life anxiety. It starts with an overview, providing a definition of culture and a theoretical model for understanding the role of culture in late-life anxiety. It then presents a summary of recent research on cross-cultural differences in various aspects of late-life anxiety, including perceptions of mental disorders, prevalence, symptom presentation, screening and diagnosis, risk and protective factors, and intervention. This chapter concludes with some recommendations for future research.

Overview

The term "culture" is used in a broad way within this chapter to refer to "a system of common heritage and shared beliefs, norms and values that unite a group of people" (Marques & Robinaugh, 2011). It encompasses several common terms used for categorizing social groups, such as ethnicity, race, nationality, and value systems. In the cross-cultural literature, the different types of cultures are usually categorized into two contrasting groups: Western versus non-Western cultures. Although there is great variation within these cultures, the term "Western cultures" generally refers to a set of cultures with their origin in Europe and that have an individualistic focus, such as those in European and North American countries (Oyserman et al., 2002). In contrast, the term "non-Western cultures" refers to a group of cultures that originate outside of the European continent and have a collectivist focus, such as those in African, Asian, and Middle Eastern countries (Oyserman et al., 2002).

It has long been argued that current definitions of mental disorders, including those in the Diagnostic and Statistical Manual of Mental Disorders, Fifth Edition (DSM-5; American Psychiatric Association, 2013) and the International Classification of Diseases, 10th Revision (ICD-10; World Health Organization, 1992), mainly reflect the Western biomedical perspective, which considers mental disorders as universal diseases with discrete diagnostic entities (e.g., Deacon, 2013; Halbreich et al., 2007; Thakker et al., 1999). The cross-cultural literature, however, reveals that there are significant differences across cultural groups in how mental disorders are perceived, experienced, and responded to. These differences have been observed among people living in different countries (e.g., cross-national studies), as well as in people living in the same country but from different cultural backgrounds (e.g., cultural studies including Caucasians and immigrants). Many of the studies discussed in this chapter come from studies with immigrants. It is important to highlight that, compared to studies with older people living in their countries of origin, the findings from those studies reflect the impact of culture as well as the impact of immigration on mental health, such as the reasons for immigration (e.g., civil war and refugee status) and the process of acculturation in the new country.

The Mandala of Health (Hancock, 1985; Hancock & Perkins, 1985) – an ecological model of health – has been used extensively in the teaching and program development of public health-promotion initiatives. It also serves as a theoretical model in this chapter to understand the role of culture in mental health. This model was developed following a shift in the understanding of health and disease from "a simplistic, reductionist cause-and-effect" medical view, which is time and cultural specific, to "a complex, holistic, interactive, hierarchic system view" (Hancock, 1985). It presents the determinants of an individual's health as a set of nested ecosystems, ranging from the biological and personal to the family, the broader community and its built environment, and the wider society and culture (see Figure 5.1). These hierarchic ecosystems continuously interact with each other, and together they influence an individual's physical, spiritual, and mental health (Hancock, 1985).

There are a number of features of the Mandala of Health that need to be highlighted. First, it is a holistic model of health in that it recognizes not only the multiple dimensions (body, mind, and spirit) of health, but also the interdependence between people, their health, and their physical and social environments. This holistic perception of health is particularly relevant to the cross-cultural literature because it is well documented that, compared to people from Western cultures, those from non-Western cultures have a more holistic view of health (Good & Kleinman, 1985; Grandbois, 2005; Martin, 2009; Torsch &

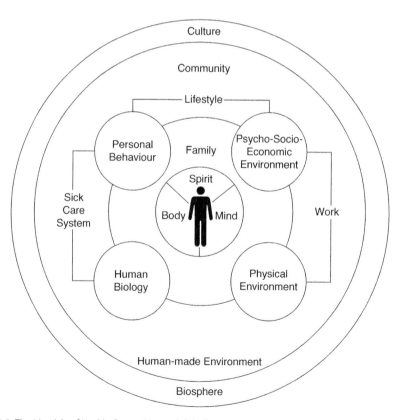

Figure 5.1 The Mandala of Health. *Source:* Hancock (1985).

Ma, 2000). Second, this model is not static, but rather it is fluid and dynamic, in that the ecosystems change and interact with each other all of the time (Hancock, 1985). This feature is consistent with a contemporary view of culture, which considers cultures as dynamic systems rather than static entities (e.g., D'Andrade, 2001; Kitayama, 2002). Such an orientation is important when interpreting findings from the cross-cultural literature so as to avoid cultural stereotyping. Finally, it is clear from the model that culture is only one of the various factors that affect an individual's health and that we need to consider the whole person in context when understanding his or her health.

Perception of Mental Disorders

There is evidence of cross-cultural differences in perceptions of mental health and mental disorders. Compared to Western cultures, non-Western cultures, such as those of Asia, the Middle East, Latin America, and indigenous groups in North America and Australia, have a more holistic view of health that does not distinguish between physical and mental health (Good & Kleinman, 1985; Grandbois, 2005; Martin, 2009; Torsch & Ma, 2000). Consistently, people from these cultures often make limited distinctions between thoughts, feelings, and bodily experiences, and in some cultures, mental health or mental disorders are not within their vocabulary (Good & Kleinman, 1985; Martin, 2009).

Many of these non-Western cultures also have supernatural or religious explanations for mental disorders (Grandbois, 2005; Kramer et al., 2002; Lee, 2012; Martin, 2009; Torsch & Ma, 2000). For example, Lee (2012) explored perceptions of mental disorders among ethnic communities in Scotland and found that there is a common belief among the Muslim, Hindu, and Sikh communities that mental disorders are not illnesses "but are caused by factors such as the will of God, inheritance, 'black magic' or 'spirits'" (p. 293). Historically, these perceptions were also present in some Western cultures, such as was seen during the Salem witch trials of the late seventeenth century in Massachusetts, USA. Due to this perception, people with mental disorders are often seen as crazy, unpredictable, and dangerous and are strongly stigmatized in these cultures (Chen et al., 2013; Grandbois, 2005; Kramer et al., 2002; Lee, 2012; Martin, 2009; Torsch & Ma, 2000).

Although stigma against people with mental disorders is, in fact, common throughout the world (World Health Organization, 2010), it is often more intense among people from non-Western cultures (e.g., Conner et al., 2009; Jimenez et al., 2013) and among older people (e.g., Jang et al., 2009; Lee, 2012). For instance, Jang et al. (2009) explored age differences in attitudes towards mental health services among younger (aged between 20 and 45 years) and older (aged 60 years and older) Korean Americans. They found that, compared to younger people, who were likely to accept the medical conceptualization of mental disorders, older people were more subject to cultural-specific perceptions and stigma of mental disorders (Jang et al., 2009).

Furthermore, as non-Western cultures have a more collectivist focus as compared to Western cultures, stigma against mental disorder is attached not only to the affected individuals, but often their family as well (Grandbois, 2005; Jang et al., 2009; Kramer et al., 2002; Lee, 2012; Martin, 2009; Torsch & Ma, 2000; Wynaden et al., 2005). In other words, the impact of stigma is amplified in these cultures, and an individual's mental health problems are perceived not only as a personal matter, but also as a shame and dishonor to the whole family (Grandbois, 2005; Jang et al., 2009; Kramer et al., 2002; Lee, 2012; Martin, 2009; Torsch & Ma, 2000; Wynaden et al., 2005). This strong stigma towards mental disorders has been found to be associated with many negative outcomes, including negative attitudes towards mental health services and treatment among older people from non-Western cultures (Carpenter-Song et al., 2010; Conner et al., 2009; Jang et al., 2009; Jimenez et al., 2012; Lee, 2012; Martin, 2009; Wynaden et al., 2005).

One limitation of this research is that most studies consider mental disorders as a whole and do not explore possible differences in perceptions towards different types of mental disorder. However, Lee's (2012) study with Pakistani, Indian, and Chinese communities in Scotland found that participants limited their view of mental disorders to more severe and enduring problems, such as schizophrenia and bipolar disorder, and considered more common problems, such as anxiety and depression, as "responses to social problems, crises of faith or just 'part of life'" (p. 292). Similarly, Li et al.'s (2014) study with older Chinese immigrants in Britain revealed that older migrant Chinese immigrants do not consider depression and anxiety as mental disorders, but rather as personality problems or responses to life stresses and pressures. As both of these studies are limited to older immigrants living in the UK, there is a need for future studies to explore whether this finding can be generalized to the general older population of people from non-Western cultures. These studies also need to include older people from Western communities to enable direct cross-cultural comparison.

Prevalence

This section focuses on the prevalence of anxiety rather than its incidence because there are currently limited data with respect to incidence. The general conclusion is that older people from non-Western cultures report a lower prevalence of anxiety than those from Western cultures (Asnaani et al., 2010; Bauer et al., 2012; Baxter et al., 2013; Burnett-Zeigler et al., 2013; Jimenez et al., 2010; Marques & Robinaugh, 2011). For example, Jimenez et al. (2010) examined the prevalence of anxiety disorders among older people living in the USA and found that, after adjusting for gender, older Caucasians reported a 19% lifetime prevalence of any anxiety disorder compared to 18% for older Latinos, 16% for older African Americans and older Asians, and 12% for older Afro-Caribbean people. Importantly, similar differences existed between overseas-born and US-born people from the same cultural group, with the latter reporting a higher prevalence (Jimenez et al., 2010). For instance, the lifetime prevalence rates of any anxiety disorder were 16% and 10% for US-born Afro-Caribbean and overseas-born Afro-Caribbean people and 16% and 14% for US-born African Americans and overseas-born African Americans (Jimenez et al., 2010).

This trend has also been observed in anxiety prevalence across countries. In a systematic review of anxiety disorder prevalence from 87 studies across 44 countries, Baxter et al. (2013) found that individuals from non-Western cultures are 20–50% less likely to experience anxiety disorders compared to those from Western cultures. Specifically, the prevalence of anxiety disorder appears to be similar across Indo/Asian and African cultures (5.3%), Central/Eastern European, Ibero/Latin, and North Africa/Middle East cultures (7.2%, 7.3%, and 8.0%, respectively), and Euro/Anglo cultures (10.4%) (Baxter et al., 2013). There are two potential explanations for the findings of lower prevalence among older people from non-Western cultures (Baxter et al., 2013). First, there might be true differences in the prevalence of late-life anxiety across cultures. Although it is unclear why this is the case in cross-national studies, the "immigrant paradox" has been used to comprehend the differences between Caucasians older people and older immigrants (Alegria et al., 2008; Baxter et al., 2013; Burnett-Zeigler et al., 2013; Escobar et al., 2000;

Lau et al., 2013; Marques & Robinaugh, 2011). The "immigrant paradox" states that although immigrants face more discrimination than the general population, their ethnicity serves as a protective factor against mental health problems. In other words, immigrants from non-Western cultures use their ethnic identity as a protective factor against discrimination and mental health problems (Burnett-Zeigler et al., 2013; Escobar et al., 2000). Consistent with this view, there is evidence that within the immigrant population, the more acculturated the individuals are, the more susceptible they are to anxiety (Burnett-Zeigler et al., 2013; Escobar et al., 2000). However, the difference in prevalence may reflect culture-based differences in perceptions (as noted earlier), presentations of mental disorders, and expression of emotions, as well as variations across languages and systematic bias due to the translation of screening and diagnostic instruments (Baxter et al., 2013). These differences are discussed in the following sections.

Symptom Presentation

It is generally believed that individuals from non-Western cultures are more likely to express mental health problems through somatic symptoms rather than psychological ones. This belief is supported by a recent review by Marques and Robinaugh (2011) on cross-cultural variation across different types of anxiety, which found that individuals from these cultures are significantly more likely to present somatic symptoms (e.g., dizziness or indigestion) rather than psychological symptoms (e.g., scared or nervous), particularly in generalized anxiety disorder, than those from Western cultures. This difference is believed to be associated with stronger stigma towards mental illness in non-Western cultures and that expressing mental health problems through physical symptoms might be socially less disadvantageous in these cultures (Chung, 2002; Lee, 2012; Marques & Robinaugh, 2011). It might also be related to cross-cultural variation in expression of emotion. Although emotions themselves are universal phenomena, the culture in which we live has a profound impact on how they are experienced, expressed, perceived, and regulated (Markus & Kitayama, 1991; Oyserman et al., 2002). The term "display rules" has therefore been used to refer to socially learned norms that dictate the management and modification of emotional displays depending on social circumstances (Ekman & Friesen, 1969). It is generally believed that people from non-Western cultures are more likely to consider public display of one's emotions as being in conflict with the maintenance of interdependent, cooperative social interaction (Markus & Kitayama, 1991; Oyserman et al., 2002). This view is consistent with Confucianism, a dominant philosophy in East Asia that discourages open displays of emotions in order to maintain harmony and to avoid exposure of personal weakness (Jang et al., 2009; Kramer et al., 2002). Consequently, emotions are often internally tolerated rather than expressed, and stoic approaches are encouraged in response to emotional distress among Asian cultures (Jang et al., 2009; Kramer et al., 2002). In contrast, people from Western cultures value personal feelings and their free expression above social relationships, and thus they are more expressive in their emotions (Markus & Kitayama, 1991; Oyserman et al., 2002).

One limitation of this literature is that most studies included participants of all ages and few studies focused on older people specifically. However, there is evidence that the difference in somatization might be less obvious among older people. For example, in a study with older Mexican Americans, Letamendi et al. (2013) found that few participants reported experiencing physical symptoms that they believed were associated with their psychological distress. One possible reason for this is that the current cohort of older people, regardless of their cultural backgrounds, are less comfortable in discussing feelings and take a somewhat stoic approach towards emotional problems (Bryant, 2010; Pachana, 2008). The other reason for this might be altered neurophysiology as people age, leading to lower levels of neuroticism and a reduced likelihood of becoming distressed (Donnellan & Lucas, 2008; Wortman et al., 2012). Given these characteristics, cross-cultural differences in the somatization of mental health problems might become less obvious among older people.

The other line of research on cross-cultural differences in the presentation of anxiety focuses on cultural or culture-specific syndromes. The term "cultural syndrome" was used in the DSM-5, and it refers to "a cluster or group of co-occurring, relatively invariant symptoms found in a specific cultural group, community, or context" (American Psychiatric Association, 2013). The DSM-5 included a glossary of cultural syndromes of distress that have been well researched, of which *ataque de nervios* is closely related to anxiety disorders. *Ataque de nervios* (literally "an attack of the nerves") is a cultural syndrome among people from Latino cultures and involves typical symptoms of panic disorder, such as uncontrollable displays of emotion, shaking, and heart palpitations (Marques & Robinaugh, 2011; Thakker et al., 1999). As Thakker et al. (1999) noted, one important distinction between *ataque de nervios* and a panic disorder is "the intense fear and apprehension which characterize a panic attack are absent" in *ataque de nervios*, which is "usually associated with a specific precipitating event" (p. 851).

The term "culture-specific disorder" was used in the ICD-10 rather than the term "cultural syndrome." Furthermore, unlike the DSM-5, the ICD-10 does not have a separate category for culture-specific disorders because it argues that there is no strong evidence that culture-specific disorders are clinically distinguishable from other disorders that have been included in the ICD-10 (World Health Organization, 1992). Consequently, the ICD-10 proposes that these culture-specific disorders should be "regarded as local variants of anxiety, depression, somatoform disorder, or adjustment disorder," and that "the nearest equivalent code should therefore be used if required, together with an additional note of which culture-specific disorder is involved" (World Health Organization, 1992).

Like the research on the cultural variation of somatization, very few studies have focused on culturally specific symptoms of anxiety among older people. Of this limited literature, Diefenbach et al. (2004) reported a positive association between *ataque de nervios* and somatization in a sample of Puerto Rican primary care patients in the USA. This finding highlights the need for further research on the possible link between somatization and culture-bound syndromes.

Similarly to the research on prevalence, cross-cultural differences in the presentation of anxiety disorders can be considered as superficial differences in the presentation of the same underlying disorder or as unique and discrete disorders that are culturally constructed (Marques & Robinaugh, 2011; Thakker et al., 1999). This chapter does not aim to comment on this debate. Rather, it highlights the need for further research to clarify the extent to which the differences in presentation across cultures reflect genuine differences between groups.

Screening and Diagnosis

In research studies and in clinical practice, it is common to use assessment tools such as questionnaires, inventories, or scales to screen for and to rate the severity of symptoms of any disorders. Almost all of these tools were developed in Western countries using the

English language. This raises a number of issues when these tools are used in people from non-English-speaking cultures and/or from non-Western countries. First, as noted earlier, there are significant cross-cultural differences in the presentation of anxiety disorders. However, culturally specific symptoms are generally not included in current screening and diagnosis tools. There are also indications that older people from non-Western cultures describe their anxious and depressive symptoms using terms that are different from those of common Western terminology (Letamendi et al., 2013; Martin, 2009). For these reasons, there are concerns that anxiety symptoms among older people from non-Western cultures might not be detected using current tools, which are based on Western terminology (Dana, 2002; Friedman, 2001; Vinson et al., 2014).

When using translated tools, reliability and validity are the two most commonly examined issues. However, other issues also need to be considered. The first is how culturally appropriate and equivalent are the translations. In a review of cross-cultural use of the Hospital Anxiety and Depression Scale (HADS; Zigmond & Snaith, 1983), Maters et al. (2013) found that information on translation is often lacking, indicating an inattention to the translation process among researchers. This finding is concerning because the quality of the translation ultimately influences the reliability and validity of the tool, and translating mental health tools is not a simple and straightforward process. For instance, it is not always possible to find identical words for items in the tool. In particular, colloquial and metaphorical terms are commonly used in Western languages when describing emotions. However, these terms are difficult to translate. For example, "butterflies in my stomach" is a phrase commonly used in screening tools for anxiety, such as the HADS and the Geriatric Anxiety Inventory (GAI; Pachana et al., 2007). This phrase has been found to be difficult to translate into many languages (Maters et al., 2013; Pachana & Byrne, 2012), and was translated into "feelings seven up and eight downs in the chest" in Chinese (Yan et al., 2014), "feelings of tightness in the chest" in Portuguese (Ribeiro et al., 2011), and "feeling like ants are in one's stomach" in Spanish (Marquez-Gonzalez et al., 2012). This example highlights that literal translation is not always possible or desirable and that it is not easy to have culturally equivalent and culturally appropriate translations for mental health measures.

The second issue is whether the same cutoff scores are valid across cultures and languages. The GAI (Pachana et al., 2007) is one of the most commonly used anxiety screening measures for older people and has been translated into many different languages (Pachana & Byrne, 2012). In a study by Ribeiro et al. (2011) with older people in Portugal, the authors reported a cutoff point of a score >8 for the Portuguese version of the GAI for detecting severe anxiety symptoms, which is the same as that proposed by the authors for any anxiety disorder (Pachana et al., 2007). However, Massena et al. (2015) used the Brazilian Portuguese version in Brazil and reported a cutoff score of 13 for generalized anxiety disorder, which was four points higher than that suggested by the authors (Pachana et al., 2007). Similar findings have also been found in the review by Maters et al. (2013) on the cross-cultural use of the HADS. These authors believed that these findings might be, in part, related to the fact that different translated versions of the HADS have been used across studies.

Risk and Protective Factors

The literature suggests that there are both similarities and differences in risk and protective factors for anxiety among older people from different cultural backgrounds. Most of the research with older people from non-Western cultures has been conducted with older immigrants and focuses on factors associated with their experience as immigrants. With regard to biological risk factors, similarly to the general population, biological risk factors for anxiety among older people from non-Western cultures include poor physical health and cognitive impairments (Braun et al., 2004; Joshi et al., 2003; Manson, 2000; Ribeiro et al., 2015). As some physical health issues might be more prominent among certain cultural groups, this might lead to increased risk for anxiety among this group. For example, among Native Hawaiians, heart disease and stroke are the principal causes of death within the community (Braun et al., 2004). Thus, some ethnic groups such as Native Hawaiians are more susceptible to cardiovascular health problems than Caucasians, which may lead to increased anxiety (Braun et al., 2004; Joshi et al., 2003; Manson, 2000; Ribeiro et al., 2015).

In terms of psychological risk factors, various such factors are associated with the immigration process, such as a traumatic event (e.g., war, torture, terrorism, or a natural disaster) during the per-migration stage, or aspects of the trip that could cause death or near-death experiences during the migration stage (Pumariega et al., 2005). However, most of the risk factors are present during post-migration stage (Pumariega et al., 2005). These include culture shock (Lerner et al., 2008), which can lead to cultural bereavement: that is, the process of an individual feeling that they are losing key pieces of their ethnic identity and/or memories from their country of origin (Agorastos et al., 2012; Burnett-Zeigler et al., 2013; Lerner et al., 2008). Other risks factors at this stage include lower socioeconomic status, low English proficiency, and experiences of discrimination, racism, and ageism (Bhugra et al., 2011; Lee & Yoon, 2011; Pumariega et al., 2005).

Cultural pride and ethnic identity serve as protective factors for older immigrants (Breslau et al., 2009; Burnett-Zeigler et al., 2013; Chatters et al., 2008; Guo et al., 2015; Krause & Bastida, 2012; Marin & Huber, 2011; Moberg, 2005; Yip et al., 2008). The protective effect of these factors was found in Yip et al.'s (2008) study with Asian immigrants aged between 41 and 50, where participants who had a strong ethnic identity and experienced high discrimination were less likely to self-report feelings of distress. This protective effect of ethnic identity has been explained by the buffering hypothesis, which states that individuals with high ethnic identity use their identity as a buffer against discrimination (Burnett-Zeigler et al., 2013; Yip et al., 2008). Essentially, the buffering hypothesis is similar to the "immigrant paradox" in that both theories state that ethnic identity works as a protective factor against mental health problems (Breslau et al., 2009; Burnett-Zeigler et al., 2013).

As individuals age, there is a trend to become more spiritual or religious to curb death anxiety (Moberg, 2005). Because spirituality and religiosity are often embedded within non-Western cultures, their protective effects might be more obvious among older people from non-Western cultures (Chatters et al., 2008; Krause & Bastida, 2012; Moberg, 2005). In a study with older Mexican Americans on the relationship among perceived contact with the dead, feelings of gratefulness, and anxiety, Krause and Bastida (2012) found that those who identified themselves as having contact with the dead were more likely to endorse connectedness with the community, which was related to thankfulness to God, leading to fewer symptoms of anxiety.

Intervention

Psychological interventions have been recommended as the first line of treatment for older people with minor and moderate symptoms of anxiety disorders (Hendriks et al., 2008; Wetherell et al., 2005b). Whereas most of these interventions were developed in Western countries, there is evidence that, once modified and adapted, they are effective for older people from non-Western countries. Hwang (2006) introduced the steps that clinicians can take to modify and adapt evidence-based treatments, including the clinician increasing their understanding of cultural beliefs, being mindful of cultural variations concerning expression, understanding cultural complexities, as well as orienting the client towards the stages of therapy. In his study with older Chinese people, Hwang (2006) found that a modified version of cognitive behavior therapy (CBT) was comparable to Chinese beliefs of the *wise mind*, which is related to aspects of Zen, Buddhism, and Taoism, and this was effective among older Chinese people.

CBT has been identified as an evidence-based treatment for anxiety disorders, and there is strong support within the research that these modalities reduce symptomology (Borkovec et al., 2002; Ladouceur et al., 2004). Other evidence-based treatments include acceptance-based approaches such as acceptance and commitment therapy (ACT). Wetherell et al. (2011) explored the feasibility of ACT in their pilot study with 16 participants. They found that all of the participants who received ACT ($n = 7$) completed all of the treatment sessions, whereas only half of the individuals who started CBT ($n = 9$) completed the sessions. Furthermore, participants in both groups showed improvements in their depressive and anxiety symptoms (Wetherell et al., 2011). The study suggested that ACT may be well suited to older people with anxiety disorders (Wetherell et al., 2011). Importantly, 38% of the participants in this study were members of minority groups, suggesting that ACT might also be effective for older people from non-Western cultures and that future studies with anxious older adults from non-Western cultures are required to explore this further.

The other psychological treatments that might be of particular use to older people from non-Western cultures are mindfulness approaches, such as progressive muscle relaxation, meditation, and controlled and deep breathing (Szanton et al., 2011). These different types of mindfulness-based practices have been found to significantly reduce anxiety symptoms among older people (Klainin-Yobas et al., 2015). The use of relaxation and other mindfulness techniques is commonly incorporated into traditional healing or religious practices in non-Western cultures (Oulanova & Moodley, 2010). However, researchers noted that, in a sample of Chinese middle-aged adults, mindfulness-based cognitive therapy and psychoeducation proved to be equally beneficial for reducing symptoms of anxiety (Wong et al., 2016). This suggests that further research is required to gain a greater understanding of mindfulness techniques, as they have great potential as treatments for anxiety among older people from non-Western cultures.

The importance of involving family members in treatment for people with mental health problems has been highlighted by many researchers (Abramson et al., 2002; Manson, 2000). Understanding family dynamics can help clinicians offer clients more support and build an effective therapeutic relationship (Abramson et al., 2002). In some cases, it would be beneficial if family members were involved in some sessions (Abramson et al., 2002). As people from non-Western cultures have a more collectivist focus (Oyserman et al., 2002), family might play an even more important role among this group. This is particularly true for older immigrants, who are likely to have smaller social networks compared to nonimmigrants (e.g., Warburton et al., 2009). Working with the client's family members can also be beneficial in terms of gaining collateral information, as well as for providing psychoeducation to the family so that they can provide better care to the clients. When delivering psychological treatment to older immigrants, the use of telepsychiatry could be considered if there is a shortage of bilingual clinicians in the area (Ye et al., 2012; Yeung et al., 2009).

There is evidence that pharmacological interventions are effective for older people with anxiety disorders; however, there are precautions that must be considered, such as the adverse effects that medications may have, including dependence, sedation, cognitive impairment, and other side effects (Baldwin et al., 2005; Pinquart & Duberstein, 2007). Additionally, providers should be aware of the possible interactions with other medications. When prescribing psychotropic medications to older people from non-Western cultures, there are several additional issues that need to be considered. First, herbal remedies are often used by people from non-Western cultures as a means to alleviate somatic symptoms related to anxiety (Chung, 2002; Dole et al., 2000; Zeilmann et al., 2003), and clinicians need to be aware of such uses of herbal remedies and possible pharmacological interactions between these herbal remedies and psychotropic medications. Specifically, in Asian and Latino cultures, the use of herbal medicines and healers is considered the norm and part of the mainstream culture (Chung, 2002; Dole et al., 2000). In a study concerning the use of herbal remedies among older Caucasians and older Latinos, Zeilmann et al. (2003) found that 61% of Latinos used herbal remedies compared to 40% among Caucasians.

Second, psychotropic medications such as tricyclic antidepressants (TCAs) need to be carefully dosed (Bhugra & Bhui, 1999; Bhugra et al., 2011). There is some evidence that older people from some ethnic groups might need a different dose of psychotropic medication compared to older Caucasians (Bhugra & Bhui, 1999; Bhugra et al., 2011). For example, Latinos and Asians might require a lower dose of TCAs (Bhugra et al., 2011), whereas Caucasians need a higher dose to receive therapeutic benefits. Concerning benzodiazepines, African Americans have higher concentrations of its metabolites and need less of the medication to receive therapeutic benefits (Bhugra & Bhui, 1999). In addition to psychotherapy and pharmacological interventions, it is important that a regular diet, exercise, and maintenance of sleep hygiene is sustained among older people (Nelson et al., 2007). According to the American College of Sports Medicine and the American Heart Association, it is recommended that older people participate in aerobic and muscle-building activities (Nelson et al., 2007). Such activities and practices can help alleviate symptoms of anxiety and can act as a source of safe coping by leading to exposure and habituation to interoceptive and exteroceptive stimuli (Nelson et al., 2007).

Conclusion

There is clear evidence from the literature that there are significant cross-cultural differences in various aspects of late-life anxiety, such as lower levels of prevalence among older people from non-Western cultures and different perceptions and symptom presentations. These cross-cultural differences present great challenges when screening, diagnosing, and treating anxiety among older people from non-Western cultures, and they highlight the importance of culturally competent practice, which includes understanding the historical background and complexities within the cultural group, recognizing role of the family and family systems, learning their cultural perspective of mental health, and developing culturally appropriate clinical interviewing skills (Abramson et al., 2002; Alvarez et al., 2013; Bhugra et al., 2014; Chung, 2002; Hwang, 2006; Vinson et al., 2014).

In spite of these important findings, there are a number of limitations in current cross-cultural research. First, similar to the research on other areas of late-life anxiety (Flint, 2005;

Haralambous et al., 2009; Riedel-Heller et al., 2006; Wetherell et al., 2005a), cross-cultural research on anxiety is far less developed when compared to that on depression. In particular, whereas several large cross-cultural studies have been undertaken for depression among older people (Dewey et al., 1993), such studies are largely absent for anxiety (Pachana & Byrne, 2012). Second, much of this cross-cultural research has been conducted in the USA and Europe, and there is a need for more attention being paid to cross-cultural issues for studies conducted in other countries. There are also barriers and challenges when accessing and integrating current cross-cultural literature. On the one hand, there are research and clinical findings published in non-English languages that are not easily accessible and/or understandable to clinicians who do not speak that language. On the other hand, researchers in the developing world might have difficulty accessing the literature published in English. Finally, it is unclear whether these cross-cultural differences reflect superficial differences in the same underlying disorder or unique anxiety disorders that are related to biological and/or socio-cultural differences across cultures. Future research on cultural variation in risk factors associated with late-life anxiety would shed light on these issues (Baxter et al., 2013; Marques & Robinaugh, 2011), which will ultimately lead to culturally appropriate screening, diagnosis, and treatment for older people from non-Western cultures.

References

Abramson, T. A., Trejo, L. and Lai, D. W. L. (2002). Culture and mental health: providing appropriate services for a diverse older population. *Generations*, **26**, 21–27.

Agorastos, A., Haasen, C. and Huber, C. G. (2012). Anxiety disorders through a transcultural perspective: implications for migrants. *Psychopathology*, **45**, 67–77.

Alegria, M., Canino, G., Shrout, P. E., et al. (2008). Prevalence of mental illness in immigrant and non-immigrant U.S. Latino groups. *American Journal of Psychiatry*, **165**, 359–369.

Alvarez, P., Rengifo, J., Emrani, T. and Gallagher-Thompson, D. (2013). Latino older adults and mental health: a review and commentary. *Clinical Gerontologist*, **37**, 33–48.

American Psychiatric Association (2013). *Diagnostic and Statistical Manual of Mental Disorders*, 5th ed. Washington, DC: American Psychiatric Association.

Asnaani, A., Richey, J. A., Dimaite, R., Hinton, D. E. and Hofmann, S. G. (2010). A cross-ethnic comparison of lifetime prevalence rates of anxiety disorders. *Journal of Nervous & Mental Disease*, **198**, 551–555.

Baldwin, D. S., Anderson, I. M., Nutt, D. J., et al. (2005). Evidence-based guidelines for the pharmacological treatment of anxiety disorders: recommendations from the British Association for Psychopharmacology. *Journal of Psychopharmacology*, **19**, 567–596.

Bauer, A. M., Chen, C.-N. and Alegría, M. (2012). Prevalence of physical symptoms and their association with race/ethnicity and acculturation in the United States. *General Hospital Psychiatry*, **34**, 323–331.

Baxter, A. J., Scott, K. M., Vos, T. and Whiteford, H. A. (2013). Global prevalence of anxiety disorders: a systematic review and meta-regression. *Psychological Medicine*, **43**, 897–910.

Bhugra, D. and Bhui, K. (1999). Ethnic and cultural factors in psychopharmacology. *Advances in Psychiatric Treatment*, **5**, 89–95.

Bhugra, D., Gupta, S., Bhui, K., et al. (2011). WPA guidance on mental health and mental health care in migrants. *World Psychiatry*, **10**, 2–10.

Bhugra, D., Gupta, S., Schouler-Ocak, M., et al. (2014). EPA guidance mental health care of migrants. *European Psychiatry*, **29**, 107–115.

Borkovec, T. D., Newman, M. G., Pincus, A. L. and Lytle, R. (2002). A component analysis of cognitive–behavioral therapy for generalized anxiety disorder and the role of interpersonal problems. *Journal of Consulting and Clinical Psychology*, 70, 288–298.

Braun, K., Yee, B., Browne, C. V. and Mokuau, N. (2004). Native Hawaiian and

Pacific Islander elders. In K. E. Whitfield, ed., *Closing the Gap: Improving the Health of Minority Elders in the New Millennium*. Washington, DC: Gerontological Society of America, pp. 55–67.

Breslau, J., Borges, G., Hagar, Y., Tancredi, D. and Gilman, S. (2009). Immigration to the USA and risk for mood and anxiety disorders: variation by origin and age at immigration. *Psychological Medicine*, **39**, 1117–27.

Bryant, C. (2010). Anxiety and depression in old age: challenges in recognition and diagnosis. *International Psychogeriatrics*, **22**, 511–513.

Burnett-Zeigler, I., Bohnert, K. M. and Ilgen, M. A. (2013). Ethnic identity, acculturation and the prevalence of lifetime psychiatric disorders among Black, Hispanic, and Asian adults in the US. *Journal of Psychiatric Research*, **47**, 56–63.

Carpenter-Song, E., Chu, E., Drake, R. E., Ritsema, M., Smith, B. and Alverson, H. (2010). Ethno-cultural variations in the experience and meaning of mental illness and treatment: implications for access and utilization. *Transcultural Psychiatry*, **47**, 224–251.

Chatters, L. M., Bullard, K. M., Taylor, R. J., Woodward, A. T., Neighbors, H. W. and Jackson, J. S. (2008). Religious participation and DSM-IV disorders among older African Americans: findings from the National Survey of American Life. *American Journal of Geriatric Psychiatry*, **16**, 957–965.

Chen, F.-P., Ying-Chi Lai, G. and Yang, L. (2013). Mental illness disclosure in Chinese immigrant communities. *Journal of Counseling Psychology*, **60**, 379–391.

Chung, H. (2002). The challenges of providing behavioral treatment to Asian Americans: Identifying the challenges is the first step in overcoming them. *Western Journal of Medicine*, **176**, 222–223.

Conner, K. O., Koeske, G. and Brown, C. (2009). Racial differences in attitudes toward professional mental health treatment: the mediating effect of stigma. *Journal of Gerontological Social Work*, **52**, 695–712.

D'Andrade, R. (2001). A cognitivist's view of the units debate in cultural anthropology. *Cross-cultural Research*, **35**, 242–257.

Dana, R. H. (2002). Mental health services for African Americans: a cultural/racial perspective. *Cultural Diversity & Ethnic Minority Psychology*, **8**, 3–18.

Deacon, B. J. (2013). The biomedical model of mental disorder: a critical analysis of its validity, utility, and effects on psychotherapy research. *Clinical Psychology Review*, **33**, 846–861.

Dewey, M. E., de la Camara, C., Copeland, J. R., Lobo, A. and Saz, P. (1993). Cross-cultural comparison of depression and depressive symptoms in older people. *Acta Psychiatrica Scandinavica*, **87**(6), 369–373.

Diefenbach, G. J., Robison, J. T., Tolin, D. F. and Blank, K. (2004). Late-life anxiety disorders among Puerto Rican primary care patients: impact on well-being, functioning, and service utilization. *Journal of Anxiety Disorders*, **18**, 841–858.

Dole, E. J., Rhyne, R. L., Zeilmann, C. A., Skipper, B. J., McCabe, M. L. and Low Dog, T. (2000). The influence of ethnicity on use of herbal remedies in elderly Hispanics and non-Hispanic whites. *Journal of the American Pharmaceutical Association (Washington, DC: 1996)*, **40**, 359–365.

Donnellan, M. B. and Lucas, R. E. (2008). Age differences in the Big Five across the life span: evidence from two national samples. *Psychology and Aging*, **23**, 558–566.

Ekman, P. and Friesen, W. V. (1969). The repertoire of nonverbal behavior: categories, origins, usage, and coding. *Semiotica*, **1**, 49–98.

Escobar, J. I., Hoyos Nervi, C. and Gara, M. A. (2000). Immigration and mental health: Mexican Americans in the United States. *Harvard Review of Psychiatry*, **8**, 64–72.

Flint, A. (2005). Anxiety and its disorders in late life: moving the field forward. *American Journal of Geriatric Psychiatry*, **13**, 3–6.

Friedman, S. (2001). Cultural issues in the assessment of anxiety disorders. In M. Antony, S. Orsillo and L. Roemer, eds., *Practitioner's Guide to Empirically Based Measures of Anxiety*. New York: Springer US, pp. 37–42.

Good, B. and Kleinman, A. (1985). Culture and anxiety: cross-cultural evidence for the patterning of anxiety disorders. In A. H. Tuma and J. P. Maser, eds., *Anxiety and the Anxiety Disorders*. Hillsdale, NJ: Lawrence Earlbaum, pp. 297–324.

Grandbois, D. (2005). Stigma of mental illness among American Indian and Alaska Native nations: historical and contemporary perspectives. *Issues in Mental Health Nursing*, **26**, 1001–1024.

Guo, M., Li, S., Liu, J. and Sun, F. (2015). Family relations, social connections, and mental health among Latino and Asian older adults. *Research on Aging*, **37**, 123–147.

Halbreich, U., Alarcon, R. D., Calil, H., et al. (2007). Culturally-sensitive complaints of depressions and anxieties in women. *Journal of Affective Disorders*, **102**, 159–176.

Hancock, T. (1985). The Mandala of Health: a model of the human ecosystem. *Family & Community Health*, **8**, 1–10.

Hancock, T. and Perkins, F. (1985). The Mandala of Health: a conceptual model and teaching tool. *Health Education*, **24**, 8–10.

Haralambous, B., Lin, X., Dow, B., Jones, C., Tinney, J. and Bryant, C. (2009). *Depression in Older Age: A Scoping Study*. Melbourne: National Ageing Research Institute.

Hendriks, G., Oude Voshaar, R., Keijsers, G., Hoogduin, C. and Van Balkom, A. (2008). Cognitive–behavioural therapy for late-life anxiety disorders: a systematic review and meta-analysis. *Acta Psychiatrica Scandinavica*, **117**, 403–411.

Hwang, W. C. (2006). The psychotherapy adaptation and modification framework: application to Asian Americans. *American Psychologist*, **61**, 702–715.

Jang, Y., Chiriboga, D. A. and Sumie, O. (2009). Attitudes toward mental health services: age-group differences in Korean American adults. *Aging & Mental Health*, **13**, 127–134.

Jimenez, D. E., Alegria, M., Chen, C. N., Chan, D. and Laderman, M. (2010). Prevalence of psychiatric illnesses in older ethnic minority adults. *Journal of the American Geriatrics Society*, **58**, 256–64.

Jimenez, D. E., Bartels, S. J., Cardenas, V. and Alegría, M. (2013). Stigmatizing attitudes towards mental illness among racial/ethnic older adults in primary care. *International Journal of Geriatric Psychiatry*, **28**, 1061–1068.

Jimenez, D. E., Bartels, S. J., Cardenas, V., Daliwal, S. S. and Alegría, M. (2012). Cultural beliefs and mental health treatment preferences of ethnically diverse older adult consumers in primary care. *American Journal of Geriatric Psychiatry*, **20**, 533–542.

Joshi, K., Kumar, R. and Avasthi, A. (2003). Morbidity profile and its relationship with disability and psychological distress among elderly people in Northern India. *International Journal of Epidemiology*, **32**, 978–87.

Kitayama, S. (2002). Culture and basic psychological processes – toward a system view of culture: comment on Oyserman et al. (2002). *Psychological Bulletin*, **128**, 89–96.

Klainin-Yobas, P., Oo, W. N., Suzanne Yew, P. Y. and Lau, Y. (2015). Effects of relaxation interventions on depression and anxiety among older adults: a systematic review. *Aging & Mental Health*, **19**, 1043–1055.

Kramer, E. J., Kwong, K., Lee, E. and Chung, H. (2002). Cultural factors influencing the mental health of Asian Americans. *Western Journal of Medicine*, **176**, 227–231.

Krause, N. and Bastida, E. (2012). Contact with the dead, religion, and death anxiety among older Mexican Americans. *Death Studies*, **36**, 932–948.

Ladouceur, R., Léger, É., Dugas, M. and Freeston, M. H. (2004). Cognitive–behavioral treatment of generalized anxiety disorder (GAD) for older adults. *International Psychogeriatrics*, **16**, 195–207.

Lau, A. S., Tsai, W., Shih, J., Liu, L. L., Hwang, W.-C. and Takeuchi, D. T. (2013). The immigrant paradox among Asian American women: are disparities in the burden of depression and anxiety paradoxical or explicable? *Journal of Consulting and Clinical Psychology*, **81**, 901–911.

Lee, K. (2012). Understanding and addressing the stigma of mental illness with ethnic minority communities. *Health Sociology Review*, **21**, 287–298.

Lee, K. and Yoon, D. P. (2011). Factors influencing the general well-being of low-income Korean immigrant elders. *Social Work*, **56**, 269–279.

Lerner, V., Kanevsky, M. and Witztum, E. (2008). The influence of immigration on the mental health of those seeking psychiatric care in southern Israel: a comparison of new immigrants to veteran residents. *Israel Journal of Psychiatry and Related Science*, **45**, 291–298.

Letamendi, A. M., Ayers, C. R., Ruberg, J. L., et al. (2013). Illness conceptualizations among older rural Mexican–Americans with anxiety and depression. *Journal of Cross-cultural Gerontology*, **28**, 421–433.

Li, S., Hatzidimitriadou, E. and Psoinos, M. (2014). "Tangled wires in the head": older migrant Chinese's perception of mental illness in Britain. *Journal of Aging Studies*, **30**, 73–86.

Manson, S. M. (2000). Mental health services for American Indians and Alaska Natives: need, use, and barriers to effective care. *Canadian Journal of Psychiatry*, **45**, 617–626.

Marin, M. R. and Huber, C. H. (2011). Mexican American elderly: self-reported anxiety and the mediating influence of family protective factors. *Family Journal*, **19**, 63–72.

Markus, H. R. and Kitayama, S. (1991). Culture and the self: Implications for cognition, emotion, and motivation. *Psychological Review*, **98**, 224–253.

Marques, L. and Robinaugh, D. J. (2011). Cross-cultural variations in the prevalence and presentation of anxiety disorders. *Expert Review of Neurotherapeutics*, **11**, 313–322.

Marquez-Gonzalez, M., Losada, A., Fernandez-Fernandez, V. and Pachana, N. A. (2012). Psychometric properties of the Spanish version of the Geriatric Anxiety Inventory. *International Psychogeriatrics*, **24**(1), 137–144.

Martin, S. S. (2009). Illness of the mind or illness of the spirit? Mental health-related conceptualization and practices of older Iranian immigrants. *Health & Social Work*, **34**, 117–126.

Massena, P. N., De Araujo, N. B., Pachana, N., Laks, J. and De Padua, A. C. (2015). Validation of the Brazilian Portuguese version of Geriatric Anxiety Inventory –

GAI-BR. *International Psychogeriatrics*, **27**, 1113–1119.

Maters, G. A., Sanderman, R., Kim, A. Y. and Coyne, J. C. (2013). Problems in cross-cultural use of the Hospital Anxiety and Depression Scale: "no butterflies in the desert". *PLoS ONE*, **8**, e70975.

Moberg, D. O. (2005). Research in spirituality, religion, and aging. *Journal of Gerontological Social Work*, **45**, 11–40.

Nelson, M. E., Rejeski, W. J., Blair, S. N., et al. (2007). Physical activity and public health in older adults: recommendation from the American College of Sports Medicine and the American Heart Association. *Circulation*, **116**, 1094–1105.

Oulanova, O. and Moodley, R. (2010). Navigating two worlds: experiences of counsellors who integrate aboriginal traditional healing practices. *Canadian Journal of Counselling and Psychotherapy/Revue canadienne de counseling et de psychothérapie*, **44**, 346–362.

Oyserman, D., Coon, H. M. and Kemmelmeier, M. (2002). Rethinking individualism and collectivism: evaluation of theoretical assumptions and meta-analyses. *Psychological Bulletin*, **128**, 3–72.

Pachana, N. A. (2008). Ageing and psychological disorders. In E. Rieger, ed., *Abnormal Psychology*. Sydney: McGraw Hill, pp. 421–457.

Pachana, N. A. and Byrne, G. J. (2012). The Geriatric Anxiety Inventory: international use and future directions. *Australian Psychologist*, **47**, 33–38.

Pachana, N. A., Byrne, G. J., Siddle, H., Koloski, N., Harley, E. and Arnold, E. (2007). Development and validation of the Geriatric Anxiety Inventory. *International Psychogeriatrics*, **19**, 103–114.

Pinquart, M. and Duberstein, P. R. (2007). Treatment of anxiety disorders in older adults: a meta-analytic comparison of behavioral and pharmacological interventions. *American Journal of Geriatric Psychiatry*, **15**, 639–651.

Pumariega, A. J., Rothe, E. and Pumariega, J. B. (2005). Mental health of immigrants and refugees. *Community Mental Health Journal*, **41**, 581–597.

Ribeiro, O., Paul, C., Simoes, M. R. and Firmino, H. (2011). Portuguese version of the Geriatric Anxiety Inventory: transcultural adaptation and psychometric validation. *Aging & Mental Health*, **15**, 742–748.

Ribeiro, O., Teixeira, L., Araújo, L., Afonso, R. M. and Pachana, N. (2015). Predictors of anxiety in centenarians: health, economic factors, and loneliness. *International Psychogeriatrics*, **27**, 1167–1176.

Riedel-Heller, S. G., Busse, A. and Angermeyer, M. C. (2006). The state of mental health in old-age across the "old" European Union – a systematic review. *Acta Psychiatrica Scandinavica*, **113**, 388–401.

Szanton, S. L., Wenzel, J., Connolly, A. B. and Piferi, R. L. (2011). Examining mindfulness-based stress reduction: perceptions from minority older adults residing in a low-income housing facility. *BMC Complementary and Alternative Medicine*, **11**, 44.

Thakker, J., Ward, T. and Strongman, K. T. (1999). Mental disorder and cross-cultural psychology: a constructivist perspective. *Clinical Psychology Review*, **19**, 843–874.

Torsch, V. L. and Ma, G. X. (2000). Cross-cultural comparison of health perceptions, concerns, and coping strategies among Asian and Pacific Islander American elders. *Qualitative Health Research*, **10**, 471–489.

Vinson, L. D., Crowther, M. R., Austin, A. D. and Guin, S. M. (2014). African Americans, mental health, and aging. *Clinical Gerontologist*, **37**, 4–17.

Warburton, J., Bartlett, H. and Rao, V. (2009). Ageing and cultural diversity: policy and practice issues. *Australian Social Work*, **62**(2), 168–185.

Wetherell, J. L., Liu, L., Patterson, T. L., et al. (2011). Acceptance and commitment therapy for generalized anxiety disorder in older adults: a preliminary report. *Behavior Therapy*, **42**, 127–134.

Wetherell, J. L., Maser, J. D. and van Balkom, A. (2005a). Anxiety disorders in the elderly: outdated beliefs and a research agenda. *Acta Psychiatrica Scandinavica*, **111**, 401–402.

Wetherell, J. L., Sorrell, J. T., Thorp, S. R. and Patterson, T. L. (2005b). Psychological interventions for late-life anxiety: a review and early lessons from the CALM study. *Journal of Geriatric Psychiatry and Neurology*, **18**, 72–82.

Wong, S. Y. S., Yip, B. H. K., Mak, W. W. S., et al. (2016). Mindfulness-based cognitive therapy v. group psychoeducation for people with generalised anxiety disorder: Randomised controlled trial. *British Journal of Psychiatry*, **209**, 68–75.

World Health Organization (1992). *The ICD-10 Classification of Mental and Behavioural Disorders: Clinical Descriptions and Diagnostic Guidelines*. Geneva: World Health Organization.

World Health Organization (2010). *Mental Health and Development: Targeting People with Mental Health Conditions as a Vulnerable Group*. Geneva: World Health Organization.

Wortman, J., Lucas, R. E. and Donnellan, M. B. (2012). Stability and change in the Big Five personality domains: evidence from a longitudinal study of Australians. *Psychology and Aging*, **27**, 867–874.

Wynaden, D., Chapman, R., Orb, A., McGowan, S., Zeeman, Z. and Yeak, S. (2005). Factors that influence Asian communities' access to mental health care. *International Journal of Mental Health Nursing*, **14**, 88–95.

Yan, Y., Xin, T., Wang, D. and Tang, D. (2014). Application of the Geriatric Anxiety Inventory-Chinese Version (GAI-CV) to older people in Beijing communities. *International Psychogeriatrics*, **26**(3), 517–523.

Ye, J., Shim, R., Lukaszewski, T., Yun, K., Kim, S. H. and Ruth, G. (2012). Telepsychiatry services for Korean Immigrants. *Telemedicine Journal and e-Health*, **18**, 797–802.

Yeung, A., Johnson, D. P., Trinh, N. H., Weng, W. C., Kvedar, J. and Fava, M. (2009). Feasibility and effectiveness of telepsychiatry services for Chinese immigrants in a nursing home. *Telemedicine Journal and e-Health*, **15**, 336–341.

Yip, T., Gee, G. C. and Takeuchi, D. T. (2008). Racial discrimination and psychological distress: the impact of ethnic identity and age among immigrant and United States-born Asian adults. *Developmental Psychology*, **44**, 787–800.

Zeilmann, C. A., Dole, E. J., Skipper, B. J., McCabe, M., Low Dog, T. and Rhyne, R. L. (2003). Use of herbal medicine by elderly Hispanic and non-Hispanic white patients. *Pharmacotherapy*, **23**, 526–532.

Zigmond, A. S. and Snaith, R. P. (1983). The Hospital Anxiety and Depression Scale. *Acta Psychiatrica Scandinavica*, **67**, 361–370.

Clinical Assessment of Late-Life Anxiety

Christine E. Gould, Brian C. Kok, Vanessa K. Ma, and Barry A. Edelstein

Introduction

The assessment of older adult anxiety requires the mindset and skills of a detective, ideally those of Sherlock Holmes. In *The Sign of Four* (Doyle, 1890), Holmes offered the following quip regarding the investigation of a crime that is of considerable value for the clinician in the assessment process: "How often have I said to you that when you have eliminated the impossible, whatever remains, however improbable, must be the truth?" (p. 111). As with the investigation of crimes, much of the assessment of older adult anxiety involves first accounting for, and oftentimes ruling out, multiple factors that can contribute to anxiety symptoms. In our chapter, we explore the complexities of assessing older adult anxiety symptoms and disorders. We begin with a discussion of age-related diagnostic issues and differences in symptom experience and presentation that contribute to diagnostic complexity. This is followed by discussions of various assessment methods and instruments, including consideration of their psychometric properties with older adults, defined as adults aged 65 and older. We end with discussions of special assessment considerations.

Diagnostic Issues and the Experience and Presentation of Anxiety

Anxiety disorders represent a diverse group of disorders that include generalized anxiety disorder (GAD), social anxiety disorder (SAD), panic disorder (PD), agoraphobia, and specific phobia (SP). In the development of the Diagnostic and Statistical Manual of Mental Disorders, 5th edition (DSM-5; American Psychiatric Association, 2013), late-life anxiety researchers proposed changes to the definitions of anxiety disorder criteria (Mohlman et al., 2012; Wolitsky-Taylor et al., 2010). Older adults are less likely to describe their anxiety symptoms as excessive or uncontrollable and tend to use words such as "concerns" or "issues" when describing their worries (Mohlman et al., 2012). The older adult's conceptualization of anxiety, in addition to age-specific symptom presentations (to be discussed later), can contribute to the presentation of anxiety symptoms that fail to meet diagnostic criteria (i.e., are subthreshold), but that still result in significant social and functional impairment (i.e., anxiety disorder other specified or unspecified). Furthermore, there is mounting evidence that older adults experience anxiety differently from younger adults and may present with a different constellation of symptoms. Older adults report fewer negative emotions than young and middle-aged adults and lower levels of depression, anxiety, guilt, hostility, and shyness (Lawton et al., 1993).

The differences in emotional experience of anxiety for older adults compared with young adults appears to be due, in part, to age-related differences in physiological activity and reactivity (Lau et al., 2001) and self-regulation (Uchino et al., 2010). For example, older adults exhibit lower heart rate reactivity and higher systolic blood pressure reactivity in response to emotion-evoking tasks than young adults (Uchino et al., 2010). Older adults are less likely than young adults to report negative emotionally arousing experiences and are less likely to attend to negative stimuli compared with neutral or positive stimuli (e.g., Isaacowitz et al., 2006). In addition, memory for emotionally arousing events appears to be age related such that, in general, older adults are more likely than young adults to recall positive experiences (Reed et al., 2014).

The nature of worries also varies across the lifespan, with older adults worrying more than young adults about health, world issues, and family concerns (Hunt et al., 2003). Older adults report lower levels of uncontrollable worry than young adults (e.g., Gould & Edelstein, 2010). In addition to age-related differences in the content and controllability of worry, the nature of fears differs across age groups. Kogan and Edelstein (2004) identified several fears that were frequently endorsed by older adults but not by young adults (e.g., mental decline, poor well-being, inability to care for one's self, being a burden to others). The nature of situations that arouse social anxiety also varies across age groups (Ciliberti et al., 2011). Several different social situations (e.g., asking others for favors or for help, looking incompetent in front of others, forgetting information in front of others) often elicit social anxiety in older adults (Ciliberti et al., 2011). Additionally, it is easier for older adults to avoid social situations that evoke anxiety compared with young adults (Bryant et al., 2008). Older adults also experience panic attacks less frequently compared with young adults (Depp et al., 2005). Correlates of panic attack frequency also differ for the two age groups, such that cognitive symptoms are associated with greater panic attack frequency for older adults and somatic symptoms are associated with greater panic attack frequency for young adults (Depp et al., 2005). In summary, age-related changes in physiological arousal, self-regulation effectiveness, and the nature of worry, fear, and anxiety conspire to produce complex experiences and diverse symptoms that require careful consideration by the clinician.

Assessment of Anxiety Symptoms and Disorders

A thorough assessment of anxiety in older adults must cover a range of somatic, cognitive, and affective symptoms. Comprehensive geriatric assessments rely on information gathered from multiple sources: the older adult, collateral sources (e.g., family member or spouse), the interviewer, consultation with physician or other health professional, and medical records (e.g., physical examination results, screening lab tests). These multimodal assessments provide much-needed diagnostic information through the use of self-report, clinician ratings, behavioral observations, and physiological measures. A comprehensive medical record review, including consideration of medications and diseases that can cause anxiety (see Zarit & Zarit, 2007), is particularly important when formulating diagnoses. Information gathered from the multimodal assessment can be used to differentiate anxiety disorders from co-occurring depressive disorders, medical conditions, and cognitive impairment. Consultation with a physician, which may include a physical examination and screening lab tests, may be necessary for accurate assessment.

The specific approach to assessment may be dictated by the clinician's setting. For example, in outpatient clinics, time may be limited and the clinician may have less time to observe patients compared with inpatient settings or home visits. In the following, we review measures commonly used to assess late-life anxiety symptoms and disorders. We describe a variety of measures ranging from longer interviews to briefer screening measures that may be selected for use in varied settings. We review reliability and validity evidence for the anxiety measures whenever such information is available for older adult samples.

Clinician-Rated Interviews

Clinician-rated interviews may be structured interviews, semi-structured interviews, or rating scales. These interviews may supplement an unstructured clinical interview or they may be used in place of a clinical interview when structured assessments are needed, such as in research settings or clinics focused on evaluation. Some clinician-rated interviews cover all possible diagnoses, while others focus specifically on anxiety disorders. Furthermore, interviews vary in length, complexity, and amount of interviewer training needed.

Structured Clinical Interview for DSM-5 Disorders

The Structured Clinical Interview for DSM-5 Disorders (SCID-5; First et al., 2015) is a clinician-rated interview that assesses most disorders in the DSM-5. It takes approximately 90–120 minutes to administer and requires substantial interviewer training. In our study of older adults seeking treatment for anxiety, we found a mean administration time for the SCID-5 to be 91 minutes (SD = 23, range = 45–156) in 48 older adults (Kok et al., 2018). The SCID-5 assesses all of the DSM-5 anxiety disorders, including other specified anxiety disorder and unspecified anxiety disorder. Psychometric properties of previous versions of the SCID for DSM-III-R and DSM-IV have been examined in older adults. Segal and colleagues (1993) found acceptable inter-rater reliability for anxiety disorders (κ of 0.73–0.77) with the SCID for DSM-III-R. Ivan et al. (2014) reported adequate inter-rater agreement for diagnoses of GAD (κ = 0.68) and other anxiety disorders (κ = 0.75) using the SCID-IV in a late-life anxiety treatment study. No psychometric data for the SCID-5 have been reported to date for older adults.

Anxiety and Related Disorders Interview Schedule-5

The Anxiety and Related Disorders Interview Schedule-5 (ADIS-5; Brown & Barlow, 2014) is a structured interview that includes assessment of DSM-5 anxiety, mood, obsessive–compulsive, trauma, substance abuse, body dysmorphic disorder, and somatic symptom disorders. In comparison with the SCID-5, which incorporates assessment of subthreshold or threshold categorical diagnoses, the ADIS-5 uses dimensional ratings and categorical diagnoses. Administration of the ADIS-5 requires substantial training to make accurate clinician-rated dimensional ratings. Unlike the SCID, the ADIS-5 administration does not allow for discontinuing most sections (cf. "skipping out" on the SCID) if the patient does not endorse symptoms. Some researchers may choose only to administer certain sections of the ADIS-5 to reduce participant burden. Inter-rater reliability for anxiety disorder diagnoses using the ADIS-IV was good (κ = 0.85) in older adults receiving care management services (Diefenbach et al., 2009).

Mini-International Neuropsychiatric Interview

The Mini-International Neuropsychiatric Interview (MINI; Sheehan et al., 1998) is a brief structured interview that takes approximately 15–45 minutes to complete and requires minimal training to administer. The MINI includes assessment of anxiety disorders, major depressive disorder, dysthymia, alcohol abuse and dependence, substance abuse and dependence, and history of manic or psychotic episodes. The MINI (Sheehan et al.,

1998) uses DSM-IV criteria and International Classification of Diseases, 10th Revision (ICD-10) (World Health Organization, 1992) diagnostic criteria. Inter-rater reliability for current anxiety disorder diagnoses ranged from good ($\kappa = 0.88$ for SP) to excellent ($\kappa = 0.98$ for GAD). Diagnostic agreement between the MINI and other structured interviews varied by diagnostic category, with the highest agreement for PD ($\kappa = 0.76$) and the lowest for SPs ($\kappa = 0.43$) and GAD ($\kappa = 0.36$).

Hamilton Anxiety Rating Scale

The Hamilton Anxiety Rating Scale (HARS or HAM-A; Hamilton, 1959) was developed for measuring severity of anxiety symptoms (Hamilton, 1959). The 14-item measure incorporates a 5-point Likert-type rating scale. Seven items address somatic symptoms and seven address *psychic anxiety* (emotional) symptoms. Shear et al. (2001) developed a structured interview guide that can be helpful, particularly with untrained raters. The inter-rater reliability was found to be excellent ($\kappa = 0.96$) and internal consistency was good ($\alpha = 0.85$) for the HARS using the structured interview guide with older adults (Ivan et al., 2014). Diefenbach et al. (2001) found weak evidence of construct validity with a sample of older adults diagnosed with GAD, likely due to the inadequate coverage of worry symptoms. Poor convergent validity evidence was found for the HARS in a study of Parkinson's disease patients (Leentjiens et al., 2011) with a mean age of 64.8 years (range = 34–87). In that study, validity coefficients for convergent evidence ranged from 0.25 to 0.56 with measures of anxiety. In light of the evidence, the HARS may not be the best choice as a measure of older adult anxiety symptoms, particularly if one is not supplementing it with a measure of worry.

Other Clinician-Rated Instruments

The Generalized Anxiety Disorder Severity Scale (GADSS; Shear et al., 2006) is a clinician-rated measure of GAD severity, which may be useful in tracking treatment progress or comparing GAD severity among patients in research studies. The GADSS was found to have good internal consistency ($\alpha = 0.79$) and evidence of convergent validity ($r = 0.45$–0.67) with measures of worry and anxiety, but there was limited evidence of discriminant validity due to a strong association ($r = 0.57$) with a depression measure (Weiss et al., 2009). Inter-rater agreement using the GADSS was excellent ($\kappa = 0.98$) for older adults with anxiety disorders (Ivan et al., 2014). Clinician-rated instruments also may be useful when assessing PD, as suggested by Heindriks et al. (2010), but clinician-rated measures of panic, such as the Panic Disorder Severity Scale (Shear et al., 1997), have not been examined in older adults to date.

Self-Report Measures

Administering self-report measures saves clinicians' time compared with lengthy clinician-rated interviews. Self-report measures also capture the patients' perception of their symptoms, which is particularly important for unobservable anxiety symptoms (i.e., worry). Although some self-report measures assess a variety of anxiety disorders (e.g., the Beck Anxiety Inventory (BAI)), applying these measures to the geriatric population may be problematic. Older adult-specific measures were created to address concerns that most anxiety scales were created for and normed on younger, nonclinical samples and thus have questionable psychometric support with older adults (Therrien & Hunsley, 2012). The drawback of older adult-specific measures is that they make comparisons with younger samples difficult.

General Anxiety Assessment Measures

In the following, we discuss four self-report assessments of anxiety that can be used to assess heterogeneous anxiety symptoms that occur with various anxiety disorders.

Beck Anxiety Inventory

The BAI (Beck et al., 1988) is a 21-item self-report anxiety assessment created to differentiate between anxiety and depression symptoms. Respondents rate symptom severity over the past week, from 0 ("Not at all") to 3 ("Severely – I could barely stand it"). The BAI has demonstrated good internal consistency among older adults (mean $\alpha = 0.86$, 95% confidence interval (CI) $= 0.82$–0.86; Therrien & Hunsley, 2013). Convergent validity evidence with community-dwelling older adults is moderate, with coefficients of 0.47–0.73 (Morin et al., 1999) with anxiety measures. Discriminant evidence is weak with regard to measures of depression ($r = 0.44$–0.50; Morin et al., 1999). One of the main shortcomings of using the BAI in older adults is the measure's reliance on somatic symptoms of anxiety; 14 of the 21 items assess physical symptoms (Kabacoff et al., 1997). One way to address this limitation is to examine the two factors or subscales of the BAI to parse out the cognitive symptoms (7 items) from the somatic anxiety symptoms (14 items), as physical ailments may lead to more endorsement of somatic items in older adults (Wetherell & Gatz, 2005).

Geriatric Anxiety Inventory

The Geriatric Anxiety Inventory (GAI; Pachana et al., 2007) is a 20-item self-report measure that uses a dichotomous response format to assess the presence of anxiety symptoms within the past week. Diefenbach and colleagues (2009) found that, among older adults, the GAI demonstrated greater ease of use than the BAI, Penn State Worry Questionnaire (PSWQ), or Generalized Anxiety Disorder 2-item (GAD-2). A cutoff of ≥ 11 has been recommended when screening for GAD (sensitivity $= 0.74$, specificity $= 0.84$) and ≥ 9 when screening for any anxiety disorder (sensitivity $= 0.73$, specificity $= 0.80$; Pachana et al., 2007). The GAI has excellent internal consistency (mean $\alpha = 0.92$, 95% CI $= 0.90$–0.93; Therrien & Hunsley, 2013). A five-item version (Geriatric Anxiety Inventory-Short Form (GAI-SF); Byrne & Pachana, 2011) correlates with the full GAI ($r = 0.89$–0.93) and has acceptable to good internal consistency ($\alpha = 0.73$–0.84; Gerolimatos et al., 2013; Johnco et al., 2015). Strong evidence of convergent validity has been found with other measures of anxiety, with coefficients ranging from 0.28 to 0.71 (Gould et al., 2014; Yochim et al., 2010). Limitations to the GAI include its emphasis on worry symptoms and strong associations with measures of depression ($r = 0.74$; Yochim et al., 2010).

Geriatric Anxiety Scale

The Geriatric Anxiety Scale (GAS; Segal et al., 2010) is a 30-item self-report measure that assesses the frequency of anxiety symptoms in the past week, ranging from 0 ("Not at all") to 3 ("All of the time"). Only the first 25 GAS items are scored; the last 5 items are used to identify areas of clinical concern (e.g., finances, health, being a burden). The GAS provides a total score and three symptom subscales: somatic, cognitive, and affective. The GAS has demonstrated good internal consistency for the total score ($\alpha = 0.93$; Segal et al., 2010). Gould et al. (2014) found that a cutoff of 17 or greater maximized sensitivity and specificity. An abbreviated 10-item version of the scale (GAS-10; Mueller et al., 2015) has shown good internal consistency ($\alpha = 0.89$) and is strongly correlated with the full GAS ($r = 0.96$, $p < 0.001$). The GAS shows strong evidence of convergent validity with measures of anxiety and worry, with coefficients ranging from 0.57 to 0.60 (Gould et al., 2014; Segal et al., 2010; Yochim et al., 2010). Similar to the GAI, the GAS has been found to have strong associations with depression ($r = 0.74$; Yochim et al., 2010), particularly for the GAS cognitive and affective subscales. An advantage of the GAS is that it assesses more facets of anxiety than the GAI; however, the GAS scores are highly associated with depression, and more evidence of the utility of the GAS with a clinical sample is needed.

Patient-Reported Outcomes Measurement Information System Anxiety Measure

The US National Institutes of Health developed a set of freely available measures called the Patient-Reported Outcomes Measurement Information System (PROMIS; Cella et al., 2010). The PROMIS anxiety measure assess the frequency of anxiety symptoms using a five-point scale. The anxiety symptoms assessed include anxious apprehension (e.g., feeling uneasy, nervous), fear, and worry. Internal consistency for the seven-item PROMIS anxiety measure was good among older adults ($\alpha = 0.85$; Moore et al., 2016). Convergent and discriminant validity in older adult samples have not been reported to date.

Specific Anxiety Disorder Measures

Several self-report measures assess specific anxiety disorders. Typically, the items on these measures closely correspond to their respective diagnostic criteria in the DSM. Thus, clinicians should be mindful of which DSM was used in the measure's creation. Additionally, although these measures may be useful to screen for anxiety disorders, they alone should not be used as diagnostic measures.

Generalized Anxiety Disorder and Worry

GAD is one of the most common late-life anxiety disorders, affecting between 1.2% (Gum et al., 2009) and 7.3% (Beekman et al., 1998) of older adults. The Generalized Anxiety Disorder 7-item (GAD-7) was developed as one of the patient health questionnaires (Spitzer et al., 2006) to detect possible GAD. The scale assesses the frequency of seven anxiety symptoms, each rated from 0 ("Not at all") to 3 ("Nearly every day"). The first two items of the GAD-7 can be administered on their own, and together they comprise the GAD-2. The internal consistency scores (Cronbach's α) of GAD-7 and GAD-2 scores were 0.82 and 0.71, respectively (Wild et al., 2014). Some evidence of convergent validity was demonstrated with a general measure of physical ($r = -0.22$) and mental health ($r = -0.48$), and strong associations with depression measures were found ($r = 0.68$ for GAD-2 and 0.70 for GAD-7; Wild et al., 2014). The suggested cutoff for GAD-7 within the general population is a score of 10 or more (Spitzer et al., 2006); however, that cutoff yielded very low sensitivity (0.26) for adults (aged 58–82; Wild et al., 2014). The authors concluded that the optimal cutoff for older adults was a score of 5 or more (sensitivity = 0.63, specificity = 0.90). However, the low sensitivity raises concerns about using GAD-7 as a screening tool with older adults.

The PSWQ (Meyer et al., 1990) is a 16-item scale that assesses an individual's tendency to worry (cf., trait worry). The respondent rates a series of worry-related statements using a five-point Likert-type scale of 1 ("Not at all typical") to 5 ("Very typical"). The PSWQ has good internal consistency in older adult samples (mean $\alpha = 0.90$, 95% CI = 0.84–0.94; Therrein & Hunsley, 2013), good test–retest reliability ($r = 0.79$), and evidence of convergent validity with measures of GAD, anxiety, and worry, with coefficients ranging from 0.29 to 0.79 (Diefenbach et al., 2009). Concerns have been raised regarding older adults' difficulty interpreting and responding to the PSWQ's reverse-scored items (Hopko et al., 2003). To address this, Hopko and colleagues (2003) created an eight-item version (PSWQ-A) for use with older adults that omits reverse-scored items. The abbreviated version is strongly correlated with the full PSWQ ($r = 0.92$; Hopko et al., 2003).

The Worry Scale (WS; Wisocki et al., 1986) is a 35-item scale designed to assess how frequently older adults worry about various aspects of their life (e.g., social, financial, physical health). Respondents rate the frequency of worrying about different domains on a five-point scale, from 0 ("Never") to 4 ("Much of the time"). The WS has good internal consistency (mean $α = 0.86$, 95% CI = 0.83–0.89; Therrien & Hunsley, 2013). The revised version (Worry Scale – Revised; Wisocki, 1994) has 88 items and has excellent internal consistency ($α = 0.95$) and evidence of convergent validity ($r = 0.45$) with the PSWQ (Hunt et al., 2003).

Specific Phobias

SPs or fears are the most common late-life anxiety disorder (e.g., Gum et al., 2009). Fears are often overlooked, as many are perceived to be easily managed and avoidable; however, some fears may result in severely restricted functioning (e.g., fear of falling). Fear measures designed for young adults omit common fears in later adulthood such as fear of mental decline or being a burden. Kogan and Edelstein (2004) modified a commonly used measure of fear, the Fear Survey Schedule-II (FSS-II; Geer, 1965), to include age-specific fears reported by older adults. The resulting measure, FSS-II for Older Adults (FSS-II-OA), assesses 22 fears, 11 of which are age-related fears. The FSS-II-OA has excellent internal consistency ($α = 0.96$ for fear intensity and 0.98 for fear interference subscales), good convergent validity ($r = 0.40$–0.47), and good test–retest reliability ($r = 0.88$, 2–3-week interval; Kogan & Edelstein, 2004). A unique feature of the FSS-II-OA is that it includes a separate scale that measures the extent to which each fear interferes with daily functioning.

There also are measures of individual fears, chiefly fear of falling. Bower and colleagues (2015) recently revised one fear of falling measure, the Fear of Falling Questionnaire (FFQ; Dayhoff et al., 1994), to improve its psychometric properties. Experts reviewed the FFQ, revised FFQ items to improve readability for older adults, and removed FFQ items that did not directly measure fear of falling, but instead measured aspects of disability or recovery from an injury. The revised measure had excellent test–retest reliability (intraclass correlation coefficient = 0.93, 3-day interval), good to excellent internal consistency ($α = 0.83$–0.98), and evidence of convergent validity with a measure of falling and discriminant validity with measures of depression and positive and negative affect (Bower et al., 2015).

Social Anxiety Disorder

Although SAD is one of the most common anxiety disorders (with an estimated 1-year prevalence rate of 7% for the general population), prevalence rates are relatively low for older adults and range from 2% to 5% (Gum et al., 2009; Kessler et al., 2012). Despite the lower prevalence in older adults, accurate identification of social anxiety is important, as persistent social anxiety may be debilitating and cause considerable distress.

The Liebowitz Social Anxiety Scale (LSAS; Liebowitz, 1987) is a 24-item, clinician-administered screener used to assess social anxiety. The measure consists of 13 items relating to performance anxiety and 11 items relating to social interactions and situations. The clinician describes the situation and asks the examinee to rate intensity of anxiety during the situation and the frequency of their avoidance of the situation on a four-point

Likert scale. A global score can be obtained by summing the four subscale scores for Performance Fear, Performance Avoidance, Social Fear, and Social Avoidance. A score of 30–59 indicates that social anxiety is probable, and a score ≥60 suggests the presence of social anxiety in multiple social situations (i.e., generalized social phobia). The measure has excellent internal consistency ($\alpha = 0.96$) in a mixed-age sample (Heimberg et al., 1999). A self-report scale (LSAS-SR) was developed and has since become popular. The LSAS-SR was evaluated with older adults and had excellent internal consistency ($\alpha = 0.93$–0.97), evidence of convergent validity with measures of social anxiety and general anxiety ($r = 0.43$–0.83), and evidence of discriminant validity with measures of depression and general mental and physical health ($r = -0.29$ to 0.48; Gould et al., 2012).

The Social Interaction Anxiety Scale (SIAS) and the Social Phobia Scale (SPS) both consist of 20 items and are commonly administered together. The SIAS assesses social interaction anxiety, whereas the SPS assesses evaluation discomfort during routine activities (Mattick & Clarke, 1998). Both measures have good to excellent internal consistency ($\alpha = 0.88$–0.94). Convergent validity evidence was demonstrated in the initial validation study (Mattick & Clarke, 1998), but these findings should be replicated with older adult samples. The SIAS has the potential to unnecessarily challenge older adults because it contains reverse-scored items, which have been demonstrated to be problematic for older adults (Hopko et al., 2003). In fact, Rodebaugh et al. (2011) found that the associations for reverse-scored items with the total scale were attenuated in older adults compared with younger adults.

The Social Phobia and Anxiety Inventory (SPAI; Turner et al., 1989) is a 45-item screening instrument that assesses cognitive, behavioral, and somatic symptoms due to social anxiety and/or fear about social situations. Gretarsdottir and colleagues (2004) found that the SPAI had excellent internal consistency among older adults ($\alpha = 0.99$). Older adults had lower overall scores on the SPAI compared with young and middle-aged adults. Item-level analyses revealed some age differences in the types of social situations that are anxiety-evoking. The SPAI had poor convergent validity with general measures of anxiety, with coefficients ranging from 0.28 to 0.41 (Gretarsdottir et al., 2004), but it showed good evidence of convergent validity with a measure of social anxiety, the LSAS-SR ($r = 0.64$; Gould et al., 2012). The Older Adult Social Evaluative Scale (OASES; Gould et al., 2012) is a 37-item measure of social anxiety specifically designed for older adults. The examinees rate their level of anxiety in a given situation on a four-point scale ranging from 0 ("Not at all") to 3 ("Severely"), which comprises the anxiety scale. Then, examinees rate the likelihood that they would avoid that situation on a scale of 0 ("Never") to 3 ("Usually"), which comprises the avoidance subscale. The OASES demonstrated excellent internal consistency for the overall score ($\alpha = 0.97$) and for both subscales (anxiety: $\alpha = 0.94$; avoidance: $\alpha = 0.95$; Gould et al., 2012). The authors noted that the two subscales were strongly correlated ($r = 0.77$, $p < 0.001$). The OASES instrument shows good convergent validity with measures of anxiety and social anxiety ($r = 0.44$–0.77). Additional studies are underway to support the use of the clinical utility of the OASES (i.e., validation against diagnoses of SAD; Kok et al., 2018).

Panic and Agoraphobia

The prevalence of PD is lower in older adults than young adults, and it has a unique symptom presentation with less frequent panic attacks among older adults (Gum et al., 2009; Hendriks et al., 2014). Because panic attack frequency is often used as an outcome measure, assessing PD severity in older adults requires special considerations (Hendriks et al., 2014). The Agoraphobic Cognitions Questionnaire (ACQ; Chambless et al., 1984), which is a 14-item measure that assesses catastrophic panic cognitions, was found to have adequate internal consistency ($\alpha = 0.63$) with older adults with PD (Hendriks et al., 2010). The Mobility Inventory (MI; Chambless et al., 1985) is a self-report measure used to track panic and agoraphobia treatment outcomes. The MI avoidance subscales were found to have excellent internal consistency with older adults ($\alpha = 0.93$–0.94; Hendriks et al., 2010). The convergent and discriminant validity of the ACQ and MI in older adult samples have not been examined to our knowledge. Another means of assessing panic symptom severity is to administer measures of general anxiety, such as BAI (Beck & Steer, 1990) or the Anxiety Sensitivity Index (ASI; Reiss et al., 1986). The BAI, discussed earlier in detail, has demonstrated evidence of convergent validity with measures of panic in young adult samples ($r = 0.56$–0.78; de Beurs et al., 1997). The ASI is a 16-item measure that assesses concerns about anxiety and panic symptoms, as well as associated impairment, using a five-point Likert-type scale ranging from 0 ("Very little") to 4 ("Very much"). The ASI has excellent internal consistency among older adults ($\alpha = 0.91$; Gerolimatos & Edelstein, 2012) and evidence of convergent validity with measures of anxiety, somatic symptoms, and panic ($r = 0.50$–0.64; Mohlman & Zinbarg, 2000). Although the ASI has multiple subscales, Mohlman and Zinbarg (2000) recommend using the total score with older adults.

In the DSM-5, agoraphobia was separated from PD, becoming a standalone diagnosis. This reorganization created an "assessment void" for measures that specifically assess agoraphobia. Above, we discussed several measures that examine symptoms of both agoraphobia and PD. Other measures discussed above (FSS-II-OA, LSAS, OASES, SPAI) include scales that assess avoidance and may be of use for measuring agoraphobia. As evidenced by the paucity of information on this topic, more research on agoraphobia assessment and age differences in agoraphobia symptoms is needed.

Interviews and Scales for Older Adults with Dementia

Some specific measures for assessing anxiety disorders in the presence of cognitive impairment (i.e., major and minor neurocognitive disorders) include separate scales to be completed by a proxy (e.g., caregiver) and the patient. One such measure is the Rating Anxiety in Dementia Scale (RAID; Shankar et al., 1999), which assesses caregiver and patient ratings of anxiety symptoms. Limitations to this measure include: a relatively lengthy time frame (past 2 weeks) for a person with dementia to recall; and weak evidence of convergent and discriminant validity (Gibbons et al., 2006). A structured interview version of the RAID (RAID-SI) was developed by Snow and colleagues (2012). The RAID-SI had good internal consistency ($\alpha = 0.75$), inter-rater reliability ($\kappa = 0.71$), and evidence of convergent validity ($r = 0.36$–0.49; Snow et al., 2012). Other measures of psychiatric symptoms in the presence of dementia (e.g., the Neuropsychiatric Inventory; Cummings et al., 1994) assess anxiety symptoms using only caregiver or proxy ratings.

To address some of the aforementioned limitations, Gerolimatos and colleagues developed the Anxiety in Cognitive Impairment and Dementia (ACID) scales (Gerolimatos et al., 2015). The ACID consists of two 13-item scales, the patient (ACID-SR) and proxy (ACID-PR), which assess anxiety symptoms in the past 24 hours. Once a symptom is endorsed, subjective distress and interference with functioning are assessed with follow-up questions. The ACID was developed to be used across the full range of cognitive impairment such that the self-report could be completed by patients with milder impairments and the proxy report could be used for patients who are too impaired to provide accurate self-reports. Both scales could be used together for a comprehensive assessment. Initial psychometric data indicated that the ACID had excellent inter-rater reliability (κ = 1.00) and good internal consistency (ACID-PR: α = 0.73; ACID-SR: α = 0.87). Evidence of convergent validity with anxiety measures was demonstrated for the ACID-SR, with coefficients ranging from 0.27 to 0.71. Evidence of convergent validity also was found for the ACID-PR, but associations were substantially lower when proxy reports were correlated with self-report measures, with coefficients ranging from 0.08 to 0.81 for ACID-PR (Gerolimatos et al., 2015). The interested reader is referred to Chapter 8 in this volume for a detailed discussion of anxiety and cognition.

Physiological Measures

Clinicians may review physiological measures, such as blood pressure, heart rate, heart rate variability, and skin conductance, to assist with differential diagnoses and monitor treatment progress. For instance, somatic symptoms such as dizziness or feeling faint may be partially accounted for by hypotension. A thorough medical evaluation may be needed to rule out medical causes of anxiety. Researchers may also choose to measure physiological responses to exposure to anxiety-evoking stimuli as an objective measure of anxiety. However, one must consider age differences in responses when drawing conclusions across age groups. The interested reader is referred to Kogan et al. (2000) and Uchino et al. (2010) for further discussion of physiological measures.

Behavioral Observations and Informant Reports

Behavioral observations include ancillary information and observations about behavioral manifestations of anxiety. Mohlman and colleagues (2012) identified 15 maladaptive avoidance behaviors specific to older adult anxiety (e.g., excessive checking of blood pressure, avoiding exercise due to fear of falling). These behaviors might be reported by the older adult's family member(s), spouse, friend(s), or medical provider. Interviewers also can use their observations about the older adult's presentation (e.g., appearing nervous) or motor behaviors (e.g., fidgeting) to indicate the presence of excessive anxiety symptoms.

Special Assessment Considerations

Use of Technology in Assessments

As more older adults use computers, smartphones, and wearable monitors (e.g., activity monitors), these technologies can be harnessed to assess anxiety and associated symptoms in real time. One particularly robust assessment method is ecological momentary assessment (EMA), which uses repeated sampling of thoughts, emotions, or behaviors in the participant's natural environment. EMA intends to increase ecological validity, reduce recall bias, and enable examination of fine-grained changes within participants (Shiffman et al., 2008). Moore et al. (2016) compared EMA and paper-and-pencil self-report measures in an intervention study with older adults and found that the EMA assessments were more sensitive in detecting reductions in anxiety and depression. Wearable activity monitors also can be used to enhance self-report measures by providing activity and sleep information. Researchers propose several important suggestions for increasing the acceptance of technology, such as using tutorials at initial deployment (Preusse et al., 2016) and using telephone calls to promote adherence to technology-based assessments (Moore et al., 2016).

Physical Disease

In total, 90% of older adults have at least one chronic medical condition (e.g., hypertension, heart disease, diabetes, lung disease, arthritis), with almost 75% having two or more such conditions (Anderson, 2010). Specific physical diseases are associated with anxiety symptoms, yet the etiological relation between anxiety and physical disorders is complicated. Anxiety can be an early symptom of a physical disorder, can present as comorbid with a disorder, can be a reaction to the disorder, or can be an adverse effect from the treatment of a disorder. An appreciation of the presentation of anxiety with various physical disorders and the ways in which symptoms of anxiety and these disorders can be related to each other is particularly important for clinicians working with older adults. A few of the more common physical disorders associated with symptoms of anxiety are discussed.

Chronic Obstructive Pulmonary Disease

Chronic obstructive pulmonary disease (COPD) comprises a group of chronic degenerative diseases (e.g., emphysema, chronic bronchitis) of the respiratory system characterized by impaired lung function. Common symptoms include increased sputum production, dyspnea (shortness of breath; difficulty obtaining enough air), and coughing (Rycroft et al., 2012). Dyspnea is particularly likely to lead to symptoms of anxiety and panic attacks. Anxiety was found to be more than twice as common among individuals with COPD compared to controls (15% vs. 6%; Eisner et al., 2010), and greater COPD severity was associated with a greater risk of anxiety. Additionally, anxious individuals with COPD had a higher longitudinal risk of COPD exacerbation compared to non-anxious individuals with COPD.

Parkinson's Disease

Parkinson's disease is a progressive neurodegenerative disorder that impairs movement and motor control and affects approximately 1% of older adults (Prediger et al., 2012). The prevalence of clinically significant anxiety symptoms among individuals with Parkinson's disease ranges from 12.8% to 43.0% (Dissanayaka et al., 2014). The most common anxiety disorders reported in patients with Parkinson's disease are: PD (1.8–25.0%), GAD (0–30.8%), SP (16.0%), SAD (0–13.0%), and anxiety disorder not otherwise specified (NOS; 2.0–25.0%) (Dissanayaka et al., 2014). Anxiety symptoms are likely a reaction to the debilitating effects of Parkinson's disease, a consequence of the underlying neurochemical changes associated with the disease (Cummings & Masterman, 1999; Dissanayaka, et al., 2014), and possibly even a prodromal syndrome (Cosci et al., 2015). Fear of falling is particularly important to assess in Parkinson's disease due to associated impairments with psychomotor functioning and balance.

Diabetes

Diabetes is a group of metabolic diseases, with Type I and II diabetes being the most common. Adults with diabetes have a higher risk than those without diabetes for meeting criteria for an anxiety diagnosis (odds ratio (OR) = 1.21, 95% CI = 1.10–1.31) and expressing elevated anxiety symptoms (OR = 1.48, 95% CI = 1.02–1.93) (Smith et al., 2013). In their review of the literature, Grigsby and colleagues (2002) found a prevalence of 14% for GAD in patients with diabetes, which is similar to the prevalence in the general population. However, the prevalence of anxiety disorder NOS was quite high, ranging from 27% to 40%. Comorbid anxiety disorders or elevated anxiety symptoms are also associated with diabetes complications, symptom burden, pain, poorer quality of life, and greater disability (Gould et al., 2014).

Cardiovascular Disease

Cardiovascular disease (CVD) is a class of diseases that includes peripheral artery disease, ischemic heart disease, stroke, and hypertension. In a large epidemiological study, Fan and colleagues (2008) found that approximately 16.6% of adults aged 45 and older with CVD had a history of anxiety disorders as compared to 10% of individuals without CVD. A recent meta-analysis found that anxiety is associated with increased mortality in those patients with stable CVD compared with patients with acute cardiovascular events (Celano et al., 2015).

In summary, the presence of chronic medical conditions should signal the need to examine whether comorbid anxiety symptoms are present. If present, the clinician might explore the temporal relation of the onset of physical symptoms and anxiety as one step toward formulating an intervention.

Diversity and Gender Differences

For accurate assessment of late-life anxiety, it is important to consider the unique influence of culture, race and ethnicity, gender, sexual orientation, religion, level of education, and socioeconomic status, and how these factors dynamically affect symptomology. Many of these factors may overlap and interact with one another, complicating accurate assessment.

Prevalence rates for anxiety disorders in Asian, African, and Latin American countries have been estimated to be 2–4% lower than in both European countries and the USA (Lewis-Fernandez et al., 2010). Jimenez and colleagues (2010) found anxiety disorder prevalence rates among adults aged 50 years or older to be lowest in Asian Americans (9.4%), followed by African Americans (15.5%), and Latinos and non-Latino Whites (18.2% and 18.7%, respectively). Men tend to report fewer anxiety symptoms than women (Fehm et al., 2005), with the large National Comorbidity Survey Replication reporting almost twice as many older women meeting the criteria for any anxiety disorder than older men (14.7% vs. 7.6%) (Byers et al., 2010). Whether these patterns reflect lower rates among certain groups is an important area for further research. It is possible that certain cultural groups use different linguistic expressions to describe their distress or impaired functioning, have limited insight into their symptoms, are unwilling to disclose their experiences of anxiety, or use different medications or nutritional supplements that may mask symptoms. Thus, multimodal assessment is critical when working with diverse populations. For instance, we have found that some older Asian men may minimize symptoms severity or deny symptoms altogether upon direct questioning during an interview, but endorse anxiety symptoms when administered a self-report measure with a Likert-type response scale. Although the clinical field currently observes some differences in prevalence rates among various cultural groups, there is more to learn about why these differences exist and whether they affect assessment and treatment.

Conclusion

Assessment of older adult anxiety can be challenging, in part because the experience and presentation of anxiety symptoms can differ across the lifespan. Moreover, presenting symptoms are not always consistent with the current diagnostic nosologies. Assessing older adults involves navigating the medical, pharmacological, cognitive, psychometric, and diversity-related issues that challenge clinicians and benefit from multimodal assessment. We have offered brief discussions of these issues and a critical review of anxiety assessment instruments often used with, but not developed with, older adults, as well as those developed specifically for use with older adults. It is our hope that the reader will come away with the knowledge to make developmentally and psychometrically sound decisions when selecting anxiety assessment instruments and interpreting their results.

Acknowledgments

Dr. Gould is supported by a Career Development Award (IK2 RX001478) from the United States Department of Veterans Affairs and by Ellen Schapiro and Gerald Axelbaum through a 2014 National Association for Research on Schizophrenia and Depression (NARSAD) Young Investigator Grant from the Brain & Behavior Research Foundation. The views expressed in this chapter are those of the authors and not necessarily those of the Department of Veterans Affairs or the Federal Government.

References

American Psychiatric Association (2013). *Diagnostic and Statistical Manual of Mental Disorders*, 5th ed. Washington, DC: American Psychiatric Association.

Anderson, G. (2010). *Chronic Care: Making the Case for Ongoing Care*. Princeton, NJ: Robert Woods Johnson Foundation.

Beck, A. T. and Steer, R. A. (1990). *Manual for the Beck Anxiety Inventory*. San Antonio, TX: Psychological Corporation.

Beck, A. T., Epstein, N., Brown, G., et al. (1988). An inventory for measuring clinical anxiety: psychometric properties. *Journal of Consulting and Clinical Psychology*, **56**, 893–897.

Beekman, A. T., Bremmer, M. A., Deeg, D. J., et al. (1998). Anxiety disorders in later life: a report from the Longitudinal Aging Study Amsterdam. *International Journal of Geriatric Psychiatry*, **13**, 717–726.

Bower, E. S., Wetherell, J. L., Merz, C. C., et al. (2015). A new measure of fear of falling: psychometric properties of the Fear of Falling Questionnaire Revised (FFQ-R). *International Psychogeriatrics*, **27**, 1121–1133.

Brown, T. A. and Barlow, D. H. (2014). *Anxiety and Related Disorders Interview Schedule for DSM-5 (ADIS-5)*. New York: Oxford University Press.

Bryant, C., Jackson, H. and Ames, D. (2008). The prevalence of anxiety in older adults: methodological issues and a review of the literature. *Journal of Affective Disorders*, **109**, 233–250.

Byers, A. L., Yaffe, K., Covinsky, K. E., et al. (2010). High occurrence of mood and anxiety disorders among older adults: the National Comorbidity Survey Replication. *Archives of General Psychiatry*, **67**, 489–496.

Byrne, G. J. and Pachana, N. A. (2011). Development and validation of a short form of the Geriatric Anxiety Inventory – the GAI-SF. *International Psychogeriatrics*, **23**, 125–131.

Celano, C. M., Millstein, R. M., Bedoya, C. A., et al. (2015). Association between anxiety and mortality in patients with coronary artery disease: a meta-analysis. *American Heart Journal*, **170**, 1105–1115.

Cella, D., Riley, W., Stone, A. A., et al. (2010). The Patient Reported Outcomes Measurement Information System (PROMIS) developed and tested its first wave of adult self-reported health outcome item banks: 2005–2008. *Journal of Clinical Epidemiology*, **63**, 1179–1194.

Chambless, D. L., Caputo, G. C., Bright, P., et al. (1985). The mobility inventory for agoraphobia. *Behaviour Research and Therapy*, **23**, 35–44.

Chambless, D. L., Caputo, G. C., Bright, P., et al. (1984). Assessment of fear of fear in agoraphobics: the Body Sensations Questionnaire and the Agoraphobic

Cognitions Questionnaire. *Journal of Consulting and Clinical Psychology*, **52**, 1090–1097.

Ciliberti, C., Gould, C., Smith, M., et al. (2011). A preliminary investigation of developmentally sensitive items for the assessment of social anxiety in late life. *Journal of Anxiety Disorders*, **25**, 686–689.

Cosci, F., Fava, G. A. and Sonio, N. (2015). Mood and anxiety disorders as early manifestations of medical illness: a systematic review. *Psychotherapy and Psychosomatics*, **84**, 22–29.

Cummings, J. L. and Masterman, D. L. (1999). Depression in patients with Parkinson's disease. *International Journal of Geriatric Psychiatry*, **14**, 711–718.

Cummings, J. L., Mega, M., Gray, K., et al. (1994). The Neuropsychiatric Inventory: comprehensive assessment of psychopathology in dementia. *Neurology*, **44**, 2308–2314.

Dayhoff, N. E., Baird, C., Bennett, S., et al. (1994). Fear of falling: measuring fear and appraisals of potential harm. *Rehabilitation Nursing Research*, **3**, 97–104.

de Beurs, E., Wilson, K. A., Chambless, D. L., et al. (1997). Convergent and divergent validity of the Beck Anxiety Inventory for patients with panic disorder and agoraphobia. *Depression and Anxiety*, **6**, 140–146.

Depp, C., Woodruff-Borden, J., Meeks, S., et al. (2005). The phenomenology of non-clinical panic in older adults in comparison to younger adults. *Journal of Anxiety Disorders*, **19**, 503–519.

Diefenbach, G. J., Stanley, M. A., Beck, J. G., et al. (2001). Examination of the Hamilton Scales in assessment of anxious older adults: a replication and extension. *Journal of Psychopathology and Behavioral Assessment*, **23**, 117–124.

Diefenbach, G. J., Tolin, D. F., Meunier, S. A., et al. (2009). Assessment of anxiety in older home care recipients. *Gerontologist*, **49**, 141–153.

Dissanayaka, N., White, E., O'Sullivan, J. D., et al. (2014). The clinical spectrum of anxiety in Parkinson's disease. *Movement Disorders*, **29**, 966–975.

Doyle, A. C. (1890). *The Sign of Four*. New York: Penguin Random House.

Eisner, M. D., Blanc, P. D., Yelin, E. H., et al. (2010). Influence of anxiety on health outcomes in COPD. *Thorax*, **65**, 229–234.

Fan, A. Z., Strine, T. W., Jiles, R., et al. (2008). Depression and anxiety associated with cardiovascular disease among persons aged 45 years and older in 38 states of the United States, 2006. *Preventive Medicine*, **46**, 445–450.

Fehm, L., Pelissolo, A., Furmark, T., et al. (2005). Size and burden of social phobia in Europe. *European Neuropsychopharmacology*, **15**, 453–462.

First, M. B., Williams, J. B. W., Karg, R. S., et al. (2015). *Structured Clinical Interview for DSM-5 Disorders*. Arlington, VA: American Psychiatric Publishing.

Geer, J. H. (1965). The development of a scale to measure fear. *Behaviour Research and Therapy*, **3**, 45–53.

Gerolimatos, L. A. and Edelstein, B. A. (2012). Predictors of health anxiety among older and young adults. *International Psychogeriatrics*, **24**, 1998–2008.

Gerolimatos, L. A., Ciliberti, C. M., Gregg, J. J., et al. (2015). Development and preliminary evaluation of the Anxiety in Cognitive Impairment and Dementia (ACID) scales. *International Psychogeriatrics*, **27**, 1825–1838.

Gerolimatos, L. A., Gregg, J. J. and Edelstein, B. A. (2013). Assessment of anxiety in long-term care: examination of the Geriatric Anxiety Inventory (GAI) and its short form. *International Psychogeriatrics*, **25**, 1533–1542.

Gibbons, L. E., Teri, L., Logsdon, R. G., et al. (2006). Assessment of anxiety in dementia: an investigation into the association of different methods of measurement. *Journal of Geriatric Psychiatry and Neurology*, **19**, 202–208.

Go, A. S., Mozaffarian, D., Roger, V. L., et al. (2013). Heart disease and stroke statistics – 2013 update: a report from the American Heart Association. *Circulation*, **127**, e6–e245.

Gould, C. E. and Edelstein, B. (2010). Worry, emotion control, and anxiety control in older and young adults. *Journal of Anxiety Disorders*, **24**, 759–766.

Gould, C. E., Gerolimatos, L. A., Ciliberti, C. M., et al. (2012). Initial evaluation of the Older Adult Social-Evaluative Situations Questionnaire: a measure of social anxiety in older adults. *International Psychogeriatrics*, **24**, 2009–2018.

Gould, C. E., Segal, D. L., Yochim, B. P., et al. (2014). Measuring anxiety in late life: a psychometric examination of the Geriatric Anxiety Inventory and Geriatric Anxiety Scale. *Journal of Anxiety Disorders*, **28**, 804–811.

Gould, C. E., Smith, M. and Edelstein, B. A. (2015). Special considerations for assessment in older adults. In F. Andrasik, J. Goodie and A. Peterson, eds., *Biopsychosocial Assessment in Clinical Health Psychology: A Handbook*. New York: Guilford Press, pp. 450–469.

Gretarsdottir, E., Woodruff-Borden, J., Meeks, S., et al. (2004). Social anxiety in older adults: phenomenology, prevalence, and measurement. *Behaviour Research and Therapy*, **42**, 459–475.

Grigsby, A. B., Anderson, R. J., Freedland, K. E., et al. (2002). Prevalence of anxiety in adults with diabetes: a systematic review. *Journal of Psychosomatic Research*, **53**, 1053–1060.

Gum, A. M., King-Kallimanis, B. and Kohn, R. (2009). Prevalence of mood, anxiety, and substance-abuse disorders for older Americans in the National Comorbidity Survey – Replication. *American Journal of Geriatric Psychiatry*, **17**, 769–781.

Hamilton, M. (1959). The assessment of anxiety states by rating. *British Journal of Medical Psychology*, **32**, 50–55.

Heimberg, R. G., Horner, K. J., Juster, H. R., et al. (1999). Psychometric properties of the Liebowitz Social Anxiety Scale. *Psychological Medicine*, **29**, 199–212.

Hendriks, G. J., Kampman, M., Keisers, G. P. J., et al. (2014). Cognitive-behavioral therapy for panic disorder with agoraphobia in older people: a comparison with younger patients. *Depression and Anxiety*, **31**, 669–677.

Hendriks, G. J., Keijsers, G. P. J., Kampman, M., et al. (2010). A randomized controlled study of paroxetine and cognitive–behavioural therapy for late-life panic disorder. *Acta Psychiatrica Scandinavica*, **122**, 11–19.

Hopko, D. R., Reas, D. L., Beck, J. G., et al. (2003). Assessing worry in older adults: confirmatory factor analysis of the Penn State Worry Questionnaire and psychometric properties of an abbreviated model. *Psychological Assessment*, **15**, 173–183.

Hunt, S., Wisocki, P. and Yanko, B. (2003). Worry and use of coping strategies among older and younger adults. *Journal of Anxiety Disorders*, **17**, 547–560.

Isaacowitz, D. M., Wadlinger, H. A., Goren, D., et al. (2006). Is there an age-related positivity effect in visual attention? A comparison of two methodologies. *Emotion*, **6**, 511–516.

Ivan, M. C., Amspoker, A. B., Nadorff, M. R., et al. (2014). Alcohol use, anxiety, and insomnia in older adults with generalized anxiety disorder. *American Journal of Geriatric Psychiatry*, **22**, 875–883.

Jimenez, D. E., Alegria, M., Chen, C. D., et al. (2010). Prevalence of psychiatric illnesses among ethnic minority elderly. *Journal of the American Geriatric Society*, **58**, 256–264.

Johnco, C., Knight, A., Tadic, D., et al. (2015). Psychometric properties of the Geriatric Anxiety Inventory (GAI) and its short-form (GAI-SF) in a clinical and non-clinical sample of older adults. *International Psychogeriatrics*, **27**, 1089–1097.

Kabacoff, R. I., Segal, D. L., Hersen, M., et al. (1997). Psychometric properties and diagnostic utility of the Beck Anxiety Inventory and the State–Trait Anxiety Inventory with older adult psychiatric outpatients. *Journal of Anxiety Disorders*, **11**, 33–47.

Kessler, R. C., Petukhova, M., Sampson, N. A., et al. (2012). Twelve-month and lifetime prevalence and lifetime morbid risk of anxiety and mood disorders in the United States. *International Journal of Methods in Psychiatric Research*, **21**, 169–184.

Kogan, J. N. and Edelstein, B. A. (2004). Modification and psychometric examination of a self-report measure of fear in older adults. *Journal of Anxiety Disorders*, **18**, 397–409.

Kogan, J. N., Edelstein, B. A. and McKee, D. R. (2000). Assessment of anxiety in older adults: current status. *Journal of Anxiety Disorders*, **14**, 109–132.

Kok, B. C., Ma, V. K. and Gould, C. E. (2018). Validation of the Older Adult Social Evaluative Scale (OASES) as a measure of social anxiety. *International Psychogeriatrics*, **30**, 1323–1332.

Lau, A., Edelstein, B. and Larkin, K. (2001). Psychophysiological responses of older adults: a critical review with implications for assessment of anxiety disorders. *Clinical Psychology Review*, **21**, 609–630.

Lawton, M. P., Kleban, M. H. and Dean, J. (1993). Affect and age: cross sectional comparisons of structure and prevalence. *Psychology and Aging*, **8**, 165–175.

Leentjens, A. F. G., Dujardin, K., Marsh, L., et al. (2011). Anxiety rating scales in Parkinson's disease: a validation study of the Hamilton Anxiety Rating Scale, the Beck Anxiety Inventory, and the Hospital Anxiety and Depression Scale. *Movement Disorders*, **26**, 407–415.

Lewis-Fernández, R., Hinton, D. E., Laria, A. J., et al. (2010). Culture and the anxiety disorders: recommendations for DSM-V. *Depression and Anxiety*, **27**, 212–229.

Liebowitz, M. R. (1987). *Social Phobia*. New York: Karger Publishers.

Mattick, R. P. and Clarke, J. C. (1998). Development and validation of measures of social phobia scrutiny fear and social interaction anxiety. *Behaviour Research and Therapy*, **36**, 455–470.

Meyer, T. J., Miller, M. L., Metzger, R. L., et al. (1990). Development and validation of the Penn State Worry Questionnaire. *Behaviour Research and Therapy*, **28**, 487–495.

Mohlman, J. and Zinbarg, R. E. (2000). The structure and correlates of anxiety sensitivity in older adults. *Psychological Assessment*, **12**, 440–446.

Mohlman, J., Bryant, C., Lenze, E. J., et al. (2012). Improving recognition of late life anxiety disorders in Diagnostic and Statistical Manual of Mental Disorders, Fifth Edition: observations and recommendations of the Advisory Committee to the Lifespan Disorders Work Group. *International Journal of Geriatric Psychiatry*, **27**, 549–556.

Moore, R. C., Depp, C. A., Wetherell, J. L., et al. (2016). Ecological momentary assessment versus standard assessment instruments for measuring mindfulness, depressed mood, and anxiety among older adults. *Journal of Psychiatric Research*, **75**, 116–123.

Morin, C. M., Landreville, P., Colecchi, C., et al. (1999). The Beck Anxiety Inventory: psychometric properties with older adults. *Journal of Clinical Geropsychology*, **5**, 19–29.

Mueller, A. E., Segal, D. L., Gavett, B., et al. (2015). Geriatric Anxiety Scale: item response theory analysis, differential item functioning, and creation of a ten-item short form (GAS-10). *International Psychogeriatrics*, **27**, 1099–1111.

Pachana, N. A., Byrne, G. J., Siddle, H., et al. (2007). Development and validation of the Geriatric Anxiety Inventory. *International Psychogeriatrics*, **19**, 103–114.

Prediger, R. D., Matheus, F. C., Schwarzbold, M. L., et al. (2012). Anxiety in Parkinson's disease: a critical review of experimental and clinical studies. *Neuropharmacology*, **62**, 115–124.

Preusse, K. C., Mitzner, T. L., Fausset, C. B., et al. (2016). Older adults' acceptance of activity trackers. *Journal of Applied Gerontology*, **36**, 127–155.

Reed, A. E., Chan, L. and Mikels, J. A. (2014). Meta-analysis of the age-related positivity effect: age differences in preferences for positive over negative information. *Psychology and Aging*, **29**, 1–15.

Reiss, S., Peterson, R. A., Gursky, D. M., et al. (1986). Anxiety sensitivity, anxiety frequency and the prediction of fearfulness. *Behaviour Research and Therapy*, **24**, 1–8.

Rodebaugh, T. L., Heimberg, R. G., Brown, P. J., et al. (2011). More reasons to be straightforward: findings and norms for two scales relevant to social anxiety. *Journal of Anxiety Disorders*, **25**, 623–630.

Rycroft, C. E., Heyes, A., Lanza, L., et al. (2012). Epidemiology of chronic obstructive pulmonary disease: a literature review.

International Journal of Chronic Obstructive Pulmonary Disease, 7, 457–494.

Segal, D. L., June, A., Payne, M., et al. (2010). Development and initial validation of a self-report assessment tool for anxiety among older adults: the Geriatric Anxiety Scale. *Journal of Anxiety Disorders*, 24, 709–714.

Segal, D. L., Hersen, M., Van Hasselt, V. B., et al. (1993). Reliability of diagnosis in older psychiatric patients using the Structured Clinical Interview for DSM-III-R. *Journal of Psychopathology and Behavioral Assessment*, 15, 347–356.

Shankar, K. K., Walker, M., Frost, D., et al. (1999). The development of a valid and reliable scale for rating anxiety in dementia (RAID). *Aging and Mental Health*, 3, 39–49.

Shear, M. K., Belnap, B. H., Mazumdar, S., et al. (2006). Generalized Anxiety Disorder Severity Scale (GADSS): a preliminary validation study. *Depression and Anxiety*, 23, 77–82.

Shear, M. K., Brown T. A., Barlow, D. H., et al. (1997). Multicenter collaborative Panic Disorder Severity Scale. *American Journal of Psychiatry*, 154, 1571–1575.

Shear, M. K., Vander Bilt, J., Rucci, P., et al. (2001). Reliability and validity of a structured interview guide for the Hamilton Anxiety Rating Scale (SIGH-A). *Depression and Anxiety*, 13, 166–178.

Sheehan, D. V., Lecrubier, Y., Sheehan, K. H., et al. (1998). The Mini-International Neuropsychiatric Inventory (M.I.N.I.): the development and validation of a structured diagnostic psychiatric interview for DSM-IV and ICD-10. *Journal of Clinical Psychiatry*, 59, 22–33.

Shiffman, S., Stone, A. A. and Hufford, M. R. (2008). Ecological momentary assessment. *Annual Review of Clinical Psychology*, 4, 1–32.

Smith, J. S., Beland, M., Clyde, M., et al. (2013). Association of diabetes with anxiety: a systematic review and meta-analysis. *Journal of Psychosomatic Research*, 74, 89–99.

Snow, A. L., Huddleston, C., Robinson, C., et al. (2012). Psychometric properties of a structured interview guide for the rating for anxiety in dementia. *Anxiety and Mental Health*, 16, 592–602.

Spitzer, R. L., Kroenke, K., Williams, J. W., et al. (2006). A brief measure for assessing generalized anxiety disorder: the GAD-7. *Archives of Internal Medicine*, **166**, 1092–1097.

Stanley, M. A., Novy, D. M., Bourland, S. L., et al. (2001). Assessing older adults with generalized anxiety: a replication and extension. *Behaviour Research and Therapy*, 39, 221–235.

Therrien, Z. and Hunsley, J. (2012). Assessment of anxiety in older adults: a systematic review of commonly used measures. *Aging and Mental Health*, 16, 1–16.

Therrien, Z. and Hunsley, J. (2013). Assessment of anxiety in older adults: reliability generalization meta-analysis of commonly used measures. *Clinical Gerontologist*, 37, 171–194.

Turner, S. M., Beidel, D. C., Dancu, C. V., et al. (1989). An empirically derived inventory to measure social fears and anxiety: the social phobia and anxiety inventory. *Psychological Assessment: A Journal of Consulting and Clinical Psychology*, 1, 35–40.

Uchino, B. N., Birmingham, W. and Berg, C. A. (2010). Are older adults less or more physiologically reactive? A meta-analysis of age-related differences in cardiovascular reactivity to laboratory tasks. *Journal of Gerontology: Psychological Sciences*, **65B**, 154–162.

Weiss, B. J., Calleo, J., Rhoades, H. M., et al. (2009). The utility of the Generalized Anxiety Disorder Severity Scale (GADSS) with older adults in primary care. *Depression and Anxiety*, 26, E10–E15.

Wetherell, J. L. and Gatz, M. (2005). The Beck Anxiety Inventory in older adults with generalized anxiety disorder. *Journal of Psychopathology and Behavioral Assessment*, 27, 17–24.

Wild, B., Eckl, A., Herzog, W., et al. (2014). Assessing generalized anxiety disorder in elderly people using the GAD-7 and GAD-2 scales: results of a validation study. *American Journal of Geriatric Psychiatry*, 22, 1029–1038.

Wisocki, P. A. (1994). The experience of worry among the elderly. In G. Davey and F. Tallis, eds., *Worrying: Perspectives on Theory, Assessment, and Treatment.* New York: Wiley, pp. 247–261.

Wisocki, P. A., Handen, B. and Morse, C. K. (1986). The Worry Scale as a measure of anxiety among home bound and community active elderly. *Behavior Therapist,* **5**, 91–95.

Wolitzky-Taylor, K. B., Castriotta, N., Lenze, E. J., et al. (2010). Anxiety disorders in older adults: a comprehensive review. *Depression and Anxiety,* **27**, 190–211.

World Health Organization (1992). *The ICD-10 Classification of Mental and Behavioural Disorders: Clinical Descriptions and Diagnostic Guidelines.* Geneva: World Health Organization.

Yochim, B. P., Mueller, A. E., June, A., et al. (2010). Psychometric properties of the Geriatric Anxiety Scale: comparison to the Beck Anxiety Inventory and Geriatric Anxiety Inventory. *Clinical Gerontologist,* **34**, 21–33.

Zarit, S. H. and Zarit, J. M. (2007). *Mental Disorders in Older Adults: Fundamentals of Assessment and Treatment,* 2nd ed. New York: Guilford Press.

Late-Life Anxiety and Comorbid Depression
The Role of Attentional Bias

Emily S. Bower and Julie Loebach Wetherell

Cognitive Bias in Late-Life Anxiety and Depression

Attention bias is a core feature of cognitive models of anxiety and depression (Mathews & MacLeod, 2005), yet relatively little research has been devoted to this construct in older adults. In younger adults, it is well established that anxiety and depression are associated with attentional biases to negative information (Bar-Haim et al., 2007; Peckham et al., 2010). Furthermore, empirical evidence in younger adults suggests a causal role of cognitive bias in the development of emotional disorders (Mathews & MacLeod, 2005), and support for attention bias modification (ABM) as a treatment for anxiety is growing (Kuckertz & Amir, 2015). It is unclear to what extent these findings apply to older adults given age-related cognitive and emotional changes that could alter attentional processes (Beaudreau et al., 2013; Charles & Carstensen, 2010). Additionally, the combined effect of anxiety and depression on attention bias is not well understood (Teachman et al., 2012), yet depression is highly comorbid in older adults with anxiety, and comorbidity is associated with greater disability and poorer prognosis (Andreescu et al., 2007; Hek et al., 2011). Thus, elucidating the role of attentional mechanisms in comorbid anxiety and depression in later life could inform treatment targets and improve treatment outcomes.

The primary aim of this chapter is to synthesize research on the attentional mechanisms of anxiety in later life, including information about the effects of comorbid depression where literature is available. Cognitive theories of anxiety, depression, and emotional aging are presented alongside theories of attention and age-related neurophysiological change to provide a framework for interpreting the relevant literature on attention bias in late-life anxiety and depression to date. Finally, future directions in terms of theoretical and intervention studies of comorbid anxiety and depression will be discussed.

Theories of Attention, Emotional Processing, and Psychopathology

Attention and Emotion Processing

Cognitive and neurological models assume that there are bottom-up and top-down mechanisms underlying attention (Corbetta & Shulman, 2002). Bottom-up processing involves sensory input that flows from sensory organs to the associated sensory cortex to influence motor output without recruiting higher-level cognitive processes. Top-down processing begins with higher-order cognitive and neurological representations of knowledge that can override bottom-up processes to influence behavior. Visual attention is driven by a top-down, goal-directed, bilateral dorsal frontoparietal network and a bottom-up, stimulus-directed, right ventral frontoparietal network (Corbetta & Shulman, 2002). Research suggests that the stimulus-directed bottom-up network may serve as an alerting system or "circuit breaker" when unexpected, relevant stimuli are detected (Corbetta & Shulman, 2002).

A widely recognized and empirically validated model of attention involves three component networks that are influenced by both bottom-up and top-down processes (Petersen & Posner, 2012). The first – alerting – involves producing and maintaining vigilance, and it is associated with right hemisphere activation. The second – orienting – involves prioritization of sensory input toward a specific feature, such as location, and is driven by the frontoparietal networks described above. The third – executive – system of attention influences target detection, focal attention, and regulation of processing networks. It is generally agreed that the lateral prefrontal cortex and the anterior cingulate cortex are involved in executive functions (for a review, see Petersen & Posner, 2012). Additional neural networks provide more elaborative processing. In the case of emotionally salient information, processing appears to be associated with a ventral system (i.e., amygdala, insula, ventral striatum, and ventral anterior cingulate gyrus) that is activated during appraisal and affective response and a dorsal system (i.e., hippocampus, dorsal anterior cingulate gyrus, and dorsal regions of the prefrontal cortex) that is activated during modulation of the affective response (Phillips et al., 2003). These models provide a general framework for linking cognitive theories of anxiety and depression to neurobiological mechanisms.

The Tripartite Model of Anxiety and Depression

The tripartite model of anxiety and depression proposed by Clark and Watson (1991) posits that depression and anxiety share a common factor of trait negative affect and are differentiated by an anxiety factor (i.e., physiological hyperarousal) and a depression factor (i.e., apathy or lack of positive affect). The tripartite model appears to explain affective symptoms in older and younger adults, but some important age-related differences exist (Cook et al., 2004; Teachman et al., 2007). Positive and negative affect were more correlated in older compared to younger adult clinical samples (Cook et al., 2004), and older adults in the community reported greater positive affect and lower negative affect than younger adults (Teachman et al., 2007). These findings are consistent with literature suggesting that depression and anxiety may be more correlated in older adults (Wetherell et al., 2001), and that positive affect tends to increase with age (Charles & Carstensen, 2010). Therefore, although a three-factor model was found to be superior to a one- or two-factor model in both younger and older adults, there may be important differences in the experience of emotion associated with anxiety and depression in older compared to younger adults.

What are the mechanisms underlying changes in emotional experience and symptom presentation with age? There is a rich extant literature on cognitive theories of anxiety and depression and emotional aging; however, the two literatures largely exist as separate bodies. A brief review of some of the seminal and emerging theories follows.

Cognitive Theories of Anxiety and Depression

According to cognitive theories, information-processing biases play an important role in the cause and maintenance of anxiety and depression (Beck, 1979; Beck & Clark, 1997). Beck and colleagues (e.g., Beck & Clark, 1997) posit that maladaptive schemas (i.e., cognitive representations of concepts) influence automatic and top-down attentional processes, and the content of the schema distortion is a key factor differentiating disorders of anxiety and depression (e.g., "danger" vs. "hopelessness"). Conversely, the information-processing model of Williams et al. (1997) predicts that different emotional states affect information processing at different time points. According to Williams et al. (1997), high trait anxiety is associated with pre-attentive bias and resource allocation toward threat, whereas depression is characterized by resource allocation toward negative information at later stages of information processing. Despite this distinction, Williams et al. (1997) acknowledge that the co-occurrence of anxiety and depression may produce a more complex pattern of biases, although they did not predict how that might occur. Indeed, many information-processing models of anxiety do not address how co-occurring depression might influence anxious attentional bias. For example, Attentional Control Theory (ACT; Eysenck et al., 2007) assumes that anxiety increases the allocation of attentional resources toward threat and away from goal-directed processing, thereby decreasing performance efficiency, but it does not predict potential effects associated with comorbid depression. The frequent co-occurrence of anxiety and depression in later life requires theoretical models that extend to both disorders and allow for potential interactive or additive effects.

Several reviews of the literature supported some, but not all, aspects of the above theories and led to the development of revised models (Bar-Haim et al., 2007; Mathews & MacLeod, 2005; Mogg & Bradley, 2005). For example, Mathews and MacLeod (2005) hypothesized that attention biases are a function of time such that anxiety is associated with rapid, unconscious processes whereas depression is associated with later, executive processes. Additionally, there is evidence that attentional bias to threat is not present in anxious individuals with comorbid depression, leading Mogg and Bradley (2005) to posit that the low motivational state associated with depression could inhibit the ability of a threat evaluation system to allocate resources toward threat. Thus, an anxiety-related hyperactive threat evaluation system would be unable to activate an attentional response in the presence of depression.

Empirical evidence does not support the hypothesis that attentional bias in anxiety and depression is limited to one stage of processing (Bar-Haim et al., 2007; Mathews & MacLeod, 2005). Such findings prompted Bar-Haim et al. (2007) to propose a four-stage process that includes a pre-attentive threat evaluation, a resource allocation system, a conscious guided threat evaluation system, and a feedback process that either enhances state anxiety or overrides the pre-attentive system, with the implication that impairments or abnormalities at any of the four stages could contribute to anxiety.

Can we apply cognitive theories of attentional bias in anxiety and depression to older adults? Age-related changes in information processing and underlying neurological processes complicate direct application. Advancing age is associated with declines in working memory (Hasher & Zacks, 1988), reduced processing speed (Salthouse, 1996), and inability to inhibit irrelevant information (Radvansky et al., 2005). Furthermore, structural and functional changes occur both in the aging brain and in psychopathology that may exert effects on attention paid to and regulation of emotional information (Beaudreau et al., 2013). These changes may not result in reduced effectiveness, but rather reduced efficiency of information processing. For example, advancing age is associated with reduced activity in posterior perceptual processing regions of the brain and increased activity in anterior executive control regions during many types of tasks, which has been linked to the use of compensatory strategies in older adults (Davis et al., 2008). Thus, although the proposed stages of attentional processes associated with anxiety and depression may be similar across the lifespan, older adults may be recruiting additional cognitive resources or differentially activating different brain regions in comparison to younger adults.

Furthermore, it is widely theorized that age-related changes in attentional processes are a result not only of neuronal changes, but also of changing social perspectives. The socio-emotional selectivity theory (SST) is a lifespan theory of social motivation that explains age-related changes in emotional information processing (Carstensen et al., 1999). The theory suggests that aging is associated with a shift in time perspective from expansive to time-limited and that this shift in perspective causes older adults to prioritize present-focused, emotion-oriented goals over future-focused, knowledge-oriented goals. The SST has been used as a theoretical framework to explain evidence that older adults attend to and remember positive more than negative information in comparison with younger adults, a phenomenon known as *the positivity effect* (Reed et al., 2014).

Recently, researchers have begun to explore the mechanisms and boundary conditions of the positivity effect. The effect appears to be larger when participants are allowed to freely allocate cognitive resources (Reed et al., 2014). Additionally, older adults with better cognitive control appear to fixate more frequently and for longer on positive than negative pictures (Sasse et al., 2014). Late-life anxiety is associated with cognitive control deficits (Price et al., 2011); thus, anxious older adults may be less able to utilize adaptive emotion regulation strategies such as gaze preference for positive information. Importantly, some cross-cultural research suggests that the age-related positivity effect may be weakened or not present in cultures that value interdependence over independence (Fung et al., 2008, 2010), whereas other research suggests that the positivity effect generalizes across cultures (Kwon et al., 2009; Wang et al., 2015). There is a great need for additional cross-cultural research in this area to characterize the nature and extent of differences in age-related attentional processes across diverse cultures.

Healthy samples comprise the bulk of research documenting an age-related positivity effect, and there are relatively few published studies examining the influence of mood and anxiety. The positivity effect is often cited to explain higher self-rated well-being and lower rates of psychopathology in older compared to younger adults (Charles & Carstensen, 2010), yet anxiety and mood disorders are common in later life and are associated with poorer self-rated well-being (Cairney et al., 2008). Given these findings, it is not clear whether anxious older adults would behave similarly to anxious younger adults (i.e., negativity bias) or to non-anxious older adults (i.e., positivity bias). Mohlman et al. (2013) attempted to answer this question by comparing attention bias as evidenced by performance on a dot-probe task in non-anxious older adults to older adults with generalized anxiety disorder (GAD). The researchers were unable to find evidence of any attention bias to positive or threatening stimuli in either group. Methodological limitations of the dot-probe task may have reduced the power to detect an effect in this study; however, it is also possible that attention bias to threat is attenuated in older adults with anxiety compared to younger anxious adults. Such a finding, if replicated in future studies, might suggest that mechanisms of anxiety in later life differ from those in younger adulthood. To further explore this issue, a review of the literature related to attention bias in late-life anxiety and depression follows.

Empirical Evidence of Attention Bias in Late-Life Anxiety and Depression

Operational definitions of attention bias typically derive from modified versions of the dot-probe or the Stroop task. Excellent descriptions of these tasks are presented elsewhere (see Bar-Haim et al., 2007; Mathews & MacLeod, 2005) and will not be elaborated here, except to note that, in older adults, stimuli are usually presented for longer durations to adjust for the slower processing speed associated with aging (e.g., Lee & Knight, 2009). Table 7.1 lists the studies described in this section.

Anxiety

In the first published study to explore the effect of anxiety on attentional bias to threat in older adults, Fox and Knight (2005) used a mood induction task to manipulate anxious or neutral mood. Participants in the state anxious condition demonstrated an attentional bias to threat on a dot-probe task, whereas participants in a neutral mood condition displayed no bias. The authors also explored the effect of induced anxiety on inhibitory processes using the emotional Stroop paradigm and reported that reaction times were significantly slower for threat words in state anxious participants who endorsed low, but not high, trait anxiety. Overall, the results provided preliminary evidence that, in older adults, anxiety produces selective attention to threat that is similar to that found in younger adults.

Following this initial study, Lee and Knight (2009) addressed the question of whether trait anxiety moderates attention to negative information in older adults using a dot-probe paradigm. The authors compared young and older adults in addition to examining the influence of several potential moderators including trait anxiety (high, low), stimulus type (faces, pictures, words), and timing of stimulus presentation (subliminal 50 ms, supraliminal 1,500 ms). The findings varied by stimulus type, but they generally suggested that trait anxiety moderated visual attention to threat in older adults. Older adults with high trait anxiety demonstrated avoidance of threatening words during subliminal exposures but a preference for threatening words during supraliminal exposures, whereas younger and low-trait anxious older adults did not demonstrate an attentional bias to threat. The pattern of threat-related attention observed for high-trait anxious older adults has been coined an *avoidant–vigilant* response, and this may be indicative of maladaptive emotion regulation strategies (i.e., avoidance and worry).

Interestingly, Lee and Knight (2009) reported that moderate, but not high, trait anxiety was associated with a vigilant-avoidant response to sad faces. This is in contrast to Demeyer and De Raedt (2013), who reported that higher trait anxiety was associated with greater attentional avoidance of sad faces presented supraliminally (1,000 ms) to older adults during an emotional exogenous cueing task. Although speculative, depressive symptoms may have contributed to the differential findings. Empirical evidence in younger adults suggests that depression is associated with attention bias to mood-congruent stimuli during later stages of processing and may inhibit early threat vigilance (for a review, see Mathews & MacLeod, 2005), a finding that is consistent with the avoidant–vigilant response pattern found in those with high trait anxiety in the Lee and Knight (2009) study. A measure of mood or depressive symptoms should be included in future studies to clarify the unique and combined effects of depression and anxiety on attentional processes.

Table 7.1 Studies of attention bias in late-life anxiety and depression.

Study	Sample	Anxiety	Depression	Paradigm	Stimuli	Key results	Conclusion
Broomfield et al. (2007)	Older adults with MDD (n = 19) or without (n = 20)	BAI	MDD	Emotional Stroop	Words (negative, positive, neutral)	Slower RT to negative words for MDD compared to non-MDD (with or without controlling for BAI); no effect for positive or neutral words	Late-life depression associated with interference of negative words
Brown et al. (2011)	Older adults with fear of falling (n = 15) or without (n = 15)	Fear of falling (self-report)	NA	Dot-probe	Words (general threat, fall threat, neutral)	All: shorter RT to probe replacing fall threat than general threat; group difference for disengagement but not engagement	Older adults biased toward fall threat; fear of falling associated with difficulty disengaging from fall-threat words
Burgess et al. (2014)	Older and younger adults with high or low anxiety (n = 16 for both groups)	Trait anxiety (self-report)	NA	Lexical decision task	Words (negative, positive, neutral)	No effects for age and anxiety on disengagement from emotional words; high-anxiety group slower to engage with positive words than low-anxiety group	High trait anxiety associated with difficulty engaging with positive words (age invariant)
Demeyer and De Raedt (2013)	Older (n = 37) and middle-aged adults (n = 25)	Trait anxiety (self-report)	NA	Exogenous cueing task	Faces (happy, sad, neutral)	Older adults: biased away from all emotional stimuli; anxiety positively associated with bias	Greater anxiety associated with avoidance of sad faces in older adults

Study	Sample	Anxiety measure	Diagnosis	Task	Stimuli	Results	Conclusion
						away from sad faces; no bias for middle-aged adults	Late-life depression associated with interference of negative words
Dudley et al. (2002)	Older adults with MDD (n = 12) and age-matched controls (n = 12)	NA	MDD	Emotional Stroop	Words (negative, positive, neutral)	Slower RT to negative words for MDD compared to controls	
Fox and Knight (2005)	Older adults (n = 68)	State (induced) and trait (self-report)	NA	Dot-probe and emotional Stroop	Words (threat, neutral)	Dot-probe: attention bias to threat in state anxiety group; no effect for trait; no interaction. Emotional Stroop: no main effects; state × trait interaction with slower RT for high state–low trait group	Anxious state produces attention bias to threat and interference effect for threat in older adults with low trait anxiety
Lee and Knight (2009)	Older (n = 44) and younger adults (n = 103)	Trait anxiety (self-report)	NA	Dot-probe	Faces (angry, sad, neutral), pictures (threat, non-threat), and words (negative, neutral)	High anxious: avoidant–vigilant to negative words; moderate: avoidant–vigilant to sad faces; none for pictures; all older adults vigilant-	Attention bias depends on time, stimulus modality, anxiety level in older adults; trait anxiety older adults have an avoidant–

Table 7.1 (cont.)

Study	Sample	Anxiety	Depression	Paradigm	Stimuli	Key results	Conclusion
						avoidant response to angry faces; no bias in younger adults	vigilant response to threat
Livermore et al. (2007)	Older adults with COPD and panic, COPD without panic, and healthy controls (n = 20 for all groups)	Panic disorder or panic attacks	HADS	Dot-probe	Words (physical threat, positive, neutral)	Patients with panic biased away from threat and toward positive; effect reversed after controlling for depression score	Unclear; possible that COPD patients with panic have bias away from threat and toward positive information, but effect is suppressed by depression
Mohlman et al. (2013)	Older adults with GAD (n = 34) and without (n = 28)	GAD	NA	Dot-probe	Words (threat, depression, positive, neutral)	All subjects biased away from positive words; reduced preference for threat words after treatment for GAD	Reduced preference for negative information following cognitive behavioral therapy for late-life GAD
Noiret et al. (2015)	Older adults with MDD (n = 20) or without (n = 62)	NA	MDD	Eye-tracking	Faces (sad, happy, neutral)	Compared to nondepressed group, depressed group had fewer and shorter fixations for emotional features of faces when	Older adults with depression disengage from sad and neutral faces

Study	Sample			Task	Stimuli	Results	Summary
Poon and Knight (2009)	Older adults (n = 71)	NA	Sad mood (induced)	Emotional Stroop	Words (symptom, neutral)	Control group attended less to symptom words than sad mood and old-age schema groups; attention bias to symptoms when both mood and schema activated	Sad mood reduces bias away from negative information and the combination of sad mood and age-schema activation create negative bias
Price et al. (2011)	Older adults with GAD (n = 16) or without (n = 12)	GAD	NA	Emotional Stroop	Words (negative, neutral)	GAD: slower RT for negative than neutral; controls: faster RT for negative than neutral; GAD vs. controls: less activity in dlPFC and greater activity in amygdala	Late-life GAD associated with interference of negative words; associated with reduced activity in the dlPFC for anxious group
Price et al. (2012)	Older adults (n = 60)	Trait worry (self-report)	Self-report (BDI, GDS)	Emotional Stroop	Words (positive, neutral, threat)	High worry: slower RT for negative than positive; moderate worry: slower RT for positive than negative; low worry: slower RT for positive than	High worry associated with interference of negative words

Table 7.1 (cont.)

Study	Sample	Anxiety	Depression	Paradigm	Stimuli	Key results	Conclusion
						negative (NS); group × valence interaction: negative bias larger in high than low worriers; controlled for depression scores	
Steiner et al. (2013)	Older adults with GAD (n = 25)	GAD	NA	Affective go/ no-go	Words (positive, negative)	No bias change over treatment period; faster RT to negative words associated with greater reduction in GAD symptoms	Positivity bias associated with better treatment outcome for late-life GAD

BAI = Beck Anxiety Inventory; BDI = Beck Depression Inventory; COPD = chronic obstructive pulmonary disease; dlPFC = dorsolateral prefrontal cortex; GAD = generalized anxiety disorder; GDS = Geriatric Depression Scale; HADS = Hospital Anxiety and Depression Scales; MDD = major depressive disorder; NA = not applicable; NS = nonsignificant; RT = reaction time.

To determine whether there are age differences in anxiety-linked attention to emotional words, another recent study compared the performances of younger and older adults with high or low trait anxiety using a computer-based lexical decision task (Burgess et al., 2014). The authors found no effects for age or anxiety on speed of disengagement from stimuli. Conversely, individuals with high trait anxiety took longer to engage with positive words than those with low trait anxiety. Age did not modify the effect, and there was no effect of anxiety on speed of engaging with negative words. The authors suggested that their findings provided some support for an age-invariant anxious attentional bias specific to processes of attentional engagement. However, the results were inconclusive as to whether the bias was due to deficient engagement with positive stimuli or facilitated engagement with negative stimuli. Further research is needed, but the findings suggest that anxious attention bias in older adults is similar to that in younger adults.

In addition to trait and state anxiety, the effect of worry on anxious attentional bias in older adults has been explored using the emotional Stroop paradigm (Price et al., 2012). Price et al. (2012) built upon earlier research by Fox and Knight (2005) by including positive words, but they did not include a younger adult comparison group. The results indicated that high worriers were biased more toward negative than positive words, whereas moderate and low worriers were biased more toward positive than negative words. Between-group comparisons revealed a moderating effect of worry on selective attention, such that high worriers had larger negative biases than low worriers, whereas low to moderate worriers had larger positive biases than high worriers. The results were similar after controlling for depression, although participants reported only minimal to mild depressive symptoms. In general, the results support the hypothesis that anxiety moderates the age-related positivity effect such that older adults with features of anxiety will attend more toward negative than positive information.

A related study by Price et al. (2011) explored the neurological mechanisms of anxious attentional bias in older adults using functional magnetic resonance imaging (fMRI) to compare older adults with GAD to non-anxious controls while they completed the emotional Stroop task. The results confirmed the findings from Price et al. (2012), showing an interference effect of negative information for anxious older adults. Imaging data suggested that this interference was associated with top-down cognitive control deficiencies in individuals with GAD. Overall, the findings suggested that non-anxious older adults activated the dorsolateral prefrontal cortex (dlPFC) to exert top-down cognitive control over the amygdala in response to negative words, thereby decreasing activation of the amygdala and improving performance. Conversely, older adults with GAD did not show increased activation of the dlPFC when exposed to negative words, likely leading to an interference of negative words on performance, which positively correlated with amygdala activation. The authors concluded that the interference of negative information observed in older adults with GAD was likely due to deficient prefrontal top-down control mechanisms. Although this study was unable to determine whether attention biases cause anxiety, in theory deficient inhibitory processes could be a viable treatment target for late-life anxiety.

A recent model put forth by Young and Williams (2015) proposes that attention biases interact with other factors such as age and postural control to increase fall risk in older adults with fear of falling. Fear of falling is common in older adults and is associated with increased fall risk (Friedman et al., 2002), but the mechanisms underlying this relationship are not known. Research on attention bias in fear of falling is in the early stages, but there is some empirical support suggesting that information-processing biases are a feature of fear of falling in older adults. In the first published study to explore this issue, a modified dot-probe task was used to compare older adults with or without fear of falling on attention to fall-threat words (Brown et al., 2011). Compared to general threat and neutral words, older adults selectively attended to fall-threat words regardless of fear of falling; however, the results suggested that older adults with fear of falling had difficulty disengaging from fall-threat words compared to non-fearful older adults. The authors posited that difficulty disengaging from fall-relevant stimuli could increase fall risk by reducing attention to other relevant aspects of the environment that might increase fall risk. Relatedly, state anxiety is associated with changes in gaze fixation and stepping patterns that increase fall risk (Young et al., 2012). Thus, information-processing abnormalities could mediate the behavioral changes observed in older adults with fear of falling. This is an intriguing possibility that could lead to novel treatment strategies (e.g., attention training) with important public health benefits.

Depression

The empirical literature on attention bias in older adults with depression is sparse, but the results from a recent eye-tracking study are consistent with theoretical models that propose that attention biases associated with depression occur at later stages compared to anxiety. Noiret et al. (2015) compared visual strategies between older adults with and without major depressive disorder while viewing sad, happy, and neutral faces. Visual patterns during initial attention to faces did not differ for depressed and nondepressed older adults. Similarly, there was no between-group difference in fixation patterns for happy faces after initial fixation. Conversely, older adult with depression fixated less on the emotional aspects of sad and neutral portraits compared to older adults without depression in later stages of viewing. These findings suggest that depression may be associated with disengagement from emotional stimuli in older adults.

The task used by Noiret et al. (2015) allowed participants to freely allocate attention, but what happens when depressed older adults are instructed to allocate attention toward negative stimuli? As discussed earlier, empirical evidence from nonclinical samples suggests that emotional processing is modified by constraints on attention (Reed et al., 2014). The emotional Stroop task necessarily constrains gaze toward negative stimuli by requiring that individuals name the color ink of a printed word. Contrary to the findings reported by Noiret et al. (2015), evidence from two studies using the emotional Stroop task suggest that depression may be associated with difficulty disengaging from negative information (Broomfield et al., 2007; Dudley et al., 2002). Specifically, negative words interfered more with task performance for depressed than for nondepressed older adults, whereas there was no group difference for positive words. The modifying effect of depression on the information processing of negative stimuli remained after controlling for anxiety symptoms (Broomfield et al., 2007). Although these studies did not directly measure engagement or disengagement with emotional stimuli, one could speculate that longer latencies to name the color of negative words compared to neutral words could be due to difficulty disengaging with negative stimuli in depressed older adults.

An intriguing study by Poon and Knight (2009) used sad mood induction in nonde-pressed community-dwelling older adults to determine the causal effect of sad mood on attentional bias for physical symptoms (e.g., vertigo, headache). Additionally, the authors explored the potential moderating effect of old-age schema by priming some participants with age-related questions to activate old-age schema. The results indicated that, compared to controls, sad mood and old-age schema activation caused participants to attend longer to symptom words than neutral words. Despite the between-group difference, within-group attention bias to symptom words was only observed in the group that received both the sad mood and old-age schema manipulations. This finding suggests that a relevant schema activation plus sad mood may be needed to create an attentional bias in healthy samples.

Comorbid Anxiety and Depression

The nature of attention bias associated with comorbid anxiety and depression in older adults is unclear. There is some research exploring attention bias related to comorbid anxiety and depression in younger samples, but the findings are inconclusive (Mogg & Bradley, 2005). For example, Mogg et al. (2000) found that nondepressed patients with GAD selectively oriented toward threatening faces, whereas GAD patients with a comorbid depressive disorder did not selectively orient toward threatening faces, suggesting that depression might moderate attentional biases associated with anxiety. Conversely, a review by Bar-Haim et al. (2007) reported similar effect sizes for attention bias to threat in samples of nondepressed anxious adults and samples of depressed anxious adults, leading the authors to conclude that depression does not modulate the threat-related bias found in individuals with anxiety disorders.

Tentative support for an influence of depression on anxious attentional bias toward threat words was found in a sample of older adults with chronic obstructive pulmonary disease (COPD) and panic symptoms (Livermore et al., 2007). In a modified visual dot-probe task, patients with COPD and panic symptoms selectively attended toward emotion words (threat and positive), but the effect was attenuated when covarying for depression. This is consistent with the cognitive-motivational theory proposed by Mogg and Bradley (2005), which predicts that apathy associated with depression will reduce engagement with emotionally salient stimuli.

Taken together, many questions remain regarding the effect of anxiety and depression on attention bias in later life. Converging literature suggests that anxiety modifies the age-related positivity effect. There appears to be an attentional preference for negative information in older adults with anxiety that is moderated by the type of stimuli, time, and level of anxiety. Whether bias is due to difficulty disengaging from negative words or engaging with positive words is unclear. The evidence for depression is mixed, and the evidence for comorbid anxiety and depression is nonexistent.

Neuropsychology and Neurophysiology of Attention Bias in Late-Life Anxiety and Depression

Few studies have explored the neuropsychological and neurophysiological correlates of cognitive bias in late-life anxiety and depression, leaving unanswered many questions about the underlying mechanisms of cognitive bias in older adults with anxiety and depression. In community-dwelling older adults, anxiety is associated with inhibitory deficits that are worsened by comorbid depression (Beaudreau & O'Hara, 2009). The extent to which such findings are age-related, anxiety-related, or both is difficult to determine given the lack of longitudinal research and experimental paradigms that could differentiate effects (Beaudreau et al., 2013).

Disruption within the amygdala–prefrontal circuitry may underlie anxious attentional bias (Bishop, 2007). One theory is that this disruption may be due to poor structural connectivity between the amygdala and prefrontal cortex, but contrary to that theory, a recent imaging study using probabilistic tractography found that greater structural connectivity (i.e., declines in fractional anisotropy and radial diffusivity) between the ventral prefrontal cortex and the amygdala was associated with higher trait anxiety in young, middle-aged, and older adults (Clewett et al., 2014). An alternative theory proposed by the authors to explain this finding is that greater connectivity could facilitate threat-related biases initiated by the amygdala; however, controlling for age attenuated this association, so additional studies are needed to confirm the finding.

With regard to functional connectivity, anxiety was associated with abnormal functional connectivity in the default mode network (DMN) within a small sample of older adults with depression (Andreescu et al., 2011b). Based on results from fMRI, higher levels of anxiety in older adults with major depressive disorder were associated with greater connectivity in posterior regions of the DMN, but with lower functional connectivity in anterior regions of the DMN. The authors posited that this difference might be due to maintaining higher levels of alertness (associated with posterior regions) and lower levels of self-regulation (associated with anterior regions). This is consistent with the finding that non-anxious older adults have increased regional cerebral blood flow to the prefrontal cortex while attempting to regulate emotional responses, whereas older adults with GAD do not (Andreescu et al., 2011a).

One interpretation of these findings is based on the integrated model of anxious attention bias proposed by Bar-Haim et al. (2007). It is possible that anxiety is associated with a hyperactive pre-attentive threat evaluation system in both young and older adults, but that age-related declines in connectivity of the dorsal attention network and DMN (for a review, see Ferreira & Busatto, 2013) lead to differential mechanisms of attention bias. For example, greater amygdala–prefrontal cortex connectivity in younger adults could strengthen the influence of a biased guided threat evaluation system on behavior, whereas poorer connectivity in older adults could weaken the ability of the guided threat evaluation system to override the hyperactive pre-attentive evaluation.

In regard to comorbid anxiety and depression, a recent review article concluded that depressed adults with anxiety appear to have a distinct neurobiological profile compared to depressed adults without anxiety, including structural and functional asymmetries (Ionescu et al., 2013). Specifically, depression appears to be associated with left frontal lobe hypoactivation, whereas anxiety is associated with right frontal lobe hyperactivation, and comorbidity appears to contribute to greater asymmetry. Such a finding, if reliable, is consistent with hypothesized differences in the mechanisms underlying resource allocation in depression and anxiety; however, age-related changes could alter this asymmetry given findings that hemispheric asymmetry is reduced in older adults (Cabeza, 2002). Overall, there is a great need for research on the neurological correlates of comorbid anxiety and depression across the entire lifespan (Ionescu et al., 2013), and the hypothesis that age-related neurobiological changes moderate attentional biases in late-life anxiety and depression remains speculative at this stage.

Treatment of Cognitive Bias

Anxiety and depression in later life are undertreated. Older adults do not respond as well to pharmacological and psychotherapeutic treatment as younger adults (Gonçalves & Byrne, 2012; Wetherell et al., 2013). Furthermore, older adults underutilize mental health services

(Byers et al., 2012). For those who receive treatment, outcome is generally worse for comorbid anxiety and depression (e.g., Andreescu et al., 2007). Thus, it is important to consider the implications of attention bias on late-life psychiatric treatment.

The first study to explore whether cognitive behavioral therapy can change attentional bias in late-life anxiety reported that treatment reduced attention bias to threat in older adults with GAD (Mohlman et al., 2013). Although this offers some support for cognitive therapy in reducing attention bias, both a clinical and a non-anxious comparison group avoided positive words, and neither group was biased toward threat at baseline. Thus, the findings diverged from those of other studies that report a preference for positive words in healthy older adults and a bias toward threat words in anxious older adults. The authors called for clinical and cognitive psychologists to collaborate and accelerate research in this area.

In a preliminary study, Steiner et al. (2013) explored the role of information-processing bias on response to pharmacological treatment in older adults with GAD. Information-processing bias scores did not change over the course of treatment; however, older adults who were faster to respond to positive than negative words reported greater symptom reduction over 12 weeks of treatment with escitalopram. Although preliminary, these results suggest that faster processing of positive relative to negative information may facilitate response to pharmacotherapy in older adults with GAD. This raises the question of whether bias modification could improve treatment outcomes in later life.

ABM training has been used in younger adults to modify attention bias associated with anxiety (Amir et al., 2009). There are no published studies on the effectiveness of ABM for late-life anxiety and depression, but the aging brain has demonstrated plasticity in attentional abilities following cognitive training in some cases (Lampit et al., 2014). For example, older adults who completed speed of processing training demonstrated improvements in sustained attention and increased amplitudes of attentional event-related potential components (i.e., N2pc and P3b; O'Brien et al., 2013). Although speculative, cognitive training could modify attentional biases in older adults with late-life anxiety and depression.

Meditation is another form of attention training that is gaining popularity for use in older adults to reduce stress and treat anxiety and depression (e.g., Lenze et al., 2014). Empirical evidence from younger samples suggests that meditation improves attention and reduces anxiety and depression (Tang et al., 2007). Research in older adults is needed to determine whether attention training can reduce attention bias, alter brain activation, and improve anxiety and depression in later life.

Future Directions

The bulk of the literature on attentional bias in older adults focuses on emotional aging in nonclinical populations (Charles & Carstensen, 2010), leaving a wide swath of scientific territory yet to be explored. Expanding the base of empirical data in this area will help determine the characteristics of attention bias in anxiety, depression, and comorbid anxiety and depression in later life, as well as provide much-needed information about the generalizability and boundary conditions of the age-related positivity bias. Empirically supported models of late-life anxiety and comorbid depression are integral to guiding the development and dissemination of effective interventions for older adults. Given the prevalence and poor outcomes associated with comorbid anxiety and depression, the development of effective, targeted interventions could significantly reduce the burden of mental illness and improve the quality of life for many older adults. The following questions represent just some of the many potential areas for future research development with regard to attention bias in late-life anxiety, depression, and comorbid anxiety and depression.

(1) What are the cognitive and underlying neurological consequences of chronic vigilance to threatening information in older adults with anxiety disorders? There is a pressing need to develop integrated models that link multidisciplinary theories of cognition, emotion, and psychopathology across the lifespan. Chronic neuronal activation in regions associated with threat detection and attentional control may interact with age-related neurobiological changes to alter emotional processing in late-life anxiety and depression. Longitudinal studies are needed to answer this question.

(2) Is the tendency to attend to and remember more positive than negative information with age moderated by anxious and depressive symptoms later in life? Additionally, do cultural differences further moderate these effects? Research suggests that the age-related preference for positive information is not evident in older adults with anxiety and depression. Furthermore, cross-cultural research suggests that individuals who value interdependence over independence may attend to emotional information differently from those who place a higher value on independence (e.g., Fung et al., 2010). There is a great need to expand cross-cultural research in this area to clarify the generalizability of these findings and to enrich theories of emotional information processing in later life.

(3) What is the influence of comorbid anxiety and depression on emotional information processing in older adults? Mogg and Bradley (2005) found some evidence for different patterns of attentional bias in GAD and clinical depression, but there is not enough evidence in older adults to extend this finding to later life. It is unknown whether depression has an additive or interactive effect on attention bias in anxious older adults. Advances in imaging, electroencephalography, and eye-tracking technology can help us to differentiate the components of attentional processing in order to answer this question. Much more research is needed in this area.

(4) Are the physical health correlates in late-life anxiety and depression partially mediated by anxious attentional processes? Recent theoretical developments related to fear of falling suggest that this might be the case (Young & Williams, 2015). This represents an exciting area for future treatment developments.

(5) Do attention biases reduce with treatment in late-life anxiety and depression? Again, much more research is needed in this area. Meditation and computerized cognitive training have been successful at modifying attention and, in regard to meditation, reducing anxiety and depression. It is not known whether ABM is effective in older adults.

The answers to these questions have important implications for the treatment of late-life anxiety and depression, and this list is not exhaustive. There are many unknowns with regard to attention bias in late-life anxiety, depression, and comorbid anxiety and depression. Without further research in this area, we risk losing the opportunity to intervene more effectively and to improve the health and quality of life of many older adults.

References

Amir, N., Beard, C., Taylor, C. T., et al. (2009). Attention training in individuals with generalized social phobia: A randomized controlled trial. *Journal of Consulting and Clinical Psychology*, **77**, 961–973.

Andreescu, C., Gross, J. J., Lenze, E., et al. (2011a). Altered cerebral blood flow patterns associated with pathologic worry in the elderly. *Depression and Anxiety*, **28**, 202–209.

Andreescu, C., Lenze, E. J., Dew, M. A., et al. (2007). Effect of comorbid anxiety on treatment response and relapse risk in late-life depression: controlled study. *British Journal of Psychiatry*, **190**, 344–349.

Andreescu, C., Wu, M., Butters, M. A., Figurski, J., Reynolds, C. F., 3rd and Aizenstein, H. J. (2011b). The default mode network in late-life anxious depression. *American Journal of Geriatric Psychiatry*, **19**, 980–983.

Bar-Haim, Y., Lamy, D., Pergamin, L., Bakermans-Kranenburg, M. J. and van IJzendoorn, M. H. (2007). Threat-related attentional bias in anxious and nonanxious individuals: a meta-analytic study. *Psychological Bulletin*, **133**, 1–24.

Beaudreau, S. A. and O'Hara, R. (2009). The association of anxiety and depressive symptoms with cognitive performance in community-dwelling older adults. *Psychology and Aging*, **24**, 507–512.

Beaudreau, S. A., MacKay-Brandt, A. and Reynolds, J. (2013). Application of a cognitive neuroscience perspective of cognitive control to late-life anxiety. *Journal of Anxiety Disorders*, **27**, 559–566.

Beck, A. T. and Clark, D. A. (1997). An information processing model of anxiety: automatic and strategic processes. *Behaviour Research and Therapy*, **35**, 49–58.

Beck, A. T., Rush, A. J., Shaw, B. F. and Emery, G. (1979). *Cognitive Therapy of Depression*. New York: Guilford Press.

Bishop, S. J. (2007). Neurocognitive mechanisms of anxiety: an integrative account. *Trends in Cognitive Sciences*, **11**, 307–316.

Broomfield, N. M., Davies, R., MacMahon, K., Ali, F. and Cross, S. M. (2007). Further evidence of attention bias for negative information in late life depression. *International Journal of Geriatric Psychiatry*, **22**, 175–180.

Brown, L. A., White, P., Doan, J. B. and de Bruin, N. (2011). Selective attentional processing to fall-relevant stimuli among older adults who fear falling. *Experimental Aging Research*, **37**, 330–345.

Burgess, M. M., Cabeleira, C. M., Cabrera, I., Bucks, R. S. and MacLeod, C. (2014). Examining attentional biases underlying trait anxiety in younger and older adults. *Cognition & Emotion*, **28**, 84–97.

Byers, A. L., Arean, P. A. and Yaffe, K. (2012). Low use of mental health services among older Americans with mood and anxiety disorders. *Psychiatric Services*, **63**, 66–72.

Cabeza, R. (2002). Hemispheric asymmetry reduction in older adults: the HAROLD model. *Psychology and Aging*, **17**, 85–100.

Cairney, J., Corna, L. M., Veldhuizen, S., Herrmann, N. and Streiner, D. L. (2008). Comorbid depression and anxiety in later life: patterns of association, subjective well-being, and impairment. *American Journal of Geriatric Psychiatry*, **16**, 201–208.

Carstensen, L. L., Isaacowitz, D. M. and Charles, S. T. (1999). Taking time seriously. A theory of socioemotional selectivity. *American Psychologist*, **54**, 165–181.

Charles, S. T. and Carstensen, L. L. (2010). Social and emotional aging. *Annual Review of Psychology*, **61**, 383–409.

Clark, L. A. and Watson, D. (1991). Tripartite model of anxiety and depression: psychometric evidence and taxonomic implications. *Journal of Abnormal Psychology*, **100**, 316–336.

Clewett, D., Bachman, S. and Mather, M. (2014). Age-related reduced prefrontal–amygdala structural connectivity is associated with lower trait anxiety. *Neuropsychology*, **28**, 631–642.

Cook, J. M., Orvaschel, H., Simco, E., Hersen, M. and Joiner, T. (2004). A test of the tripartite model of depression and anxiety in older adult psychiatric outpatients. *Psychology and Aging*, **19**, 444–451.

Corbetta, M. and Shulman, G. L. (2002). Control of goal-directed and stimulus-driven attention in the brain. *Nature Reviews Neuroscience*, **3**, 201–215.

Davis, S. W., Dennis, N. A., Daselaar, S. M., Fleck, M. S. and Cabeza, R. (2008). Qué PASA? The posterior–anterior shift in aging. *Cerebral Cortex*, **18**, 1201–1209.

Demeyer, I. and De Raedt, R. (2013). Attentional bias for emotional information in older adults: the role of emotion and future time perspective. *PLoS ONE*, **8**, e65429.

Dudley, R., O'Brien, J., Barnett, N., McGuckin, L. and Britton, P. (2002). Distinguishing depression from dementia in later life: a pilot study employing the emotional Stroop task. *International Journal of Geriatric Psychiatry*, **17**, 48–53.

Eysenck, M. W., Derakshan, N., Santos, R. and Calvo, M. G. (2007). Anxiety and cognitive performance: Attentional Control Theory. *Emotion*, **7**, 336–353.

Ferreira, L. K. and Busatto, G. F. (2013). Resting-state functional connectivity in normal brain aging. *Neuroscience & Biobehavioral Reviews*, **37**, 384–400.

Fox, L. S. and Knight, B. G. (2005). The effects of anxiety on attentional processes in older adults. *Aging & Mental Health*, **9**, 585–593.

Friedman, S. M., Munoz, B., West, S. K., Rubin, G. S. and Fried, L. P. (2002). Falls and fear of falling: which comes first? A longitudinal prediction model suggests strategies for primary and secondary prevention. *Journal of the American Geriatrics Society*, **50**, 1329–1335.

Fung, H. H., Isaacowitz, D. M., Lu, A. Y., and Li, T. (2010). Interdependent self-construal moderates the age-related negativity reduction effect in memory and visual attention. *Psychology and Aging*, **25**, 321–329.

Fung, H. H., Lu, A. Y., Goren, D., Isaacowitz, D. M., Wadlinger, H. A. and Wilson, H. R. (2008). Age-related positivity enhancement is not universal: older Chinese look away from positive stimuli. *Psychology and Aging*, **23**, 440–446.

Gonçalves, D. C. and Byrne, G. J. (2012). Interventions for generalized anxiety disorder in older adults: systematic review and meta-analysis. *Journal of Anxiety Disorders*, **26**, 1–11.

Hasher, L. and Zacks, R. T. (1988). Working memory, comprehension, and aging: a review and a new view. In G. H. Bower, ed., *The Psychology of Learning and Motivation*. New York: Academic Press, pp. 193–225.

Hek, K., Tiemeier, H., Newson, R. S., Luijendijk, H. J., Hofman, A. and Mulder, C. L. (2011). Anxiety disorders and comorbid depression in community dwelling older adults. *International Journal of Methods in Psychiatric Research*, **20**, 157–168.

Ionescu, D. F., Niciu, M. J., Mathews, D. C., Richards, E. M. and Zarate, C. A., Jr. (2013). Neurobiology of anxious depression: a review. *Depression and Anxiety*, **30**, 374–385.

Kuckertz, J. M. and Amir, N. (2015). Attention bias modification for anxiety and phobias: current status and future directions. *Current Psychiatry Reports*, **17**, 9.

Kwon, Y., Scheibe, S., Samanez-Larkin, G. R., Tsai, J. L. and Carstensen, L. L. (2009). Replicating the positivity effect in picture memory in Koreans: evidence for cross-cultural generalizability. *Psychology and Aging*, **24**, 748–754.

Lampit, A., Hallock, H. and Valenzuela, M. (2014). Computerized cognitive training in cognitively healthy older adults: a systematic review and meta-analysis of effect modifiers. *PLoS Medicine*, **11**, e1001756.

Lee, L. O. and Knight, B. G. (2009). Attentional bias for threat in older adults: moderation of the positivity bias by trait anxiety and stimulus modality. *Psychology and Aging*, **24**, 741–747.

Lenze, E. J., Hickman, S., Hershey, T., et al. (2014). Mindfulness-based stress reduction for older adults with worry symptoms and co-occurring cognitive dysfunction. *International Journal of Geriatric Psychiatry*, **29**, 991–1000.

Livermore, N., Sharpe, L. and McKenzie, D. (2007). Selective attention to threatening information in anxious patients with chronic obstructive pulmonary disease. *Cognitive Therapy and Research*, **31**, 885–895.

Mathews, A. and MacLeod, C. (2005). Cognitive vulnerability to emotional disorders. *Annual Review of Clinical Psychology*, **1**, 167–195.

Mogg, K. and Bradley, B. (2005). Attentional bias in generalized anxiety disorder versus depressive disorder. *Cognitive Therapy and Research*, **29**, 29–45.

Mogg, K., Millar, N. and Bradley, B. P. (2000). Biases in eye movements to threatening facial expressions in generalized anxiety disorder and depressive disorder. *Journal of Abnormal Psychology*, **109**, 695–704.

Mohlman, J., Price, R. B. and Vietri, J. (2013). Attentional bias in older adults: effects of generalized anxiety disorder and cognitive behavior therapy. *Journal of Anxiety Disorders*, **27**, 585–591.

Noiret, N., Carvalho, N., Laurent, É., et al. (2015). Visual scanning behavior during processing of emotional faces in older adults with major depression. *Aging & Mental Health*, **19**, 264–273.

O'Brien, J. L., Edwards, J. D., Maxfield, N. D., Peronto, C. L., Williams, V. A. and Lister, J. J. (2013). Cognitive training and selective attention in the aging brain: an electrophysiological study. *Clinical Neurophysiology*, **124**, 2198–2208.

Peckham, A. D., McHugh, R. K. and Otto, M. W. (2010). A meta-analysis of the magnitude of biased attention in depression. *Depression and Anxiety*, **27**, 1135–1142.

Petersen, S. E. and Posner, M. I. (2012). The attention system of the human brain: 20 years after. *Annual Review of Neuroscience*, **35**, 73–89.

Phillips, M. L., Drevets, W. C., Rauch, S. L. and Lane, R. (2003). Neurobiology of emotion perception I: the neural basis of normal emotion perception. *Biological Psychiatry*, **54**, 504–514.

Poon, C. Y. and Knight, B. G. (2009). Influence of sad mood and old age schema on older adults' attention to physical symptoms. *Journals of Gerontology, Series B: Psychological Sciences and Social Sciences*, **64**, 41–44.

Price, R. B., Eldreth, D. A. and Mohlman, J. 2011. Deficient prefrontal attentional control in late-life generalized anxiety disorder: an fMRI investigation. *Translational Psychiatry*, **1**, e46.

Price, R. B., Siegle, G. and Mohlman, J. 2012. Emotional Stroop performance in older adults: effects of habitual worry. *American Journal of Geriatric Psychiatry*, **20**, 798–805.

Radvansky, G. A., Zacks, R. T. and Hasher, L. 2005. Age and inhibition: the retrieval of situation models. *Journals of Gerontology, Series B: Psychological Sciences and Social Sciences*, **60**, P276–P278.

Reed, A. E., Chan, L. and Mikels, J. A. (2014). Meta-analysis of the age-related positivity effect: age differences in preferences for positive over negative information. *Psychology and Aging*, **29**, 1–15.

Salthouse, T. A. (1996). The processing-speed theory of adult age differences in cognition. *Psychological Review*, **103**, 403–428.

Sasse, L. K., Gamer, M., Büchel, C. and Brassen, S. (2014). Selective control of attention supports the positivity effect in aging. *PLoS ONE*, **9**, e104180.

Steiner, A. R., Petkus, A. J., Nguyen, H. and Loebach Wetherell, J. (2013). Information processing bias and pharmacotherapy outcome in older adults with generalized anxiety disorder. *Journal of Anxiety Disorders*, **27**, 592–597.

Tang, Y. Y., Ma, Y., Wang, J., et al. (2007). Short-term meditation training improves attention and self-regulation. *Proceedings of the National Academy of Sciences*, **104**, 17152–17156.

Teachman, B. A., Joormann, J., Steinman, S. A. and Gotlib, I. H. (2012). Automaticity in anxiety disorders and major depressive disorder. *Clinical Psychology Review*, **32**, 575–603.

Teachman, B. A., Siedlecki, K. L. and Magee, J. C. (2007). Aging and symptoms of anxiety and depression: structural invariance of the tripartite model. *Psychology and Aging*, **22**, 160–170.

Wang, J., He, L., Jia, L., Tian, J., and Benson, V. (2015). The 'positive effect' is present in older Chinese adults: evidence from an eye tracking study. *PLoS ONE*, **10**, e0121372.

Wetherell, J. L., Gatz, M. and Pedersen, N. L. (2001). A longitudinal analysis of anxiety and depressive symptoms. *Psychology and Aging*, **16**, 187–195.

Wetherell, J. L., Petkus, A. J., Thorp, S. R., et al. (2013). Age differences in treatment response to a collaborative care intervention for anxiety disorders. *British Journal of Psychiatry*, **203**, 65–72.

Williams, J. M. G., Watts, F. N., MacLeod, C. and Mathews, A. (1997). *Cognitive Psychology and Emotional Disorders*. Chichester: John Wiley & Sons.

Young, W. R. and Williams, A. M. (2015). How fear of falling can increase fall-risk in older adults: applying psychological theory to practical observations. *Gait & Posture*, **41**, 7–12.

Young, W. R., Wing, A. M. and Hollands, M. A. (2012). Influences of state anxiety on gaze behavior and stepping accuracy in older adults during adaptive locomotion. *Journals of Gerontology Series B: Psychological Sciences and Social Sciences*, **67B**, 43–51.

Anxiety and Cognitive Functioning

Sherry A. Beaudreau, Andrew J. Petkus, Nathan C. Hantke, and Christine E. Gould

Introduction

The past decade has witnessed a proliferation of studies examining anxiety in older populations. This research underscores how anxiety is not just an ancillary symptom of depression, but a clinical issue on its own. Not only does anxiety cause suffering in older adults, but anxious older adults also have more functional disability (Brenes et al., 2005) and a reduced quality of life (Wetherell et al., 2004) compared to non-anxious older adults. In conditions that are common in later life (i.e., poor physical health, depression), those older adults experiencing comorbid anxiety typically have greater disability compared to non-anxious adults with these conditions. Cognitive functioning and the presence of neurocognitive disorders are aspects of comorbidity that have garnered increasing research attention (Beaudreau & O'Hara, 2008). This exciting new research underscores the complexity of the relations between anxiety and cognitive functioning in older individuals. Research findings suggest that this association is bidirectional, which raises important questions regarding the biological pathways potentially moderating this association and the clinical implications of possessing both anxiety and cognitive impairment.

This chapter will first review the state of the science regarding cognitive functioning in older community-residing adults who report elevated anxiety. Here, we summarize late-life anxiety research examining global cognitive functioning and specific cognitive domains, particularly information processing speed, cognitive control, and memory. This work is inclusive of state and trait anxiety, anxiety symptom severity on clinical measures, and the presence of one common anxiety disorder, namely generalized anxiety disorder (GAD). Cognitive aging models relevant to these findings are reviewed. Next, we review current work on the presence and frequency of neuropsychiatric anxiety in late-life cognitive impairment and the potential pathways linking anxiety to neurocognitive disorders. Neuropsychiatric anxiety refers to one of several psychological symptoms often observed in cognitively impaired individuals with neurodegenerative disorders, such as Alzheimer's disease (AD) (Cummings, 1997; Seignourel et al., 2008). Then, we discuss the emerging science of biological models, particularly genetics, brain imaging, and neurotransmitters, as related to anxiety and cognitive functioning. Lastly, clinical issues for assessment and intervention and directions for improving late-life anxiety clinical care in the spirit of a precision medicine approach are reviewed.

Late-Life Anxiety and Cognitive Performance

Studies of anxiety and cognition in older persons fall generally into one of two categories. In the first, older individuals recruited from community samples complete assessments of anxiety and cognitive performance, and the associations between the two are examined cross-sectionally. In some of these studies, cognitive performance in older persons with an anxiety disorder is compared with cognitive performance in older, non-anxious controls. In the second, the prevalence of neuropsychiatric anxiety and other behavioral and psychological symptoms is compared in samples of older individuals with no cognitive impairment relative to those with known neurocognitive disorders, such as mild neurocognitive disorder and major neurocognitive disorder (formerly mild cognitive impairment (MCI) or dementia prior to the Diagnostic and Statistical Manual of Mental Disorders, Fifth Edition (DSM-5; American Psychiatric Association, 2013)). A few of these investigations also delineate risk of conversion to mild or major neurocognitive disorder. The overarching findings are summarized and placed in the context of existing cognitive models such as the bidirectional model of late-life anxiety and cognition proposed by Beaudreau and O'Hara (2008), with anxiety leading to cognitive impairment in some instance and cognition leading to anxiety in others. For instance, higher levels of anxiety may directly contribute to poorer cognitive performance and decline by taxing cognitive resources. Alternatively, poorer cognitive performance could become a source of worry and anxiety. Anxiety could also be a prodromal neuropsychiatric symptom of an underlying neurodegenerative disorder. Whatever the cause or direction of the association, both anxiety symptoms and cognitive impairment likely exacerbate each other.

With regard to global cognitive functioning, investigations generally support the view that elevated symptoms of anxiety are associated with decrements in cognitive performance, including in later life (Beaudreau & O'Hara, 2008). The declines in cognitive performance associated with anxiety are above and beyond those seen in normal cognitive aging (Beaudreau & O'Hara, 2008). Relative to same aged peers reporting few anxiety symptoms, older adults with elevated anxiety symptoms have poorer performance on global measures of cognitive functioning (Schultz et al., 2005; Sinoff & Werner, 2003). Longitudinal studies also generally demonstrate that, in cognitively intact older adults, anxiety severity is positively associated with risk of future global cognitive decline (Potvin et al., 2011; Schultz et al., 2005; Sinoff & Werner, 2003) and future diagnosis of major cognitive disorder (Burton et al., 2013; Gallacher et al., 2009; Petkus et al., 2016b; Potvin et al., 2011; Sinoff & Werner, 2003).

Research has also found negative associations between anxiety and specific cognitive abilities. Older adults with higher anxiety have been observed to exhibit slower information processing speed and attention on symbol digit transcription tasks (Beaudreau & O'Hara, 2009; Wetherell et al., 2002). This association was not unique to anxiety in the Beaudreau and O'Hara (2009) study, with variance in information processing speed and attention accounted for by an interaction between greater anxiety and greater depressive symptom severity. In addition, older adults reporting greater severity of anxiety symptoms perform worse than those reporting minimal anxiety on tasks of divided attention (Hogan, 2003).

Furthermore, anxiety is associated with impacting more complex cognitive abilities such as memory and aspects of executive functioning (sometimes referred to as "cognitive control"). Poorer episodic memory has been reported in older individuals carrying a diagnosis of GAD relative to controls (Mantella et al., 2007). In addition, a critical review identified elevated anxiety as a common correlate of worse cognitive control on Stroop interference tasks (Beaudreau et al., 2013). Consistent with these findings, Butters and colleagues (2011) found poorer complex cognitive abilities (i.e., poorer working memory, cognitive control abilities, and memory) in older adults with GAD compared with older nonpsychiatric controls. They also found slower speed of information processing in the late-life GAD group relative to controls, which raises the possibility that anxiety competes for attentional resources allocated to simple cognitive processes that underlie late-life anxiety. The overall negative impact of anxiety on cognitive control and other cognitive abilities has been explained by their mutual reliance on prefrontal networks in the brain (Eysenck et al., 2007; Mohlman et al., 2009). This finding is supported by studies of older adults with GAD who are deficient relative to non-anxious older controls in recruiting prefrontal regions when faced with negatively valenced stimuli (Price et al., 2011).

Yet, the story of anxiety and cognitive control might not be so straightforward. More recently, worry symptoms have been gaining attention in relation to late-life cognition. Often viewed as a component of anxiety, worry involves perseverative negative thinking about future events (Borkevec et al., 1983). A recent investigation of community-dwelling older adults found evidence that greater worry symptom severity modulated negative associations between anxiety severity symptoms on cognitive control (Beaudreau et al., 2017). Specifically, higher worry in addition to anxiety was associated with fewer instead of more self-corrected errors on a Stroop task relative to anxiety with lower worry symptom severity. Not only does this finding challenge assumptions based on previous studies, but a similar pattern with depressive symptoms was also found. Therefore, this finding is not specific to anxiety, as there were fewer self-corrected errors when there were elevated depressive symptoms along with the presence of elevated worry symptoms. The authors provide several explanations for this unexpected finding, including worry as a trait marker of greater internally focused self-monitoring and perfectionism.

The influence of anxiety or worry on cognition may depend upon the coexistence of depressive symptoms or disorders. There is evidence that anxiety has a dose effect on older adults with depression, accelerating cognitive decline over a period of 4 years (DeLuca et al., 2005). Hence, anxiety symptoms likely interact with other mood symptoms in their influence on cognition. Decreased available cognitive resources as a function of anxiety may also contribute to the accelerated cognitive decline seen in individuals with co-occurring mood disorders and major neurocognitive disorder (Palmer et al., 2007). Though few studies have expressly examined worry in relation to cognition in older persons, there is evidence that worry could accelerate memory decline (Pietzrak et al., 2012). In contrast, greater worry symptom severity in community-dwelling older adults modulated associations between delayed verbal memory and depressive symptoms, but not in the expected direction. Those with a high severity of both depressive and worry symptoms recalled more words after a delay than those with high depressive symptoms but low worry symptoms or high worry symptoms but low depressive symptoms. Neither anxiety nor its interaction with worry had significant associations with delayed memory, suggesting that worry and anxiety might operate independently in relation to cognition (Beaudreau et al., 2017).

In summary, both anxiety symptoms and disorders have been implicated with worse cognitive functioning, both cross-sectionally and longitudinally. The domains of cognition thought to be affected by anxiety include the basic functions of processing speed and attention, but also complex cognitive abilities mediated by the frontal cortex and hippocampus, such as memory, cognitive control, and executive functioning. Models of cognition and anxiety have been developed in an attempt to explain why higher anxiety might result in worse cognitive performance.

Cognitive Models

Two cognitive models may account for the link between elevated anxiety and cognitive functioning. First, one possible explanation for the association between anxiety symptoms and lowered cognitive efficiency is proposed within Eysenck's Processing Efficiency Theory and subsequent expansion with the Attentional Control Theory (Eysenck et al., 2007). Eysenck and colleagues posit that a preoccupation with internal or external threat diverts cognitive resources toward threat information, reducing available attentional resources for performing cognitive tasks (Eysenck et al., 2007). As such, anxiety taxes both goal-directed (top-down) and stimulus-driven (bottom-up) cognitive process. This depletion of cognitive resources may especially interfere with attentional control on tasks involving inhibition of a response, shifting between tasks, and monitoring or updating information in working memory (Eysenck et al., 2007).

In an expansion of Processing Efficiency Theory, Marchant and Howard (2015) recently proposed the concept of "cognitive debt," merging Eysenck's theory with the concept of cognitive reserve (Stern, 2002). The authors propose that anxiety and future-directed negative thoughts (i.e., worry), along with several other internal and external factors, may be associated with cognitive decline. These factors deplete an individual's ability to compensate for AD-related pathology, taxing cognitive reserves and available cognitive resources in older adults. With regard to worry, the authors propose that repetitive negative thinking chronically narrows attention and diverts cognitive resources away from active tasks (Marchant & Howard, 2015). This suggests that associations between anxiety and cognitive functioning could be driven in part by worry symptoms.

These two theories offer plausible explanations for associations between anxiety and cognitive functioning in community-residing cognitively intact older adults and those with late-life mental health disorders. The next section turns to a different population of older persons: those with diagnosed neurocognitive disorders. Both the presence and frequency of anxiety are reviewed, as well as theories linking anxiety and neurodegeneration.

Neuropsychiatric Anxiety

Anxiety is one of the most common neuropsychiatric symptoms affecting older adults with major neurocognitive disorder (Teri et al., 1999). As many as 29% of older adults with mild neurocognitive disorder and 69% with major neurocognitive disorder experience clinically significant symptoms of emotional distress (Lyketsos et al., 2002). Older adults with mild neurocognitive disorder are also three times more likely to have clinically significant anxiety than those with normal cognitive functioning (Geda et al., 2008). Cognitively impaired older adults frequently report more symptoms of anxiety as compared to cognitively healthy peers, with the severity of cognitive and anxiety symptoms increasing in parallel (Hwang et al., 2004; Lyketsos et al., 2002; Tatsch et al., 2006).

Along the cognitive continuum, individuals carrying a diagnosis of mild neurocognitive disorder are significantly more likely to manifest symptoms of anxiety as compared to same-aged cognitively healthy peers (Hwang et al., 2004). Increased anxiety and agitation are often seen in individuals diagnosed with AD, with a recent study finding that 50% of older adults carrying a diagnosis of mild AD displayed three or more neuropsychiatric symptoms and reported worse quality of life (Karttunen et al., 2011). Another study utilizing both clinician and caregiver reports found a high proportion of older adults with a diagnosis of AD with subsyndromal symptoms of anxiety and worry (68–71%) over the course of a week (Ferretti et al., 2001). Furthermore, greater anxiety symptoms in these samples were associated with greater behavioral and cognitive problems (Ferretti et al., 2001). Taken together, these findings demonstrate that anxiety symptoms frequently manifest in older adults exhibiting cognitive dysfunction.

This is consistent with other research showing that anxiety is an important predictor of transitioning from mild to major neurocognitive disorder over a span of 36 months (Mah et al., 2015). Symptoms of anxiety have been shown to increase over the course of major neurocognitive disorder (Brodaty et al., 2015), although one other study found no association between the prevalence of anxiety and the severity of major neurocognitive disorder (Lyketsos et al., 2000). A recent study by Andreescu and colleagues (2014) found complex associations between anxiety symptoms and mild neurocognitive disorder. In particular, a recent onset of anxiety was associated with one form of mild neurocognitive disorder (non-amnestic), while chronic severe anxiety was associated with all of the diverse subtypes of mild neurocognitive disorder, including the amnestic subtype. This association is noteworthy because amnestic mild neurocognitive disorder has a higher rate of progression into AD. Research by Palmer and colleagues (2007) indicates that the presence of anxiety symptoms doubled the risk of conversion from mild neurocognitive disorder I to AD over a 3-year span.

Anxiety symptoms likely interact with cognitive functioning on multiple levels in older adults. Not only do anxiety symptoms seem to negatively impact cognitive efficiency, but they may also portend the insidious onset of cognitive impairment. Also likely are cases where older adults' insight into their own cognitive decline leads to anxiety symptoms; thus, anxiety could also be a psychological reaction to stress as well as a prodrome of neurodegeneration. Furthermore, older adults experiencing cognitive impairment are more likely to experience symptoms of anxiety, suggesting a complicated relationship between mood and cognition. There are several proposed mechanisms for this relationship between anxiety symptoms and cognitive functioning, including the postulation that anxiety diverts cognitive resources from task-related cognitive functioning, resulting in increased cognitive load and decreased cognitive efficiency. Taken together, this has led some authors to suggest that the association between anxiety and cognitive function is reciprocal, bidirectional, and potentially mutually exacerbating. This perspective implicates multiple pathways by which anxiety can lead to reduced or impaired cognition in older individuals, or by which cognitive impairment can lead to anxiety in older adults. The next section specifies potential biological pathways that could lead to or moderate the relationship between late-life anxiety and cognitive function.

Biological Models

The association between anxiety, cognition, and aging is complex, with much yet to be learned. In this section, we will begin with an evolutionary perspective to provide a rationale for why anxiety and cognitive functioning would be related. Next, the overlap between the genes implicated with anxiety and cognitive performance and aging will be reviewed. We will then review the physiological factors that are common to anxiety and cognitive functioning, starting at the neurotransmitter level and progressing to clinical presentations. Finally, overlaps in the biological factors between anxiety and cognitive functioning will be reviewed.

Evolutionary Basis for Anxiety

The roots of reduced or impaired cognitive abilities in anxious older adults can be explained from an evolutionary perspective. In this perspective, anxiety is an emotion that functions to prepare organisms to anticipate, escape from, and cope with future environmental threats (Mathews, 1990). This response includes activation of the sympathetic nervous system, as well as acute alterations in cognition, particularly in the domains of processing speed, attention, learning, and memory. The cognitive processes associated with acute anxiety that were developed through evolution serve as a way to protect us from threats in our environment.

While acute anxiety results in adaptive alterations to cognitive functioning, maladaptive chronic anxiety is associated with more enduring deficits in these same cognitive areas (slower processing speed, worse attention, and poor learning and memory). Chronic anxiety may lead to physiological overactivation of the brain areas associated with this anxiety response, thus leading to poorer cognitive performance in these same domains over time. Animal models show that mild manageable stress is beneficial for hippocampus neurogenesis (Lyons & Macri, 2011), while chronic unpredictable stress was associated with impaired hippocampal neurogenesis (Li et al., 2008), which could have detrimental consequences on cognitive processes later in the organism's development. Hence, chronic anxiety in an older adult could have an enduring effect on their cognitive abilities and increase the risk of cognitive decline over time.

Genetics

In addition, behavioral genetics could offer additional insight into the late-life anxiety and cognition relationship. Behavioral genetics studies with twins afford the means of distinguishing between the effects of genetics and those attributable to environmental influences. The limited studies conducted to date in this area suggest that shared genetic factors may partially explain the association between poorer cognitive performance and anxiety in later life. The heritability of anxiety symptoms (i.e., that which can be attributed to genetic variation) may increase into older adulthood (Petkus et al., 2016a). One hypothesis is that genetic factors shared with cognitive decline may increase the heritability estimate of depressive symptoms. In another study, higher anxiety symptoms were associated with worse performance on tests of processing speed, attention, and nonverbal memory (Petkus, 2014). Furthermore, shared genetic influences explained between 36% (symbol digit) and 80% (block design) of this correlation, suggesting a role of shared genetic influences. In another study with Swedish twins, symptoms of anxiety, independent of depression, measured in 1984 were associated with greater declines in processing speed and nonverbal memory, as well as increased likelihood of developing a major neurocognitive disorder over the following 28 years (Petkus et al., 2016b). Studies of twins discordant for major neurocognitive disorder have found that genetic factors common to both anxiety and major neurocognitive disorder partially mediated this association.

Given the significant overlap in genetic influences contributing to depression and anxiety (Kendler et al., 1987), the literature on depression may also be informative of the extent to which shared genetic factors explain this association. Research from the Vietnam Era Twin Study of Aging found that having greater depressive symptoms at age 20 was associated with poorer general cognitive ability 35 years later, and shared genetic influences explained 77% of this correlation (Franz et al., 2011). Another study found that neurocognitive deficits associated with depression were explained by genetic factors shared with major depressive disorder (Hsu et al., 2014).

Twin studies are valuable in providing an estimate of how much the shared genetic and environmental contributions may be mediating this association; however, twin studies do not elucidate which specific genes may be driving this association. In their review, Rodrigues et al. (2014) discuss the overlap between depression, anxiety, and AD. The authors posit that genes associated with inflammation may first increase vulnerability to depression and anxiety followed by vulnerability to AD later in life. Other genetic polymorphisms may be common to both anxiety and cognitive performance in later life. Brain-derived neuro-trophic factor (BDNF) is a protein implicated in neurogenesis and synaptic plasticity. The Val66Met polymorphism of the *BDNF* gene is associated with decreased secretion of BDNF and has been implicated as a possible risk allele for anxiety (Suliman et al., 2013) and worse cognitive functioning (Ward et al., 2014). The *APOE ε4* variant is the most studied genetic risk factor for AD and also has been implicated with anxiety (Michels et al., 2012) and stress (Petkus et al., 2012). Likewise, genes associated with serotonin reuptake and the dopamin-ergic system have been implicated in anxiety and cognitive performance (Lenze et al., 2013; Proitsi et al., 2012; Reynolds et al., 2006). The specific genetic factors common to both anxiety and cognitive performance need to be explored further to determine novel targets for both preventative and treatment interventions.

Though genes most likely account for a proportion of this association, they do not explain the entire relationship. Genetic vulnerabilities to anxiety are clearly moderated by environmental factors (Brown & Barlow, 2009). Early-life environments characterized by high stress, abuse, and decreased self-efficacy and control are linked to higher rates of anxiety in later life (Heim & Nemeroff, 2001). In addition to contributing to increased risk of anxiety, early-life adversity may have a detrimental influence on brain development. Significant early-life stress may contribute to hyper-responsiveness of the amygdala, as well as disruption to connections between the amygdala and the prefrontal cortex (Dannlowski et al., 2012). The authors of these aforementioned studies posit that brain changes increase vulnerability to continued anxiety and depression throughout adulthood.

The brain structures disrupted by early-life stress are also important for cognitive functioning throughout life. Disruptions to the hippocampus stemming from early-life stress may result in relatively mild cognitive deficits. Brain changes associated with signifi-cant early-life stress may reduce cognitive reserve. In the face of an age-related decline in cognitive resources, these individuals may be more susceptible to anxiety, but also to more severe cognitive impairments. Although more research is needed to examine this further, some studies provide support for this idea. Experiencing repeated sexual assault, primarily early in life, was associated with earlier and more severe declines in executive functioning throughout older adulthood (Petkus et al., 2012). In another study, childhood trauma exposure was associated with worse spatial memory (Majer et al., 2010). Findings have been mixed, however, with some studies reporting no association between childhood adversity and poorer cognitive functioning (Barnes et al., 2012; Feeney et al., 2013).

One explanation for these mixed results may be the presence of a gene × environment interaction. Genetic factors may moderate the association between early-life adversity and poorer cognition in later life. Carriers of the *BDNF* MET allele who are exposed to early-life stress may be at higher risk for abnormalities in the amygdala, hippocampus, and prefrontal cortex compared to noncarriers (Gatt et al., 2009). Sexual assault victims who are also *APOE ε4* carriers may be at increased risk of the negative effects of sexual assault on executive functioning (Petkus et al., 2018). Early-life stress may also cause epigenetic effects in both the *BDNF* and inflammation genes. In a rodent study, maternal separation to young rats was associated with an increase in epigenetic production of BDNF, which promoted neurogenesis and cognitive function (Suri et al., 2013). Older maternally separated rats exhibited decreased epigenetic production of BDNF as well as poor cognitive performance when compared with control rats. Human studies have also found epigenetic effects of early-life stress on inflammation genes with childhood stressors associated with increased transcription of pro-inflammatory genes in later life (Levine et al., 2015).

Neurotransmitters

Disruption of neurotransmitters is another potential biological link between anxiety and cognition in older adults. A long line of research has documented that anxiety disorders are associated with disrupted γ-aminobutyric acid (GABA) function, characterized by lower GABA levels (Nuss, 2015). The GABAergic system is the main inhibitory neurotransmitter in the brain. GABA is important for inhibition of the amygdala and for modulating connections between the amygdala and the hippocampus and prefrontal cortex (Nuss, 2015). Recent research has identified similar disruptions to the GABAergic system in AD, specifically in the dentate gyrus of the hippocampus (Wu et al., 2014). It is possible that this disruption to GABA may first manifest itself as anxiety followed by cognitive decline and AD in older adulthood, although further research is needed to support this claim.

Hormones

In addition to neurotransmitter disturbances as potential biological pathways linking anxiety and cognition, hormonal disruption is also critical and has a much stronger evidence base. The hypothalamic–pituitary–adrenal (HPA) axis produces the hormone cortisol in response to stress, which is associated with anxiety and likely affects cognition (Carlson, 2004). Chronically elevated cortisol may affect cognitive functioning. Elevated cortisol levels have been shown to damage the hippocampus (Lupien et al., 1998), which in turn may explain deficits in learning and memory. The prefrontal cortex may also be vulnerable to damage from cortisol. In one study, adults with higher cortisol levels had significantly thinner prefrontal cortices (Kremen et al., 2010). Behavioral findings from that study also show that elevated cortisol was associated with worse visuospatial ability, abstract reasoning, processing speed, and executive functioning.

Anxiety is strongly associated with dysregulation in the HPA stress response. Individuals with anxiety disorders have been shown repeatedly to exhibit chronic hyperactivation of the HPA axis and elevated cortisol levels (Mantella et al., 2008). Treatment for late-life anxiety may result in decreased HPA activation (Lenze et al., 2011). Furthermore, these decreases are correlated with improvements in memory (Lenze et al., 2012). Studies with younger adults suggest that individuals with anxiety disorders may have smaller hippocampal volumes (Stein et al., 1997) and smaller prefrontal cortices (Corbo et al., 2005; Radua et al., 2010) than those without an anxiety disorder. A study with older adults with post-traumatic stress disorder (PTSD) supports this hypothesis that chronically elevated anxiety may be damaging these brain areas (Cardenas et al., 2011). In this study, PTSD was associated with increased atrophy of the prefrontal cortex over time, and the amount of atrophy correlated with changes in cognitive functioning.

Anxiety, Cognitive Decline, Chronic Illness, and Neurodegenerative Diseases

Thus far, we have reviewed how the function of anxiety is directly related to cognitive function. We have also reviewed the overlap between the genetic, environmental, and physiological factors that are implicated as risk factors for anxiety as well as cognitive decline. Not surprisingly, a number of chronic medical conditions are associated with higher anxiety and worse cognitive performance. This review will now focus on the overlap between anxiety and cardiovascular disease, diabetes, thyroid disorders, and neurodegenerative disorders, specifically AD and Parkinson's disease (PD).

Cardiovascular disease increases in prevalence in older adulthood (Mozaffarian et al., 2015) and is associated with increased rates of anxiety, as well as being a risk factor for decreased cognitive performance. The physical symptoms of cardiovascular disease such as high blood pressure, racing heart, and shortness of breath are all also physical symptoms of anxiety. These physical symptoms may trigger and prolong the cognitive and behavioral symptoms of anxiety. Additionally, the knowledge and impact of having a diagnosis may increase hypervigilance to physical symptoms and contribute to worry about the future. Cardiovascular disease is also associated with poorer cognitive functioning. Higher blood pressure and cardiac problems are associated with increased risk of white matter changes in the brain, commonly leading to slower processing speed and executive dysfunction (Carmichael, 2014). Higher pulse pressure has also been associated with neurodegeneration and progression to AD (Nation et al., 2015). Physiological changes associated with cardiovascular disease may contribute to both anxiety and cognitive problems. It is also possible that maladaptive health behaviors commonly used to cope with anxiety and stress, such as overeating foods high in carbohydrates and fat, smoking, and alcohol, may subsequently increase the risk of developing cardiovascular disease.

Thyroid diseases – both hyperthyroidism and hypothyroidism – are also implicated with both anxiety and cognitive functioning. Thyrotoxicosis and Grave's disease – both diseases of hyperthyroidism – have been associated with more severe levels of anxiety symptoms in younger (Gulseren, 2006) and older adults (Brandt et al., 2014). Hyperthyroidism may also produce cognitive problems such as worse attention, concentration, and working memory (Yudiarto, 2006), although at least one study did not find any relationship between hyperthyroidism and poorer cognitive ability (Lilesvant-Johansen, 2014). Hypothyroidism may also increase anxiety and result in poorer cognitive functioning (Ritchie & Yeap, 2015).

As noted earlier, anxiety is an important and common symptom found in individuals with mild neurocognitive disorder and AD. Amyloid-β deposition is one of the characteristic features of AD. Anxiety symptoms may moderate the effect of amyloid-β-related cognitive decline (Pietrzak et al., 2015). This study found that cognitively intact older adults with high amyloid-β concentrations experienced greater declines over the following 4 years if they were also anxious. Emerging research on biological moderators to explain the preponderance of anxiety issues in late-life neurocognitive disorders is an exciting new direction for further refining our understanding of this association.

Finally, anxiety and cognitive decline are commonly comorbid in PD. As many as 40% of patients with PD experience significant anxiety (Dissanayaka et al., 2010), and up to 50% of those with PD meet criteria for major neurocognitive disorder (Aarsland et al., 2005). Dopamine deficiency is one mechanism that may link both anxiety and cognitive decline seen in PD, although research on anxiety and cognitive functioning in PD is currently limited.

Summary of Biological Models

Common physiological processes at the cellular, hormonal, and systems levels have been implicated in both cognitive functioning and anxiety. Table 8.1 summarizes some of these different pathways. Genetic factors common to cognitive performance and anxiety may explain the covariance between these two phenotypes. Similarly, adverse environments, particularly in childhood, may negatively impact brain physiology and structure, contributing to the negative association between these phenotypes. More research is needed to elucidate the specific genetic contributions that are shared between late-life anxiety and cognition. Identifying genetic and environmental factors that are common to both anxiety and cognition is important, as these common factors may become targets for future preventative and intervention efforts. This is of upmost important because currently there are no effective treatments for mild or major neurocognitive disorder. Similarly, interventions for anxiety – both pharmacological and psychosocial – are less effective for older adults compared to younger adults. The next section reviews the assessments and recommendations for treatment for clinicians working with patients suffering from both anxiety and cognitive decline.

Clinical Implications

The previous sections establish known relations between anxiety and cognition in older adults and the biology potentially underlying these associations. This section reviews the clinical implications that the neurocognitive reductions or impairments in late-life anxiety can have on assessment and treatment delivery. For assessment, understanding cognitive impairments that may or may not result from anxiety has implications for test selection during an assessment. Furthermore, the recent emphasis on precision medicine (i.e., using the individual's unique psychological, genetic, and biological profiles to guide prevention or intervention efforts; Insel, 2014) has potential to guide efforts to optimize treatments for late-life anxiety. In particular, as this section will discuss, precision medicine has begun to guide efforts to address the diminished treatment efficacy of psychological interventions for late-life anxiety disorders, such as GAD, and anxiety-related disorders, such as hoarding behavior, by taking cognitive status and abilities into account. Implications for assessment in relation to precision medicine are also discussed.

Assessment

To date, there are no formal recommendations regarding cognitive testing as part of an anxiety assessment, despite it being an essential component of the clinical assessment of older adults. Although it is widely recognized that major neurocognitive disorder and depression share symptoms and can be misdiagnosed as one another (Kaszniak & Christenon, 1994), the level of diagnostic confusion between anxiety and cognitive impairment is less well recognized. In addition, as noted previously, anxiety issues pervade in persons with cognitive impairment. Nevertheless, the sudden appearance of anxiety could manifest as a neuropsychiatric symptom and portend future or flag current cognitive issues.

It is generally accepted that all late-life mental health assessments should include some assessment of cognitive status, through cognitive screening or neuropsychological testing if possible. The presence and degree of cognitive impairment has important implications for diagnostics and treatment planning. Evidence-based information is not currently available for identifying patient subtypes of late-life anxiety and cognitive impairment; however, future work

Table 8.1 Genetic, early environment, and hormonal conditions that have been implicated with both worse cognitive performance and higher anxiety (not an exhaustive list).

Genetics	Cognition	Anxiety
Genetics		
COMT Function: breakdown of dopamine in the frontal cortex	Worse working memory (Jasper et al., 2015) Disrupted white-matter structure (Papenberg et al., 2015) Increased neurodegeneration (Gennatas et al., 2012)	Higher rates of phobic anxiety (McGrath et al., 2004) Increased risk of panic disorder (Domschke et al., 2007)
5-HTLLPR Function: uptake of serotonin	Worse attention (Lenze et al., 2013) Increased risk of major neurocognitive disorder (Micheli et al., 2006)	Anxiety sensitivity (Klauke et al., 2011) Vulnerability to stress (Caspi et al., 2010)
BDNF Function: secretion of BDNF	Worse episodic memory (Ward et al., 2014)	Anxiety disorders (Suliman et al., 2013)
APOE ε4	Increased risk of major neurocognitive disorder (Michaelson, 2014)	Greater anxiety severity (Michels et al., 2012) *APOE* × sexual assault interaction (Petkus et al., 2012)
Early environmental		
Childhood trauma	Worse spatial memory (Majer et al., 2010) Worse verbal fluency and early-life sexual assault (Petkus et al., 2012)	Anxiety disorders (Heim & Nemeroff, 2001) Anxiety (Brown & Barlow, 2009)
Hormones		
Cortisol	Hippocampal damage (Lupien et al., 1998) Prefrontal cortex damage (Kremen et al., 2010)	Hyperactivation of cortisol response (Mantella et al., 2008) Treatment for anxiety reduces cortisol (Lenze et al., 2011)

delineating the cognitive phenotypes of late-life anxiety or specific anxiety profiles among those with late-life neurocognitive disorders could further both assessment and intervention development in this area.

Which cognitive tests or batteries would be ideal if included as part of an anxiety assessment? There are several considerations in making this decision. First, is there documented cognitive impairment already? Estimating the severity of cognitive impairment, if any, will guide the selection of a test. For example, if the patient has a diagnosis of probable mild or major neurocognitive disorder, cognitive screens suitable for less or more impaired individuals would be selected.

Two cognitive screens that are available free of charge, are brief to administer, and require minimal training are the St. Louis University Mental Status (SLUMS) Examination (www.slu.edu/medicine/internal-medicine/geriatric-medicine/aging-successfully/assessment-tools/mental-status-exam.php) and the Montreal Cognitive Assessment (MoCA; www.mocatest.org). The SLUMS is appropriate when major neurocognitive disorder is possible, whereas the MoCA is more useful for detecting different levels of MCI. The MoCA has the advantage of being available in more than 50 languages. These simple screens can indicate the possible presence of cognitive impairment. Further neuropsychological assessment could follow up on specific items of the cognitive screen on which patients have trouble, but this level of cognitive assessment would likely need to occur with a qualified clinician, such as a trained clinical neuropsychologist.

Cognitive assessments as part of a late-life anxiety study should include specific neuropsychological tests. These tests can be used for fine-grained analysis of the cognitive characteristics of late-life anxiety. Cognitive control tests have been particularly singled out, and more specifically test of inhibitory control (Beaudreau et al., 2013). Specific research recommendations for selecting inhibitory control tests are discussed by Beaudreau and colleagues (2013) to dissociate aspects of performance that are related or unrelated to anxiety in older individuals. These include experimental tasks that tap goal maintenance using memory and modifications of the standard Stroop task that impose varying levels of goal maintenance and flexibility.

What happens once cognitive impairment is detected in a patient being assessed for anxiety? One must consider the severity of the cognitive impairment and the extent to which impairment would affect the patient's ability to provide accurate retrospective report of the history of their cognitive decline and useful current history regarding self-reported information about anxiety. The assessor should consider how the individual's cognitive issues might influence the validity of anxiety measurement and thus the selection of the anxiety assessment tests. One study recently found attenuated internal consistency of self-report measures in older adults with lower scores (average vs. superior range) on delayed memory tasks (Gould et al., 2014). Other alternatives include using anxiety measures completed by a proxy or those completed both by the patient and a proxy if a traditional self-report measure would not be appropriate. Behavioral observations and interviews with family members, caregivers, or professional caregivers are critical as well. A detailed discussion of anxiety symptom assessment and decisions regarding anxiety test selection in the presence of cognitive impairment is beyond the scope of this chapter, but these issues are addressed in Chapter 6.

Treatment

Cognitive ability is a critical variable for guiding treatment selection and implementation in late-life anxiety. New research suggests that evidence-based treatments can work when there are cognitive issues in an anxious older adult, some of which might be part of the anxiety or a frank cognitive issue comorbid to anxiety. Many nonpharmacological treatments require a capacity to learn new information and some cognitive flexibility. When these cognitive abilities are compromised, the standard protocols for treatment delivery may not be effective and, even worse, could frustrate an older adult with anxiety concerns. This emerging area of research on anxiety protocols for cognitively impaired older adults shows promising results for several treatments.

Cognitive Behavioral Therapy

Cognitive behavioral therapy (CBT) has been the most widely studied approach for late-life anxiety. Support for CBT generally shows that older adults with GAD respond better to CBT than to treatment as usual or a waitlist control, but may not respond better to CBT than to an active control (Gould et al., 2012). Nevertheless, concern regarding CBT with cognitively impaired older adults with anxiety has been recently addressed. An adapted delivery of CBT – Peaceful Mind – shows promise for treating older adults with anxiety and major neurocognitive disorder (described in Paukert et al., 2013). The treatment includes a support person, such as a family member or spouse, who is present during each treatment session to help the individual with cognitive impairment learn the skills and remember to practice them between sessions. Both the patient and support person receive workbooks to support the learning of these skills. The Peaceful Mind program differs from other CBT treatments in that it is delivered over a 6-month period. The first 9–12 sessions are conducted in person along with weekly telephone check-ins. After the initial 3 months of treatment, telephone follow-up appointments continue for 3 months (weekly for 4 weeks, then biweekly for the following 8 weeks). The feasibility of Peaceful Mind and improvements in clinician ratings of patient anxiety and collateral distress were found in a pilot randomized controlled trial (Stanley et al., 2013). This is an exciting direction for treatment research, and, if found to be efficacious in this population, it could be adapted to patients with milder impairments as well. More evidence is needed, but the initial results are promising.

For specific types of cognitive impairment, such as the executive dysfunction observed in hoarding disorder, another approach that has been shown to improve effect sizes in CBT is the provision of initial cognitive rehabilitation prior to training. Ayers and colleagues (2014) worked with older patients with hoarding disorder for 22 weeks (24 sessions) to deliver cognitive rehabilitation of executive abilities alongside exposure therapy, and this was found to nearly double the effect size of CBT. A similar approach of combining cognitive rehabilitation within an existing psychological treatment protocol could be suitable for anxiety disorders where executive dysfunction is present, although there are no trials of this to date.

Problem-Solving Therapy

Problem-solving therapy (PST; Nezu et al., 2013) falls under the rubric of cognitive behavioral treatments, but it differs from traditional CBT in that it emphasizes teaching individuals to solve life problems effectively as a primary focus. PST emphasizes both the repetition and practice of skills and an experiential way of learning (Nezu et al., 2013), both of which are compatible strategies to use with older adults who may harbor both anxiety and cognitive impairment.

PST has been used in a number of populations and, most relevant to late life, has included medical populations (i.e., cancer, hospice) and those with late-life depression (Alexopoulos et al., 2003, 2011; Areán et al., 2010). At least one clinical trial has examined PST as a preventative intervention for GAD in individuals recovering from stroke, the results of which were promising (Mikami et al., 2014). Though no randomized controlled trials of PST for late-life anxiety have been published to date, PST's success in treating late-life depression with executive dysfunction (Alexopoulos et al., 2011) suggests that this could be an effective approach for treating anxiety in older adults, particularly those who may have executive function issues. Notably, a recent investigation found that older adults with depression, who had poor set-shifting ability at treatment baseline, were more likely to respond to treatment with PST or supportive therapy (Beaudreau et al., 2015). Nevertheless, it is unknown whether similar treatment responses can be expected in late-life anxiety. In PST, compared with a control condition, older homebound patients with cardiovascular disease have been shown to experience significant reductions in depressive symptoms, but not in anxiety symptoms (Gellis & Bruce, 2010). However, patients in this study only reported mild levels of anxiety relative to moderate depressive symptoms at treatment baseline. Furthermore, the PST protocol was tailored to depression (Gellis & Bruce, 2010). Studies using an older sample with moderate to severe anxiety symptoms and with a PST protocol adapted to late-life anxiety are needed.

In the absence of clinical trials of PST in late-life anxiety, clinical cases of PST for anxiety in older veterans and caregivers offer some initial support for the prospect of PST as an intervention for late-life anxiety (Beaudreau et al., 2014). Although speculative, these cases suggest the need to offer some initial relaxation training or other calming strategies to older adults with anxiety disorders in order to maximize their ability to attend to and learn problem-solving skills (Beaudreau et al., 2014). This view is consistent with modern approaches to PST (Nezu et al., 2013), which advocate for inclusion of other skills to address arousal, hopelessness, and so forth in a flexible fashion if needed for particular patients. Formal clinical trials are needed to determine whether older adults with anxiety disorders respond to PST in light of the limited evidence collected to date.

Mindfulness-Based Stress Reduction

Mindfulness-based stress reduction (MBSR; Kabat-Zinn et al., 1992) is an 8-week group-based protocol that teaches mindfulness through the practice of breathing, mindfulness meditation, yoga, and other mindfulness exercises (e.g., body scanning). MBSR has been found consistently to reduce anxiety in mixed-age adult samples (Goldin & Gross, 2010; Vøllestad et al., 2011). Lenze and colleagues (2014) examined 8-session and 12-session MBSR in older adults with elevated anxiety and cognitive dysfunction. The findings from their treatment development study demonstrated that MBSR yielded improvements in worry severity, memory, and executive functioning. No differences were found between 8- and 12-session MBSR, which contrasts with other aforementioned late-life anxiety treatments modified for use with patients with cognitive dysfunction that relied on longer protocols. This difference may be a function of the severity of the patients included in the different studies. Further studies with MBSR among older adults with anxiety and cognitive dysfunction are needed to affirm these preliminary findings of the efficacy of MBSR in this population.

Pharmacological Agents

Pharmacological treatments for anxiety also show promise both for the treatment of anxiety symptoms (for a review, see Gonçalves & Byrne, 2012) and for improving cognitive symptoms as well. Interestingly, a recent research study (Butters et al., 2011) suggests improvement in cognitive function across multiple domains following successful treatment of anxiety symptoms with escitalopram. Thus, there is potential for some treatments to improve cognition.

Conclusions

Empirical evidence to date, particularly over the past decade, generally supports the notion that greater anxiety impairs global cognitive functioning and cognitive control abilities in older adults. Furthermore, those with late-life neurocognitive disorders suffer from anxiety disproportionately compared with those with normal cognition, and those with more severe neurocognitive disorders evidence more anxiety than those with a mild neurocognitive disorder. The confluence of cognitive and biological aging underscores the multitude of processes that could link anxiety and cognition among the aged. The complexity of the relationship between anxiety and cognitive functioning in relation to worry has yet to be determined. In particular, it is unclear whether worry mediates or moderates their relationship in either a positive or negative way. Finally, improving patient care for geriatric patients through the inclusion of cognitive screens to determine whether there is a clinically significant issue can guide later anxiety treatment. Modifications of anxiety treatments are possible, and some initial protocols devised for anxiety in patients with major neurocognitive disorder demonstrate that our behavioral interventions need not exclude such individuals, but rather the protocols may need to be adapted.

References

Aarsland, D., Zaccai, J. and Brayne, C. (2005). A systematic review of prevalence studies of dementia in Parkinson's disease. *Official Journal of the Movement Disorders Society*, **20**(10), 1255–1263.

Aleopoulous, G. S., Raue, P. and Areán, P.A. (2003). Problem-solving therapy versus supportive therapy in geriatric major depression with executive dysfunction. *American Journal of Geriatric Psychiatry*, **11**, 46–52.

Alexopoulos, G. S., Raue, P. J., Kiosses, D. N., et al. (2011). Problem-solving therapy and supportive therapy in older adults with major depression and executive dysfunction: effect on disability. *Archives of General Psychiatry*, **68**, 33–41.

American Psychiatric Association (2013). *Diagnostic and Statistical Manual of Mental Disorders*, 5th ed. Washington, DC: American Psychiatric Association.

Andreescu, C., Teverovsky, E., Fu, B., Hughes, T. F., Chang, C. C. and Ganguli, M. (2014). Old worries and new anxieties: behavioral symptoms and mild cognitive impairment in a population study. *American Journal of Geriatric Psychiatry*, **22**(3), 274–284.

Areán, P. A., Raue, P., Mackin, R. S., Kanellopoulos, D., McCulloch, C. and Alexopoulos, G. S. (2010). Problem-solving therapy and supportive therapy in older adults with major depression and executive dysfunction. *American Journal of Geriatric Psychiatry*, **167**, 1391–1398.

Ayers, C. R., Saxena, S., Espejo, E., Twamley, E. W., Granholm, E. and Wetherell, J. L. (2014). Novel treatment for geriatric hoarding disorder: an open trial of cognitive rehabilitation paired with behavior therapy. *American Journal of Geriatric Psychiatry*, **22**(3), 248–252.

Barnes, L. L., Wilson, R. S., Everson-Rose, S. A., Hayward, M. D., Evans, D. A. and Mendes de Leon, C. F. (2012). Effects of early-life adversity on cognitive decline in older African Americans and whites. *Neurology*, **79**(24), 2321–2327.

Beaudreau, S. A. and O'Hara, R. (2008). Late-life anxiety and cognitive impairment: a review. *American Journal of Geriatric Psychiatry*, **16**(10), 790–803.

Beaudreau, S. A. and O'Hara, R. (2009). The association of anxiety and depressive symptoms with cognitive performance in community-dwelling older adults. *Psychology and Aging*, **24**(2), 507–512.

Beaudreau, S. A., Gould, C. E., Fairchild, J. K., Rideaux, T., Huh, J. and O'Hara, R. (2014). A pilot comparison of problem solving therapy and cognitive behavioral therapy for generalized anxiety disorder in older adults.

Symposium conducted at the meeting of the Gerontological Society of America, Washington, DC.

Beaudreau, S. A., Hantke, N. C., Mashal, N., Gould, C. E., Henderson, V. W. and O'Hara, R. (2017). Unlocking neurocognitive substrates of late-life affective symptoms using the Research Domain Criteria: worry is an essential dimension. *Frontiers in Aging Neuroscience*, 9, 380.

Beaudreau, S. A., MacKay-Brant, A. and Reynolds, J. (2013). Application of a cognitive neuroscience perspective of cognitive control to late life anxiety. *Journal of Anxiety Disorders*, 27(6), 559–566.

Beaudreau, S. A., Rideaux, T., O'Hara, R. and Arean, P. (2015). Does cognition predict treatment response and remission in psychotherapy for late-life depression? *American Journal of Geriatric Psychiatry*, 23 (2), 215–219.

Bellander, M., Backman, L., Liu, T., et al. (2015). Lower baseline performance but greater plasticity of working memory for carriers of the Val allele of the *COMT* Val(1)(5)(8)Met polymorphism. *Neuropsychology*, 29, 247–254.

Borkovec, T. D., Robinson, E., Pruzinsky, T., and DePree, J. A. (1983). Preliminary exploration of worry: some characteristics and processes. *Behaviour Research and Therapy*, 21, 9–16.

Bower, E. S., Wetherell, J. L., Mon, T. and Lenze, E. J. (2015). Treating anxiety disorders in older adults: current treatments and future directions. *Harvard Review of Psychiatry*, 23 (5), 329–342.

Brandt, F., Thvilum, M., Almind, D., et al. (2014). Hyperthyroidism and psychiatric morbidity: evidence from a Danish nationwide register study. *European Journal of Endocrinology/European Federation of the Endocrinological Society*, 170, 341–348.

Brenes, G. A., Guralnik, J. M., Williamson, J. D., Fried, L. P., Simpson, C. and Penninx, B. W. (2005). The influence of anxiety on the progression of disability. *Journal of the American Geriatrics Society*, 53(1), 34–39.

Brodaty, H., Connors, M. H., Xu, J., Woodward, M. and Ames, D. (2015). The course of neuropsychiatric symptoms in dementia: a 3-year longitudinal study. *Journal of the American Medical Directors Association*, 16(5), 380–387.

Brown, T. A. and Barlow, D. H. (2009). A proposal for a dimensional classification system based on the shared features of the DSM-IV anxiety and mood disorders: implications for assessment and treatment. *Psychological Assessment*, 21(3), 256–271.

Burton, C., Campbell, P., Jordan, K., Strauss, V. and Mallen, C. (2013). The association of anxiety and depression with future dementia diagnosis: a case–control study in primary care. *Family Practice*, 30 (1), 25–30.

Butters, M. A., Bhalla, R. K., Andreescu, C., et al. (2011). Changes in neuropsychological functioning following treatment for late-life generalised anxiety disorder. *British Journal of Psychiatry*, 199(3), 211–218.

Cardenas, V. A., Samuelson, K., Lenoci, M., et al. (2011). Changes in brain anatomy during the course of posttraumatic stress disorder. *Psychiatry Research: Neuroimaging*, 193(2), 93–100.

Carlson, N. (2004). *Physiology of behavior*, 8th ed. New York: Pearson.

Carmichael, O. (2014). Preventing vascular effects on brain injury and cognition late in life: knowns and unknowns. *Neuropsychology Review*, 24(3), 371–387.

Caspi, A., Hariri, A. R., Holmes, A., Uher, R. and Moffitt, T. E. (2010). Genetic sensitivity to the environment: the case of the serotonin transporter gene and its implications for studying complex diseases and traits. *American Journal of Psychiatry*, 167, 509–527.

Coles, M. E. and Heimberg, R. G. (2002). Memory biases in the anxiety disorders: current status. *Clinical Psychology Review*, 22 (4), 587–627.

Corbo, V., Clement, M. H., Armony, J. L., Pruessner, J. C. and Brunet, A. (2005). Size versus shape differences: contrasting voxel-based and volumetric analyses of the anterior cingulate cortex in individuals with acute posttraumatic stress disorder. *Biological Psychiatry*, 58(2), 119–124.

Cummings, J. L. (1997). The Neuropsychiatric Inventory: assessing psychopathology in dementia patients. *Neurology*, **48**(5), 10S–16S.

Dannlowski, U., Stuhrmann, A., Beutelmann, V., et al. (2012). Limbic scars: long-term consequences of childhood maltreatment revealed by functional and structural magnetic resonance imaging. *Biological Psychiatry*, **71**(4), 286–293.

DeLuca, A. K., Lenze, E. J., Mulsant, B. H., et al. (2005). Comorbid anxiety disorder in late life depression: association with memory decline over four years. *International Journal of Geriatric Psychiatry*, **20**(9), 848–854.

Dissanayaka, N. N., Sellbach, A., Matheson, S., et al. (2010). Anxiety disorders in Parkinson's disease: prevalence and risk factors. *Official Journal of the Movement Disorder Society*, **25**(7), 838–845.

Domschke, K., Deckert, J., O'Donovan M. C. and Glatt, S. J. (2007). Meta-analysis of *COMT* Val158Met in panic disorder: Ethnic heterogeneity and gender specificity. *American Journal of Medical Genetics Part B: Neuropsychiatric Genetics*, **144B**, 667–673.

Drag, L. L. and Bieliauskas, L. A. (2010). Contemporary review 2009: cognitive aging. *Journal of Geriatric Psychiatry and Neurology*, **23**(2), 75–93.

Eysenck, M. W., Derakshan, N., Santos, R. and Calvo, M. G. (2007). Anxiety and cognitive performance: Attentional Control Theory. *Emotion*, **7**(2), 336–353.

Feeney, J., Kamiya, Y., Robertson, I. H. and Kenny, R. A. (2013). Cognitive function is preserved in older adults with a reported history of childhood sexual abuse. *Journal of Traumatic Stress*, **26**(6), 735–743.

Ferretti, L., McCurry, S. M., Logsdon, R., Gibbons, L. and Teri, L. (2001). Anxiety and Alzheimer's disease. *Journal of Geriatric Psychiatry and Neurology*, **14**(1), 52–58.

Franz, C. E., O'Brien, R. C., Hauger, R. L., et al. (2011). Cross-sectional and 35-year longitudinal assessment of salivary cortisol and cognitive functioning: the Vietnam Era Twin Study of Aging. *Psychoneuroendocrinology*, **36**(7), 1040–1052.

Gallacher, J., Bayer, A., Fish, M., et al. (2009). Does anxiety affect risk of dementia? Findings from the Caerphilly Prospective Study. *Psychosomatic Medicine*, **71**(6), 659–666.

Gatt, J. M., Nemeroff, C. B., Dobson-Stone, C., et al. (2009). Interactions between *BDNF* Val66Met polymorphism and early life stress predict brain and arousal pathways to syndromal depression and anxiety. *Molecular Psychiatry*, **14**(7), 681–695.

Geda, Y. E., Roberts, R. O., Knopman, D. S., et al. (2008). Prevalence of neuropsychiatric symptoms in mild cognitive impairment and normal cognitive aging: population-based study. *Archives of General Psychiatry*, **65**(10), 1193–1198.

Gellis, Z. D. and Bruce, M. L. (2010). Problem solving therapy for subthreshold depression in home healthcare patients with cardiovascular disease. *American Journal of Geriatric Psychiatry*, **18**, 464–474.

Gennatas, E. D., Cholfin, J. A., Zhou, J., et al. (2012). *COMT* Val158Met genotype influences neurodegeneration within dopamine-innervated brain structures. *Neurology*, **78**, 1663–1669.

Goldin, P. R. and Gross, J. J. (2010). Effects of mindfulness-based stress reduction (MBSR) on emotion regulation in social anxiety disorder. *Emotion*, **10**(1), 83–91.

Gonçalves, D. C. and Byrne, G. J. (2012). Interventions for generalized anxiety disorder in older adults: systematic review and meta-analysis. *Journal of Anxiety Disorders*, **26**(1), 1–11.

Gould, R. L., Coulson, M. C. and Howard, R. J. (2012). Efficacy of cognitive behavioral therapy for anxiety disorders in older people: a meta-analysis and meta-regression of randomized controlled trials. *Journal of American Geriatrics Society*, **60**(2), 218–229.

Gould, C. E., Segal, D. L., Yochim, B. P., Pachana, N.A., Byrne, G. J. and Beaudreau, S. A. (2014). Measuring anxiety in late life: a psychometric examination of the Geriatric Anxiety Inventory and Geriatric Anxiety Scale. *Journal of Anxiety Disorders*, **28**(8), 804–811.

Gulseren, S., Gulseren, L., Hekimsoy, Z., Cetinay, P. and Tokatlioglu, B. (2006). Depression, anxiety, health-related quality of life, and disability in patients with overt and subclinical thyroid dysfunction. *Archives of Medical Research*, **37**(1), 133–139.

Heim, C. and Nemeroff, C. B. (2001). The role of childhood trauma in the neurobiology of mood and anxiety disorders: preclinical and clinical studies. *Biological Psychiatry*, **49**(12), 1023–1039.

Hogan, M. J. (2003). Divided attention in older but not younger adults is impaired by anxiety. *Experimental Aging Research*, **29**(2), 111–136.

Hsu, K. J., Young-Wolff, K. C., Kendler, K. S., Halberstadt, L. J. and Prescott, C. A. (2014). Neuropsychological deficits in major depression reflect genetic/familial risk more than clinical history: a monozygotic discordant twin-pair study. *Psychiatry Research*, **215**(1), 87–94.

Hwang, T. J., Masterman, D. L., Ortiz, F., Fairbanks, L. A. and Cummings, J. L. (2004). Mild cognitive impairment is associated with characteristic neuropsychiatric symptoms. *Alzheimer Disease and Associated Disorders*, **18**(1), 17–21.

Insel, T. R. (2014). The NIMH Research Domain Criteria (RDoC) Project: precision medicine for psychiatry. *American Journal of Psychiatry*, **171**(4), 395–397.

Jaspar, M., Dideberg, V., Bours, V., Maquet, P. and Collette, F. (2015). Modulating effect of COMT Val(158)Met polymorphism on interference resolution during a working memory task. *Brain and Cognition*, **95**, 7–18.

Kabat-Zinn J., Massion A. O., Kristeller J., et al. (1992). Effectiveness of a meditation-based stress reduction program in the treatment of anxiety disorders. *American Journal of Psychiatry*, **149**(7), 936–943.

Karttunen, K., Karppi, P., Hiltunen, A., et al. (2011). Neuropsychiatric symptoms and quality of life in patients with very mild and mild Alzheimer's disease. *International Journal of Geriatric Psychiatry*, **26**(5), 473–482.

Kaszniak, A. W. and Christenson, G. D. (1994). Differential diagnosis of dementia and depression. In M. Storandt and G. R. VandenBos, eds., *Neuropsychological Assessment of Dementia and Depression in Older Adults: A Clinician's Guide.* Washington, DC: American Psychological Association, pp. 81–119.

Kendler, K. S., Heath, A. C., Martin, N. G. and Eaves, L. J. (1987). Symptoms of anxiety and symptoms of depression. Same genes, different environments? *Archives of General Psychiatry*, **44**(5), 451–457.

Klauke, B., Deckert, J., Reif, A., et al. (2011). Serotonin transporter gene and childhood trauma – a G × E effect on anxiety sensitivity. *Depression and Anxiety*, **28**, 1048–1057.

Kremen, W. S., O'Brien, R. C., Panizzon, M. S., et al. (2010). Salivary cortisol and prefrontal cortical thickness in middle-aged men: a twin study. *Neuroimage*, **53**(3), 1093–1102.

Lee, L. O. and Knight, B. G. (2009). Attentional bias for threat in older adults: moderation of the positivity bias by trait anxiety and stimulus modality. *Psychological Aging*, **24**, 741–747.

Lenze, E. J., Dixon, D., Mantella, R. C., et al. (2012). Treatment-related alteration of cortisol predicts change in neuropsychological function during acute treatment of late-life anxiety disorder. *International Journal of Geriatric Psychiatry*, **27**(5), 454–462.

Lenze, E. J., Dixon, D., Nowotny, P., et al. (2013). Escitalopram reduces attentional performance in anxious older adults with high-expression genetic variants at serotonin 2A and 1B receptors. *International Journal of Neuropsychopharmacology*, **16**(2), 279–288.

Lenze, E. J., Hickman, S., Hershey, T., et al. (2014). Mindfulness-based stress reduction for older adults with worry symptoms and co-occurring cognitive dysfunction. *International Journal of Geriatric Psychiatry*, **29**(10), 991–1000.

Lenze, E. J., Mantella, R. C., Shi, P., et al. (2011). Elevated cortisol in older adults with generalized anxiety disorder is reduced by treatment: a placebo-controlled evaluation of escitalopram. *American Journal of Geriatric Psychiatry*, **19**(5), 482–490.

Levine, M. E., Cole, S. W., Weir, D. R. and Crimmins, E. M. (2015). Childhood and later life stressors and increased inflammatory gene expression at older ages. *Social Science & Medicine*, 130, 16–22.

Li, S., Wang, C., Wang, W., Dong, H., Hou, P. and Tang, Y. (2008). Chronic mild stress impairs cognition in mice: from brain homeostasis to behavior. *Life Science*, 82 (17–18), 934–942.

Lillevang-Johansen, M., Petersen, I., Christensen, K., Hegedüs, L. and Brix, T. H. (2014). Is previous hyperthyroidism associated with long-term cognitive dysfunction? A twin study. *Clinical Endocrinology (Oxford)*, 80(2), 290–295.

Lupien, S. J., de Leon, M., de Santi, S., et al. (1998). Cortisol levels during human aging predict hippocampal atrophy and memory deficits. *Nature Neuroscience*, 1(1), 69–73.

Lyketsos, C. G., Lopez, O., Jones, B., Fitzpatrick, A. L., Breitner, J. and DeKosky, S. (2002). Prevalence of neuropsychiatric symptoms in dementia and mild cognitive impairment: results from the cardiovascular health study. *Journal of the American Medical Association*, 288(12), 1475–1483.

Lyketsos, C. G., Steinberg, M., Tschanz, J. T., et al. (2000). Mental and behavioral disturbances in dementia: findings from the Cache County Study on Memory in Aging, *American Journal of Psychiatry*, 157(5), 708–714.

Lyons, D. M. and Macri, S. (2011). Resilience and adaptive aspects of stress in neurobehavioral development. *Neuroscience and Biobehavioral Reviews*, 35(7), 1451.

Mah, L., Binns, M. A., Steffens, D. C. (2015). Anxiety symptoms in amnestic mild cognitive impairment are associated with medial temporal atrophy and predict conversion to Alzheimer disease. *American Journal of Geriatric Psychiatry*, 23(5), 466–476.

Majer, M., Nater, U. M., Lin, J. M., Capuron, L. and Reeves, W. C. (2010). Association of childhood trauma with cognitive function in healthy adults: a pilot study. *BMC Neurology*, 10, 61.

Mantella, R. C., Butters, M. A., Amico, J. A., et al. (2008). Salivary cortisol is associated with diagnosis and severity of late-life generalized anxiety disorder. *Psychoneuroendocrinology*, 33(6), 773–781.

Mantella, R. C., Butters, M. A., Dew, M. A., et al. (2007). Cognitive impairment in late-life generalized anxiety disorder. *American Journal of Geriatric Psychiatry*, 15(8), 673–679.

Marchant, N. L. and Howard, R. J. (2015). Cognitive debt and Alzheimer's disease. *Journal of Alzheimer's Disease*, 44(3), 755–770.

Mathews, A. (1990). Why worry? The cognitive function of anxiety. *Behaviour Research Therapy*, 28(6), 455–468.

McGrath, M., Kawachi, I., Ascherio, A., Colditz, G. A., Hunter, D. J. and De Vivo, I. (2004). Association between catechol-O-methyltransferase and phobic anxiety. *American Journal of Psychiatry*, 161, 1703–1705.

Michaelson, D. M. (2014). APOE ε4: the most prevalent yet understudied risk factor for Alzheimer's disease. *Alzheimer's & Dementia*, 10(6), 861–868.

Micheli, D., Bonvicini, C., Rocchi, A., et al. (2006). No evidence for allelic association of serotonin 2A receptor and transporter gene polymorphisms with depression in Alzheimer disease. *Journal of Alzheimer's Disease*, 10, 371–378.

Michels, A., Multhammer, M., Zintl, M., Mendoza, M. C. and Klunemann, H. H. (2012). Association of apolipoprotein E epsilon4 (APOE epsilon4) homozygosity with psychiatric behavioral symptoms. *Journal of Alzheimer's Disease*, 28(1), 25–32.

Mikami, K., Jorge, R. E., Moser, D. J., et al. (2014). Prevention of post-stroke generalized anxiety disorder, using escitalopram or problem-solving therapy. *Journal of Neuropsychiatry and Clinical Neurosciences*, 26, 323–328.

Mohlman, J., Price, R. B., Eldreth, D. A., Chazin, D., Glover, D. M. and Kates, W. R. (2009). The relation of worry to prefrontal cortex volume in older adults with and without generalized anxiety disorder. *Psychiatry Research*, 173(2), 121–127.

Mozaffarian, D., Benjamin, E. J., Go, A. S., et al. (2015). Heart disease and stroke statistics – 2015 update: a report from the American Heart Association. *Circulation*, 131(4), e29–e322.

Nation, D. A., Edmonds, E. C., Bangen, K. J., et al. (2015). Pulse pressure in relation to tau-mediated neurodegeneration, cerebral amyloidosis, and progression to dementia in very old adults. *JAMA Neurology*, 72(5), 546–553.

Nezu, A. M., Nezu, C. M. and D' Zurilla, T. J. (2013). *Problem-Solving Therapy: A Treatment Manual*. New York: Springer Publishing Company.

Nuss, P. (2015). Anxiety disorders and GABA neurotransmission: a disturbance of modulation. *Neuropsychiatric Disease and Treatment*, 11, 165–175.

Palmer, K., Berger, A. K., Monastero, R., Winblad, B., Bäckman, L. and Fratiglioni, L. (2007). Predictors of progression from mild cognitive impairment to Alzheimer disease. *Neurology*, 68(19), 1596–1602.

Papenberg, G., Lovden, M., Laukka, E. J., et al. (2015). Magnified effects of the *COMT* gene on white-matter microstructure in very old age. *Brain Structure and Function*, 220, 2927–2938.

Paukert, A. L., Kraus-Schuman, C., Wilson, N., et al. (2013). The peaceful mind manual: A protocol for treating anxiety in persons with dementia. *Behavior Modification*, 37(5), 631–664.

Petkus, A. J. (2014). *Anxiety and Cognition in Swedish Twins: Genetic and Environmental Contributions*. Doctoral dissertation, University of California, San Diego.

Petkus, A. J., Gatz, M., Reynolds, C. A., Kremen, W. S. and Wetherell, J. L. (2016a). Stability of genetic and environmental contributions to anxiety symptoms in older adulthood. *Behavior Genetics*, 46(4), 492–505.

Petkus, A. J., Lenze, E. J., Butters, M. A., Twamley, E. W. and Wetherell, J. L. (2018). Childhood trauma is associated with poorer cognitive performance in older adults. *Journal of Clinical Psychiatry*, 79(1), 16m11021.

Petkus, A. J., Reynolds, C., Wetherell, J. L., Kremen, W. S., Pedersen, N. and Gatz, M. (2016b). Anxiety is associated with increased risk of dementia in older Swedish twins. 12 (4), 399–406.

Petkus, A. J., Wetherell, J. L., Stein, M. B., Liu, L. and Barrett-Connor, E. (2012). History of sexual assault is associated with greater declines in executive functioning in older adults with APOE epsilon4. *Journal of Gerontology: Series B: Psychology Sciences and Social Sciences*, 67(6), 653–659.

Pietrzak, R. H., Lim, Y. Y., Neumeister, A., et al. (2015). Amyloid-beta, anxiety, and cognitive decline in preclinical Alzheimer disease: a multicenter, prospective cohort study. *JAMA Psychiatry*, 72(3), 284–291.

Pietrzak, R. H., Maruff, P., Woodward, M., et al. (2012). "Mild worry symptoms predict decline in learning and memory in healthy older adults: a 2-year prospective cohort study": erratum. *American Journal of Geriatric Psychiatry*, 20(7), 634.

Potvin, O., Forget, H., Grenier, S., Préville, M. and Hudon, C. (2011). Anxiety, depression, and 1-year incident cognitive impairment in community-dwelling older adults. *Journal of American Geriatrics Society*, 59(8), 1421–1428.

Price, R. B., Eldreth, D. A. and Mohlman, J. (2011). Deficient prefrontal attentional control in late-life generalized anxiety disorder: an fMRI investigation. *Translational Psychiatry*, 1, e46.

Proitsi, P., Lupton, M. K., Reeves, S. J., et al. (2012). Association of serotonin and dopamine gene pathways with behavioral subphenotypes in dementia. *Neurobiology of Aging*, 33(4), 791–803.

Radua, J., van den Heuvel, O. A., Surguladze, S. and Mataix-Cols, D. (2010). Meta-analytical comparison of voxel-based morphometry studies in obsessive-compulsive disorder vs other anxiety disorders. *Archives of General Psychiatry*, 67(7), 701–711.

Reynolds, C. A., Jansson, M., Gatz, M. and Pedersen, N. L. (2006). Longitudinal change in memory performance associated with *HTR2A* polymorphism. *Neurobiology of Aging*, 27(1), 150–154.

Ritchie, M. and Yeap, B. B. (2015). Thyroid hormone: influences on mood and cognition in adults. *Maturitas*, 81(2), 266–275.

Rodrigues, R., Petersen, R. B. and Perry, G. (2014). Parallels between major depressive disorder and Alzheimer's disease: role of oxidative stress and genetic vulnerability. *Cellular and Molecular Neurobiology*, 34(7), 925–949.

Salthouse, T. A. (1996). The processing-speed theory of adult age differences in cognition. *Psychological Review*, 103(3), 403–428.

Schultz, S. K., Moser, D. J., Bishop, J. R. and Ellingrod, V. L. (2005). Phobic anxiety in late-life in relationship to cognition and *5HTTLPR* polymorphism. *Psychiatric Genetics*, 15(4), 305–306.

Seignourel, P. J., Kunik, M. E., Snow, L., Wilson, N. and Stanley, M. (2008). Anxiety in dementia: a critical review. *Clinical Psychology Review*, 28, 1071–1082.

Sinoff, G. and Werner, P. (2003). Anxiety disorder and accompanying subjective memory loss in the elderly as a predictor of future cognitive decline. *International Journal of Geriatric Psychiatry*, 18(10), 951–959.

Stanley, M. A., Calleo, J., Bush, A. L., et al. (2013). The Peaceful Mind program: a pilot test of a cognitive–behavioral therapy-based intervention for anxious patients with dementia. *American Journal of Geriatric Psychiatry*, 21(7), 696–708.

Stein, M. B., Koverola, C., Hanna, C., Torchia, M. G. and McClarty, B. (1997). Hippocampal volume in women victimized by childhood sexual abuse. *Psychological Medicine*, 27(4), 951–959.

Stern, Y. (2002). What is cognitive reserve? Theory and research application of the reserve concept. *Journal of the International Neuropsychological Society*, 8(3), 448–460.

Suliman, S., Hemmings, S. J. and Seedat, S. (2013). Brain-derived neurotrophic factor (BDNF) protein levels in anxiety disorders: systematic review and meta-regression analysis. *Frontiers in Integrative Neuroscience*, 7, 55.

Suri, D., Veenit, V., Sarkar, A., et al. (2013). Early stress evokes age-dependent biphasic changes in hippocampal neurogenesis, BDNF expression, and cognition. *Biological Psychiatry*, 73(7), 658–666.

Tatsch, M. F., Bottino, C. M., Azevedo, D., et al. (2006). Neuropsychiatric symptoms in Alzheimer disease and cognitively impaired, nondemented elderly from a community-based sample in Brazil: prevalence and relationship with dementia severity. *American Journal of Geriatric Psychiatry*, 14(5), 438–445.

Teri, L., Ferretti, L. E., Gibbons, L. E., et al. (1999). Anxiety of Alzheimer's disease: prevalence, and comorbidity. *Journals of Gerontology. Series A, Biological Sciences and Medical Sciences*, 54(7), M348–M352.

Vøllestad, J., Sivertsen, B. and Nielsen, G. H. (2011). Mindfulness-based stress reduction for patients with anxiety disorders: evaluation in a randomized controlled trial. *Behaviour Research and Therapy*, 49, 281–288.

Ward, D. D., Summers, M. J., Saunders, N. L., Janssen, P., Stuart, K. E. and Vickers, J. C. (2014). *APOE* and *BDNF* Val66Met polymorphisms combine to influence episodic memory function in older adults. *Behavioural Brain Research*, 271, 309–315.

Wetherell, J. L., Reynolds, C. A., Gatz, M. and Pedersen, N. L. (2002). Anxiety, cognitive performance, and cognitive decline in normal aging. *Journals of Gerontology. Series B: Psychological Sciences and Social Sciences*, 57B(3), P246–P255.

Wetherell, J. L., Thorp, S. R., Patterson, T. L., Golshan, S., Jeste, D. V. and Gatz, M. (2004). Quality of life in geriatric generalized anxiety disorder: a preliminary investigation. *Journal of Psychiatric Research*, 38(3), 305–312.

Wu, Z., Guo, Z., Gearing, M. and Chen, G. (2014). Tonic inhibition in dentate gyrus impairs long-term potentiation and memory in an Alzheimer's disease model. *Nature Communications*, 5, 4159.

Yochim, B. P., Mueller, A. E. and Segal, D. L. (2013). Late life anxiety is associated with decreased memory and executive functioning in community dwelling older adults. *Journal of Anxiety Disorders*, **27**(6), 567–575.

Yudiatro, F. L., Muliadi, L., Moeljanto, D. and Hartono, B. (2006). Neuropsychological findings in hyperthyroid patients. *Acta Medica Indonesiana*, **38**(1), 6–10.

Anxiety in Parkinson's Disease

Chapter
9

Nadeeka N. W. Dissanayaka

Introduction

Parkinson's disease (PD) is a chronic, progressive, and disabling neurological disorder. The incidence of PD increases with age, and therefore the disease is predominantly observed in later life. The prevalence of PD is estimated at 1% in individuals aged 60 years and over, 2–3% in those aged 65 years and over, and 10% in those aged 80 years and over (de Rijk et al., 1997). In clinical practice, PD is classified as a *movement* disorder and is characterized by motor symptoms such as tremor, rigidity, bradykinesia, postural instability, and gait dysfunction. However, there are a large number of non-motor symptoms observed in PD, including neuropsychiatric complications, sleep disorders, fatigue, sensory symptoms, autonomic dysfunction, and gastrointestinal symptoms (Chaudhuri et al., 2011). Both motor and non-motor symptoms of PD negatively impact patients' quality of life (Chaudhuri et al., 2011; Schrag et al., 2000; Weintraub et al., 2004).

Anxiety is a prominent neuropsychiatric disturbance in PD and often coexists with depression (Dissanayaka et al., 2014). In comparison with depression, anxiety has received less attention in the medical scientific literature and is an emerging topic that has attracted increasing recognition within PD research. This chapter outlines the prevalence, symptomatology, assessment, characteristics, chronology, neurobiology, and treatment of anxiety in PD.

Prevalence and Anxiety Subtypes

The reported prevalence of anxiety disorders is variable due to differences in study samples and the methodology used to assess anxiety. Overall, the prevalence of current anxiety disorder according to diagnostic criteria such as the Diagnostic and Statistical Manual of Mental Disorders (DSM), the International Classification of Diseases (ICD), or by estimation from scores above published cut-off values on rating scales in general ranges between 12.8% and 43.0% (Chen et al., 2010; Dissanayaka et al., 2010; Hu et al., 2011; Khedr et al., 2012; Kulisevsky et al., 2008; Leentjens et al., 2011; Marinus et al., 2002; Menza et al., 1993; Negre-Pages et al., 2010; Ozdilek & Gunal, 2012; Pontone et al., 2009; Rodriguez-Blazquez et al., 2009; Shulman et al., 2001; Solla et al., 2011; Stefanova et al., 2013; Stein et al., 1990). A recent review estimated a point prevalence of 31% for anxiety in PD (Broen et al., 2016).

Subtypes of anxiety in PD include syndromal DSM disorders (those disorders that meet strict diagnostic criteria) and other clinically significant anxiety. Common DSM anxiety disorders observed in PD include generalized anxiety disorder (GAD), panic disorder with or without agoraphobia, and social phobia. The reported point prevalence of current GAD ranges between 0% and 30.8% (Chen & Marsh, 2014; Dissanayaka et al., 2010; Kummer et al., 2010; Lauterbach et al., 2003, 2004; Leentjens et al., 2011, 2012; Menza et al., 1993; Pontone et al., 2009; Qureshi et al., 2012; Stein et al., 1990). While some researchers have used hierarchical criteria when assessing GAD, others have included GAD symptoms as a disorder when they are considered to be secondary to another anxiety disorder (Dissanayaka et al., 2010; Leentjens et al., 2011). The prevalence of current panic disorder ranges between 1.8% and 25.0% (Chen et al., 2010; Dissanayaka et al., 2010; Lauterbach et al., 2003, 2004; Leentjens et al., 2011; Menza et al., 1993; Pontone et al., 2009; Qureshi et al., 2012; Stein et al., 1990), and current social phobia ranges between 0% and 50% (Bolluk et al., 2010; Chen et al., 2010; Dissanayaka et al., 2010; Lauterbach et al., 2004; Leentjens et al., 2011; Pontone et al., 2009). A recent study demonstrated the average prevalence rates of anxiety subtypes in PD as 14.0% GAD, 13.8% social phobia, 13.0% specific phobia, and 6.8% panic disorder with or without phobia (Broen et al., 2016).

Anxiety disorder not otherwise specified (NOS) in the DSM-IV criteria is another common subtype of clinically significant anxiety often described in the PD literature (Dissanayaka et al., 2014). The reported point prevalence of this DSM residual category of anxiety ranges between 2.0% and 26.7% (Chen et al., 2010; Dissanayaka et al., 2015b; Lauterbach et al., 2004; Leentjens et al., 2011; Menza et al., 1993; Pontone et al., 2009; Qureshi et al., 2012). On average, 13.3% experience anxiety disorder NOS (Broen et al., 2016). In DSM-5, this category is redefined as 'Unspecified Anxiety Disorder'. The DSM classifications of 'Anxiety due to a general medical condition', the medical condition being PD (or, in DSM-5, 'Anxiety due to another medical condition'), and 'Adjustment disorder with anxiety or adjustment disorder with mixed anxiety and depression' (i.e., adjustment to PD illness and its associated impairment and disability) are disregarded in PD research studies when diagnosing anxiety disorders. In the extant PD literature, significant anxiety that does not conform to a diagnosable anxiety disorder has been classified as anxiety disorder NOS rather than as anxiety due to a general medical condition or as medication-induced anxiety. To clarify the diagnosis of anxiety in PD, a revision of the anxiety diagnostic criteria would be useful, and a standardized set of criteria for PD-related anxiety should be developed in the future.

Symptomatology

Symptomatology of anxiety in PD is complex and relates to both general anxiety and anxiety due to PD-specific symptoms (Table 9.1) (Dissanayaka et al., 2016b). General anxiety symptoms commonly identified in PD include 'inability to relax' (Matheson et al., 2012; Mondolo et al., 2007), 'restlessness' (Brown et al., 2011; Marinus et al., 2002; Mondolo et al., 2007), 'feeling tense' (Brown et al., 2011; Leentjens et al., 2011; Marinus et al., 2002; Mondolo et al., 2007), and 'worrying thoughts' (Brown et al., 2011; Marinus et al., 2002; Matheson et al., 2012; Mondolo et al., 2007). Overlapping symptoms between PD and anxiety disorders such as sleep disturbance, fatigue, and autonomic symptoms of anxiety are also reported in PD (Brown et al., 2011; Leentjens et al., 2011, 2012; Macht et al., 2005). It is recommended that clinicians use an inclusive approach when a patient presents with overlapping symptoms. A large multicentre cross-sectional study in PD patients noted that social phobia is often associated with fear of losing control, while PD patients with GAD also present with panic-like symptoms such as palpitations, shortness of breath, sweating, trembling, and fears of dying or choking (Leentjens et al., 2011).

Anxiety symptoms relating to the disease can be explained by many PD-specific factors, including: (1) having a chronic, disabling, and incurable condition; (2) motor symptoms; (3)

Table 9.1 General and Parkinson's disease (PD)-specific anxiety symptoms commonly observed in people living with PD.

Anxiety	Symptoms
General anxiety symptoms	Inability to relax
	Restlessness
	Feeling tense
	Worrying thoughts
	Sleep disturbances
	Fatigue
	Autonomic symptoms of anxiety
PD-specific anxiety symptoms	
Chronic, incurable, and disabling disease	Distress
	Insecurity/fear
	Worry about future
Motor symptoms	Worry
	Embarrassment and withdrawal
	Fear of postural instability and falling
	Panic associated with freezing of gait
Non-motor symptoms	Worry due to non-motor symptoms
	Frustrations and fear about cognitive impairment
Complications of medication	Worry due to motor fluctuations and dyskinesias
	Enhanced anxiety at 'off' times
	Worry and fear of 'off' periods
	Anxiety relating to impulse control disorders, dopamine dysregulation syndrome, and dopamine agonist withdrawal syndrome
Neurosurgical treatment	Anxiety relating to expectations and reality
	Dopamine agonist withdrawal syndrome

non-motor symptoms; (4) complications of pharmacotherapy; and (5) neurosurgical treatment (Table 9.1). A high proportion (68%) of PD patients reports an association between enhanced motor symptoms and arousal. Patients have also indicated stress due to disability and needing help (38%) (Macht et al., 2005). Fear of falling is also common within PD patients and makes a significant contribution towards a poorer quality of life (Bloem et al., 2001; Pontone et al., 2009; Rahman et al., 2011).

Anxiety relating to motor fluctuations is complex, and often anxiety is exacerbated during motor 'off' periods (Leentjens et al., 2012). Excessive and recurrent situational anxiety associated with the wearing off of PD medication is observed in patients with anxiety disorder NOS (Kulisevsky et al., 2007; Pontone et al., 2009). Anxiety in PD is also linked to iatrogenic addictive behaviours such as impulse control disorders (ICDs) and dopamine dysregulation syndrome (DDS), as well as being associated with dopamine agonist withdrawal syndrome (DAWS) (Ambermoon et al., 2011, 2012). High levels of stress can occur leading up to invasive neurosurgical therapy such as deep brain stimulation (DBS), which is increasingly common as a treatment for PD. Withdrawal of dopaminergic medication post-surgical treatment can result in DAWS and contribute to a risk of developing anxiety (Castrioto et al., 2014).

A recent study evaluated the frequency of 30 disease-specific symptoms of anxiety in 90 persons with PD (Dissanayaka et al., 2016b). Common PD-specific anxiety symptoms found at >25% frequency included distress, worry, fear, agitation, embarrassment, and social withdrawal due to motor symptoms and PD medication complications. These symptoms were experienced commonly in patients meeting DSM-IV criteria for an anxiety disorder, suggesting the need to evaluate PD-specific anxiety symptomatology for targeted treatment.

Assessment of Anxiety Using Rating Scales

Despite the high prevalence of anxiety disorders in PD, assessment of anxiety remains a challenge in clinical practice. As a consequence, anxiety is often under-diagnosed and under-treated in PD (Dissanayaka et al., 2014). As discussed earlier, a high proportion of PD patients experience significant levels of anxiety, which often cannot adequately be captured by existing diagnostic criteria for anxiety disorders. The overlap between anxiety symptoms and PD symptoms such as autonomic dysfunction, fatigue, and sleep disturbances complicates assessment of anxious patients. Moreover, the current rating scales available to assess anxiety do not adequately capture the unique characteristics of PD-specific anxiety, and there remains the need to develop a new validated PD-specific scale for better identification of anxiety in this highly vulnerable patient group.

Researchers have examined the validity of general anxiety scales for use in PD (Dissanayaka et al., 2015a). The Hamilton Anxiety Rating Scale (HAM-A) and the Hospital Anxiety and Depression Scale (HADS) are widely studied scales within PD (Forjaz et al., 2013; Kummer et al., 2010; Leentjens et al., 2011; Marinus et al., 2002; Mondolo et al., 2007; Rodriguez-Blazquez et al., 2009; Stefanova et al., 2013). Overall, both scales have demonstrated good reliability but poor discriminant validity. While the HAM-A is suggested as an appropriate scale to assess GAD in PD, the HADS is not recommended for use as a diagnostic or screening tool in PD. Likewise, the Beck Anxiety Inventory (BAI) is not recommended for use in PD due to limitations in item content and validity (Forjaz et al., 2013; Leentjens et al., 2011). While the validity of the Zung Self-Rated Anxiety Scale (SAS) and the Anxiety Status Inventory (ASI) in PD has not been investigated (Leentjens et al., 2008), a few studies have examined the validity of the Spielberger State–Trait Anxiety Inventory (STAI), the Liebowitz Social Anxiety Scale (LSAS), the Neuropsychiatric Inventory – Anxiety subscale (NPI-Anxiety), and the Movement Disorders Society Unified Parkinson's Disease Rating Scale (MDS-UPDRS) – Anxiety item; all of these scales have shown at least some evidence for discriminant validity, suggesting the need for further investigation (Gallagher et al., 2012; Kummer et al., 2008; Leentjens et al., 2011; Matheson et al., 2012; Mondolo et al., 2007; Stefanova et al., 2013).

There are two new anxiety scales validated in PD and deemed appropriate to use in this patient population: the Geriatric Anxiety Inventory (GAI) and the Parkinson's Disease Anxiety Scale (PAS) (Leentjens et al., 2014; Matheson et al., 2012). The GAI is a 20-item self-report scale with a dichotomous response set for easy administration (Pachana et al., 2007). It was designed for the purposes of evaluating the severity of current anxiety and largely avoids somatic symptoms that overlap between anxiety and PD. The PAS is a 12-item scale that is available in two versions: self-report and observer report. The item response set includes a five-point Likert scale ranging from 0 ('Not or never') to 4 ('Severe or almost always'). The scale is divided into three subsections of persistent anxiety, episodic anxiety, and avoidance behaviour. Both the GAI and the PAS have demonstrated good validity and reliability in non-demented patients with PD (Leentjens et al., 2014; Matheson et al., 2012). However, both of these validity studies included a DSM-IV diagnosis of syndromal anxiety disorders and did not consider the residual, highly prevalent category of anxiety disorder NOS. Research is required to investigate the usefulness of rating scales to identify this sub-syndromal anxiety in PD. In addition, the majority of validity studies have excluded PD patients with dementia, and research focused on assessing anxiety in this group is required.

Characteristics and Chronology

Identifying general and PD-specific characteristics of syndromal and sub-syndromal anxiety in PD may assist with both clinical diagnosis and management. Many studies have suggested that female gender (Dissanayaka et al., 2015b; Leentjens et al., 2011; Mondolo et al., 2007; Negre-Pages et al., 2010; Picillo et al., 2013; Solla et al., 2011, 2012), younger age (Bolluk et al., 2010; Dissanayaka et al., 2010, 2015b; Negre-Pages et al., 2010; Pontone et al., 2009), a previous history of anxiety (Dissanayaka et al., 2010; Jacob et al., 2010; Leentjens et al., 2011; Richard et al., 2004,), a younger age of PD onset (Burn et al., 2012; Chen et al., 2010; Dissanayaka et al., 2010), longer duration of PD (Bogdanova & Cronin-Golomb, 2012; Khedr et al., 2012; Kulisevsky et al., 2008; Kummer et al., 2010; Siemers et al., 1993; Stefanova et al., 2013), more severe stages of PD (Bolluk et al., 2010; Dissanayaka et al., 2010, 2015b; Khedr et al., 2012; Kulisevsky et al., 2008; Manor et al., 2009; Stefanova et al., 2013), and the presence of complications of PD therapy are associated with anxiety in PD. The presence of motor fluctuations is one of the strongest predictors of anxiety in PD (Burn et al., 2012; Dissanayaka et al., 2010; Erdal, 2001; Leentjens et al., 2011, 2012; Menza et al., 1993; Solla et al., 2011; Stefanova et al., 2013). Anxious patients are likely to report a greater number of life stressors and a poorer PD-related quality of life compared to those without anxiety (Dissanayaka et al., 2010, 2015b; Rodriguez-Violante et al., 2013) (Table 9.2).

Onset of anxiety in PD can occur before or after a diagnosis of PD (Figure 9.1). While the onset of anxiety can occur at different stages during the course of PD, some research has suggested that anxiety may be a risk factor or an early non-motor marker for PD (Bower et al., 2010; Shiba et al., 2000; Weisskopf et al., 2003). A high proportion (64%) of PD patients also develop significant anxiety after their diagnosis of PD (Dissanayaka et al., 2016b). Both psychological and neurobiological factors may influence the onset of anxiety following a diagnosis of PD. Psychological explanations stem from disease-specific anxious symptoms due to motor disability and complications of medications such as motor fluctuations, dyskinesias, and ICDs (Table 9.1). Neurobiological explanations demonstrate common pathological mechanisms between anxiety and PD motor symptoms (Ceravolo et al., 2013; Moriyama et al., 2011).

Table 9.2 General and disease-specific characteristics of anxiety in Parkinson's disease (PD).

General	Female gender
	Younger age
	Previous history of anxiety
	More life stressors
PD-specific	Younger age of PD onset
	Longer duration of PD
	More severe stages of PD
	Motor fluctuations

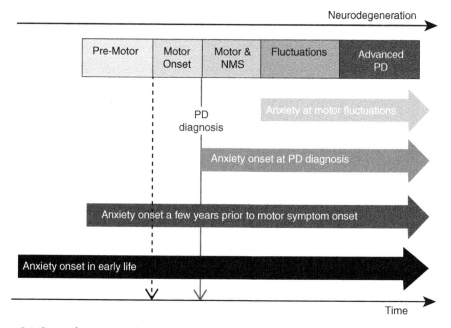

Figure 9.1 Onset of anxiety in relation to a diagnosis of Parkinson's disease. NMS = non-motor symptoms; PD = Parkinson's disease. *Source:* Adapted from Dissanayaka et al. (2016b).

Neurobiology

Alterations in the dopaminergic neurotransmitter system, which is the primary neurotransmitter system implicated in PD, can be directly linked to a high risk of anxiety in PD. Involvement of the dopaminergic system is clinically demonstrated by having high levels of anxiety when dopaminergic medication is withdrawn following DBS or the development of ICDs and during the wearing-off period of dopaminergic medication (Ambermoon et al., 2011, 2012; Castrioto et al., 2014; Leentjens et al., 2012). While plasma levodopa levels are positively correlated with anxiety (Kulisevsky et al., 2007), neuroanatomical alterations in PD such as the degeneration of the mesolimbic and mesocortical dopaminergic pathways can also be associated with a high prevalence of anxiety in PD (Peron et al., 2012).

Single-photon emission computed tomography studies have demonstrated upregulation (Ceravolo et al., 2013; Moriyama et al., 2011) and downregulation (Erro et al., 2012; Weintraub et al., 2005) of striatal dopamine transporter densities in PD, which may explain fluctuations of anxiety symptoms along with motor fluctuations in PD. Positron emission tomography studies have suggested an inverse correlation between anxiety and binding value in the left ventral striatum, caudate, locus coeruleus, inferior thalamic region, bilateral amygdala, and medial thalamus (Huang et al., 2013; Remy et al., 2005). However, an imaging study did not find any significant relationship between anxiety in PD and the caudate and putamen (Tinaz et al., 2011).

The amygdala is a key brain structure involved in the anxious phenotype, and a dysfunctional amygdala is seen in PD (Peron et al., 2012). Tessitore et al. (2002) suggested a significantly lower level of amygdala activity in PD within a functional magnetic resonance imaging study, and they demonstrated that dopaminergic therapy only partially restores this loss of amygdala activity. A post-mortem study has demonstrated degeneration of the amygdala in PD (Harding et al., 2002), which may account for the reduction in amygdala activity in PD. A T1-weighted imaging study further supported the existence of an inverse relationship between anxiety and volume of the left amygdala in PD (Vriend et al., 2016).

While a diffusion tensor imaging (DTI) study has shown degeneration of projections to anterior cingulate bundles with depression in PD (Matsui et al., 2007), at the time of writing there have been no DTI studies focused on anxiety in PD (Wen et al., 2016). Other dysfunctional neural networks associated with anxiety disorders in general, such as the cingulo-opercular, frontoparietal, ventral attention, and default mode, suggest an association with anxiety disorders (Sylvester et al., 2012), which could be further studied in the context of PD in the future.

Apart from the dopaminergic system, there are a number of other neurotransmitter systems implicated in PD (Prediger et al., 2012). Serotonergic and noradrenergic systems are additional primary neurotransmitter systems suggested to be altered in PD, and they are also the systems that play a primary role in anxiety. The Braak staging of PD suggests that brainstem structures such as the serotonergic raphe nucleus and the noradrenergic locus coeruleus are degenerated in the early stages of PD (Braak et al., 2004). Such early deficits may help to explain the development of anxiety during the pre-motor stages of PD (Jacob et al., 2010). The locus coeruleus is also a key brain area that has been recently linked to the progression of PD and cognitive deficits in advanced PD (Del Tredici & Braak, 2013), and therefore it may be implicated in the development of anxiety during the motor phase of PD. Further research is required to advance understanding of neuroanatomical alterations in anxiety in the context of PD.

There is limited research investigating the genetic associations of anxiety in PD. Menza et al. (1999) showed an association between PD anxiety and the serotonin transporter gene, *5HTT*, long/short polymorphism. The G196A polymorphism of brain-derived neurotrophic factor (*BDNF*) is another genetic polymorphism studied in the context of PD and anxiety. BDNF is important in neural cell growth and survival, and it has been shown to protect dopaminergic neurons from degeneration (Hyman et al., 1991). However, no association was found between the G196A polymorphism and anxiety in PD (Svetel et al., 2013). Studies replicating these genetic findings are required to confirm these results.

Interestingly, rodent studies have shown anxiety-like behaviours in models expressing mutant (A53T) human α-synuclein, a protein that has been linked to the pathology of PD. By using the elevated-plus maze and the open field test, these studies have indicated an increase (Kim et al., 2014; Marxreiter et al., 2013), decrease (George et al., 2008; Graham & Sidhu, 2010; Rothman et al., 2013; Yamakado et al., 2012), or no difference (Pena-Oliver et al., 2010) in anxious behaviour in transgenic as compared with wild-type rodents. An increase in anxiety-like behaviour was also observed in another study with transgenic mice overexpressing A30P α-synuclein. Of particular interest is that treatment with doxycycline has been shown to reverse anxiety-like behaviours in these transgenic mice (Marxreiter et al., 2013). The role of α-synuclein in the pathology of anxiety in PD warrants future research.

Treatment

There is a paucity of both pharmacological and non-pharmacological treatment trials focused on anxiety in PD, and currently there is no gold standard of treatment that can be recommended to treat anxiety in PD. In clinical practice, the management of PD is primarily directed towards control of physical symptoms rather than management of psychological symptoms, and therefore common psychological symptoms like anxiety are often poorly treated (Pachana et al., 2013). When psychological issues are addressed, pharmacotherapy is typically focused on co-morbid depression, and anxiety is often treated secondarily (Chen & Marsh, 2014).

Despite limited supporting evidence, benzodiazepines and selective serotonin reuptake inhibitors (SSRIs) are generally preferred as the pharmacological treatments of choice for anxiety in PD (Casacchia et al., 1975; Chen & Marsh, 2014; Connolly & Fox, 2014; Djamshidian & Friedman, 2014). The only randomized controlled trial (RCT) focused on the drug treatment of anxiety in PD used the benzodiazepine bromazepam and demonstrated improvement in anxious symptoms (Casacchia et al., 1975). In addition, there has been a case report suggesting clonazepam as an effective treatment for a patient with panic disorder who was refractory to alprazolam, lorazepam, and a number of antidepressants (Chuang & Fahn, 2001). Although benzodiazepines can be useful for PD patients with anxiety and co-morbid sleep disturbances, they can cause unfavourable effects on alertness, cognition, and gait and elevate the risk of falls (Cumming & Le Couteur, 2003).

A number of case studies have reported SSRIs including citalopram (Menza et al., 2004), paroxetine (Tarczy & Szombathelyi, 1998), and sertraline (Shulman et al., 1996) as effective for anxiety in PD. However, a recent large ($n = 115$) RCT focused on treatment for depression did not show improvement in secondary anxiety with paroxetine or the selective noradrenaline reuptake inhibitor venlafaxine extended release (Richard et al., 2012). SSRIs are relatively well tolerated, although adverse effects such as agitation, akathisia, nausea, diarrhoea, insomnia, and somnolence can occur. Use of SSRIs can result in hyponatremia, sexual dysfunction, and weight gain (Chen & Marsh, 2014). Importantly, higher levels of anxiety are associated with poorer responses to antidepressant treatment in depressed PD patients, and therefore more intensive and targeted alternative treatment strategies are required for such severe and treatment-resistant patients (Moonen et al., 2014).

Psychotherapeutic approaches are likely to be critical for the effective treatment of anxiety in PD (Pachana et al., 2013). Cognitive behavioural therapy (CBT) has been the primary psychotherapy approach trialled in PD. However, these CBT studies have mainly focused on depression, and anxiety has been examined only as a secondary outcome measure (Armento et al., 2012). There are two case studies using one patient each focused on GAD and social phobia. Both studies showed improvement in anxiety following treatment (Heinrichs et al., 2001; Mohlman et al., 2010). A recent uncontrolled CBT study using 12 PD patients with anxiety demonstrated a significant reduction in anxiety after 6 weeks of CBT sessions (Dissanayaka et al., 2017). The primary outcome of reducing anxiety was maintained at 3 and 6 months of follow-up. This manualized and tailored CBT protocol for PD patients included a dyadic approach in which caregivers were included when delivering CBT to patients, and outcomes for caregivers were also assessed. A significant reduction in carer burden was observed post-CBT.

Two small telephone-based CBT studies investigating anxiety and depression demonstrated reductions in anxiety in PD (Dobkin et al., 2011b; Veazey et al., 2009). The first, a study by Veazey et al. (2009), randomly allocated 14 PD patients into treatment or support groups and used the BAI to measure change in anxiety pre- and post-treatment. The second, an uncontrolled study by Dobkin et al. (2011b), included both PD patients and caregivers (21 each) and used the HAM-A to assess anxiety.

There is one large RCT by Dobkin et al. (2011a) including 80 depressed PD patients in which 10 weekly individualized CBT sessions modified for PD were applied. In this study, anxiety measured by the HAM-A as a secondary outcome demonstrated significant improvement in patients who received the treatment compared to the clinical monitoring control group. Gains were sustained at the 14-week follow-up. Interestingly, a second study was conducted using caregivers of these patients where caregivers received four weekly treatment sessions. In this study, the involvement of a caregiver was a strong predictor of treatment outcomes, highlighting the need for psychotherapy for the caregivers of PD patients (Dobkin et al., 2012).

Troeung et al. (2014) conducted a waitlist-controlled trial focusing on depression and anxiety in 18 PD patients. Using the Depression, Anxiety and Stress Scale (DASS-21), this study demonstrated a significant reduction in anxiety following an 8-week group CBT treatment, and the benefits were sustained at the 6-month follow-up. Although the validity of the DASS-21 has not been explored (Dissanayaka et al., 2015a), Troeung et al. (2014) were the first to demonstrate the efficacy of group CBT for PD. Okai et al. (2013) also conducted a waitlist-controlled CBT study in 27 PD patients with impulse control behaviours in PD. A significant reduction in secondary anxiety (measured by the BAI) was observed after 12 CBT sessions. Two other small CBT studies that used the STAI to assess anxiety showed no significant change in anxiety post-treatment in comparison to baseline (Dobkin et al., 2007; Feeney et al., 2005). The STAI has not demonstrated satisfactory psychometric properties when used in PD, and the four-point response options of this scale may be difficult for PD patients to complete because the majority of patients are older adults who present with some cognitive problems (Dissanayaka et al., 2015a).

A study by Kraepelien et al. (2015) explored the usefulness of Internet-based CBT (ICBT) for the treatment of depression and anxiety in nine PD patients. Using the HADS, they showed a reduction in anxiety symptoms; however, patients found the ICBT method too complex and preferred more input from therapists. This was the first study to explore the usefulness of Internet-based therapy for PD patients with co-morbid depression and anxiety. Such low-cost approaches are useful for persons living in rural areas who have limited access to psychologists and for those who are unable to travel (e.g., due to disability or transportation barriers stemming from PD) to receive treatment. However, the co-morbid cognitive impairment commonly observed in PD patients may limit the effectiveness of ICBT.

Apart from CBT, there are other psychotherapy approaches trialled for anxiety in PD (Yang et al., 2012). While group psychodrama (Sproesser et al., 2010) and Patient Education Program Parkinson's (PEPP) (A'Campo et al., 2010) suggested improvements in anxiety, a multidisciplinary rehabilitation approach showed no change in anxious symptoms (Trend et al., 2002; Wade et al., 2003). Mindfulness-based stress reduction is another psychological intervention trialled in PD (Advocat et al., 2013, 2016; Birtwell et al., 2017; Bogosian et al., 2017; Dissanayaka et al., 2016a; Fitzpatrick et al., 2010; McLean et al., 2017; Pickut et al., 2015). The majority of these studies did not include a validated measure of anxiety in PD and did not directly focus on PD patients with anxiety. Mindfulness was tested as a lifestyle program in PD rather than an intervention to reduce anxiety in PD. However, recent studies demonstrated significant reductions in anxiety following mindfulness interventions in PD (Advocat et al., 2016; Dissanayaka et al., 2016a).

Overall, CBT appears to be an effective treatment for anxiety in PD when examined secondarily to depression or impulse control behaviours. Therefore, studies primarily focused on anxiety are required. The effectiveness of other psychotherapy approaches such as the mindfulness therapy and acceptance and commitment therapy also warrant future investigations. Such new studies should be carefully designed to enhance the effectiveness of the intervention. This can be achieved by (Figure 9.2):

(1) Modifying the content of sessions tailored for the specific needs of PD patients;

(2) Developing more targeted treatments for subgroups of PD patients such as those with dementia or who have had functional neurosurgery (e.g., DBS);

(3) Inclusion of follow-up and booster sessions for longer periods such as 6-month and 12-month reviews for examination of the long-term sustainability of the treatment;

(4) Inclusion of caregivers in patient treatment sessions;

(5) Randomization of participants with an appropriate control group;

(6) Including cost-effective group therapy sessions while designing individualized therapy for treatment-resistant patients who require more targeted intervention;

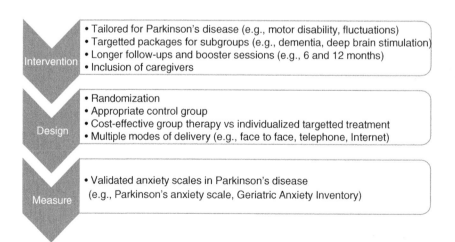

Figure 9.2 Items to consider when developing psychotherapy studies for Parkinson's disease.

(7) Trialling various delivery modes such as the telephone and Internet to allow access to therapy for those living in rural and remote areas with limited psychologists and PD patients with severe disability who are unable to travel;

(8) Using an anxiety measure with appropriate validity and reliability in PD such as the PAS or the GAI to evaluate the efficacy of the treatment.

Conclusion

Over 50% of PD patients experience significant anxiety symptoms that contribute to a detrimental impact on patients' quality of life. According to conventional diagnostic criteria such as the DSM, GAD, panic disorder, and social phobia are common syndromal anxiety disorders observed in PD. Moreover, a DSM-IV residual category of anxiety disorder NOS is often described in PD. Patients within this group present with significant anxiety that cannot be described as a subtype of a syndromal DSM-IV disorder. Symptomatology of anxiety in PD is complex and consists of characteristics unique to PD such as anxiety relating to the wearing off of PD medications and related motor fluctuations and episodic anxiety, including panic attacks, associated with motor impairment (e.g., freezing of gait). Such complex symptomatology makes diagnosis of anxiety difficult, and there is a need to develop standardized criteria for a diagnosis of anxiety disorders in PD. On the other hand, this unique symptomatology of anxiety in PD results in difficulties in assessing anxiety using rating scales developed for measuring anxiety in general, non-neurological populations. Validity studies of anxiety rating scales in PD suggest that popular anxiety rating instruments such as the HAM-A and the BAI are inappropriate for the assessment of anxiety in PD. A new PD anxiety scale (i.e., PAS) was recently developed and validated; however, this scale is general and does not address PD-specific anxiety symptoms. A need remains to develop a disease-specific anxiety scale that can capture both general and PD-specific symptomatology, ensuring all significant anxiety is captured and appropriately treated.

Anxiety in PD is positively associated with female gender, younger age, previous history of anxiety, younger age of PD onset, longer duration of PD, more severe stages of PD, having complications of PD therapy including motor fluctuations and iatrogenic addictive behaviours, and more reporting of life stressors. Investigations focused on the chronology of anxiety in relation to a diagnosis of PD and the neurobiological contributions to the risk of anxiety are important when conceptualizing the phenomenology of this neuropsychiatric manifestation in PD. There is a consensus that PD and anxiety may have shared neurobiological factors and that anxiety may be a first symptom of PD appearing prior to the onset of motor symptoms. Further research is required to advance our understanding of the neurobiological and genetic contributions to anxiety in PD.

There is a lack of clinical trials investigating the treatment of anxiety in PD. Anxiety is often examined secondarily to depression, although in PD a large proportion of patients experience significant anxiety without co-morbid depression. Despite limited trials, pharmacological treatments such as benzodiazepines and SSRIs are currently deemed favourable for the treatment of PD anxiety. In addition to pharmacotherapy, psychotherapy approaches may prove effective in alleviating anxiety in PD. Well-controlled and long-term psychotherapy studies tailored for PD-specific anxiety symptoms warrant further research in order to develop efficient, effective, and targeted treatment for anxiety in PD.

References

A'Campo, L. E., Wekking, E. M., Spliethoff-Kamminga, N. G., Le Cessie, S. and Roos, R. A. (2010). The benefits of a standardized patient education program for patients with Parkinson's disease and their caregivers. *Parkinsonism & Related Disorders*, **16**, 89–95.

Advocat, J., Enticott, J., Vandenberg, B., Hassed, C., Hester, J. and Russell, G. (2016). The effects of a mindfulness-based lifestyle program for adults with Parkinson's disease: a mixed methods, wait list controlled randomised control study. *BMC Neurology*, **16**, 166.

Advocat, J., Russell, G., Enticott, J., Hassed, C., Hester, J. and Vandenberg, B. (2013). The effects of a mindfulness-based lifestyle programme for adults with Parkinson's disease: protocol for a mixed methods, randomised two-group control study. *BMJ Open*, **3**, e003326.

Ambermoon, P., Carter, A., Hall, W., Dissanayaka, N. and O'Sullivan, J. (2011). Impulse control disorders in patients with Parkinson's disease receiving dopamine replacement therapy: evidence and implications for the addictions field. *Addiction*, **106**, 283–293.

Ambermoon, P., Carter, A., Hall, W., Dissanayaka, N. and O'Sullivan, J. (2012). Compulsive use of dopamine replacement therapy: a model for stimulant drug addiction? *Addiction*, **107**, 241–247.

Armento, M. E. A., Stanley, M. A., Marsh, L., et al. (2012). Cognitive behavioral therapy for depression and anxiety in Parkinson's disease: a clinical review. *Journal of Parkinson's Disease*, **2**, 135–151.

Birtwell, K., Dubrow-Marshall, L., Dubrow-Marshall, R., Duerden, T. and Dunn, A. (2017). A mixed methods evaluation of a mindfulness-based stress reduction course for people with Parkinson's disease. *Complementary Therapies in Clinical Practice*, **29**, 220–228.

Bloem, B. R., Grimbergen, Y. A., Cramer, M., Willemsen, M. and Zwinderman, A. H. (2001). Prospective assessment of falls in Parkinson's disease. *Journal of Neurology*, **248**, 950–958.

Bogdanova, Y. and Cronin-Golomb, A. (2012). Neurocognitive correlates of apathy and anxiety in Parkinson's disease. *Parkinson's Disease* **2012**, 793076.

Bogosian, A., Hurt, C. S., Vasconcelos, E. S. D., Hindle, J. V., McCracken, L. and Cubi-Molla, P. (2017). Distant delivery of a mindfulness-based intervention for people with Parkinson's disease: the study protocol of a randomised pilot trial. *Pilot and Feasibility Studies*, **3**, 4.

Bolluk, B., Ozel-Kizil, E. T., Akbostanci, M. C. and Atbasoglu, E. C. (2010). Social anxiety in patients with Parkinson's disease. *Journal of Neuropsychiatry and Clinical Neurosciences*, **22**, 390–394.

Bower, J. H., Grossardt, B. R., Maraganore, D. M., et al. (2010). Anxious personality predicts an increased risk of Parkinson's disease. *Movement Disorders*, **25**, 2105–2113.

Braak, H., Ghebremedhin, E., Rub, U., Bratzke, H. and Del Tredici, K. (2004). Stages in the development of Parkinson's disease-related pathology. *Cell and Tissue Research*, **318**, 121–134.

Broen, M. P., Narayen, N. E., Kuijf, M. L., Dissanayaka, N. N. and Leentjens, A. F. (2016). Prevalence of anxiety in Parkinson's disease: a systematic review and meta-analysis. *Movement Disorders*, **31**, 1125–1133.

Brown, R. G., Landau, S., Hindle, J. V., et al. (2011). Depression and anxiety related subtypes in Parkinson's disease. *Journal of Neurology, Neurosurgery, and Psychiatry*, **82**, 803–809.

Burn, D. J., Landau, S., Hindle, J. V., et al. (2012). Parkinson's disease motor subtypes and mood. *Movement Disorders*, **27**, 379–386.

Casacchia, M., Zamponi, A., Squitieri, G. and Meco, G. (1975). Treatment of anxiety in Parkinson's disease with bromazepam. *Rivista di Neurologia*, **45**, 326–338.

Castrioto, A., Lhommee, E., Moro, E. and Krack, P. (2014). Mood and behavioural effects of subthalamic stimulation in Parkinson's disease. *Lancet Neurology*, **13**, 287–305.

Ceravolo, R., Frosini, D., Poletti, M., et al. (2013). Mild affective symptoms in *de novo* Parkinson's disease patients: relationship with dopaminergic dysfunction. *European Journal of Neurology*, **20**, 480–485.

Chaudhuri, K. R., Odin, P., Antonini, A. and Martinez-Martin, P. (2011). Parkinson's disease: the non-motor issues. *Parkinsonism & Related Disorders*, **17**, 717–723.

Chen, J. J. and Marsh, L. (2014). Anxiety in Parkinson's disease: identification and management. *Therapeutic Advances in Neurological Disorders*, **7**, 52–59.

Chen, Y. K., Lu, J. Y., Chan, D. M., et al. (2010). Anxiety disorders in Chinese patients with Parkinson's disease. *International Journal of Psychiatry in Medicine*, **40**, 97–107.

Chuang, C. and Fahn, S. (2001). Dramatic benefit with clonazepam treatment of intractable anxiety and panic attacks in Parkinson's disease [abstract]. *Movement Disorders*, **16**, S35.

Connolly, B. and Fox, S. H. (2014). Treatment of cognitive, psychiatric, and affective disorders associated with Parkinson's disease. *Neurotherapeutics*, **11**, 78–91.

Cumming, R. G. and Le Couteur, D. G. (2003). Benzodiazepines and risk of hip fractures in older people: a review of the evidence. *CNS Drugs*, **17**, 825–837.

de Rijk, M. C., Tzourio, C., Breteler, M. M., et al. (1997). Prevalence of Parkinsonism and Parkinson's disease in Europe: the EUROPARKINSON Collaborative Study. European Community Concerted Action on the Epidemiology of Parkinson's disease. *Journal of Neurology, Neurosurgery, and Psychiatry*, **62**, 10–15.

Del Tredici, K. and Braak, H. (2013). Dysfunction of the locus coeruleus–norepinephrine system and related circuitry in Parkinson's disease-related dementia. *Journal of Neurology, Neurosurgery, and Psychiatry*, **84**, 774–783.

Dissanayaka, N. N., Idu Jion, F., Pachana, N. A., et al. (2016a). Mindfulness for motor and nonmotor dysfunctions in Parkinson's disease. *Parkinson's Disease*, **2016**, 7109052.

Dissanayaka, N. N. W., O'Sullivan, J. D., Pachana, N. A., et al. (2016b). Disease specific anxiety symptoms in Parkinson's disease *International Psychogeriatrics*, **28**, 1153–1163.

Dissanayaka, N. N. W., Pye, D., Mitchell, L. K., et al. (2017). Cognitive behavior therapy for anxiety in Parkinson's disease: outcomes for patients and caregivers. *Clinical Gerontology*, **40**, 159–171.

Dissanayaka, N. N. W., Sellbach, A., Matheson, S., et al. (2010). Anxiety disorders in Parkinson's disease: prevalence and risk factors. *Movement Disorders*, **25**, 838–845.

Dissanayaka, N. N. W., Torbey, E. and Pachana, N. (2015a). Anxiety rating scales in Parkinson's disease: a critical review updating recent literature. *International Psychogeriatrics*, **27**, 1777–1784.

Dissanayaka, N. N. W., White, E., O'Sullivan, J. D., Marsh, R., Pachana, N. A. and Byrne, G. J. (2014). The clinical spectrum of anxiety in Parkinson's disease. *Movement Disorders*, **29**, 967–975.

Dissanayaka, N. N. W., White, E., O'Sullivan, J. D., et al. (2015b). Characteristics and treatment of anxiety disorders in Parkinson's disease. *Movement Disorders Clinical Practice*, **2**, 155–162.

Djamshidian, A. and Friedman, J. H. (2014). Anxiety and depression in Parkinson's disease. *Current Treatment Options in Neurology*, **16**, 285.

Dobkin, R. D., Allen, L. A. and Menza, M. (2007). Cognitive-behavioral therapy for depression in Parkinson's disease: a pilot study. *Movement Disorders*, **22**, 946–52.

Dobkin, R. D., Menza, M., Allen, L. A., et al. (2011a). Cognitive–behavioral therapy for depression in Parkinson's disease: a randomized, controlled trial. *American Journal of Psychiatry*, **168**, 1066–1074.

Dobkin, R. D., Menza, M., Allen, L. A., et al. (2011b). Telephone-based cognitive–behavioral therapy for depression in Parkinson disease. *Journal of Geriatric Psychiatry and Neurology*, **24**, 206–214.

Dobkin, R. D., Rubino, J. T., Allen, L. A., et al. (2012). Predictors of treatment response to cognitive–behavioral therapy for depression in Parkinson's disease. *Journal of Consulting and Clinical Psychology*, 80, 694–699.

Erdal, K. J. (2001). Depression and anxiety in persons with Parkinson's disease with and without 'on–off' phenomena. *Journal of Clinical Psychology in Medical Settings*, 8, 293–299.

Erro, R., Pappata, S., Amboni, M., et al. (2012). Anxiety is associated with striatal dopamine transporter availability in newly diagnosed untreated Parkinson's disease patients. *Parkinsonism & Related Disorders*, 18, 1034–1038.

Feeney, F., Egan, S. and Gasson, N. (2005). Treatment of depression and anxiety in Parkinson's disease: a pilot study using group cognitive behavioural therapy. *Clinical Psychologist*, 9, 31–38.

Fitzpatrick, L., Simpson, J. and Smith, A. (2010). A qualitative analysis of mindfulness-based cognitive therapy (MBCT) in Parkinson's disease. *Psychology and Psychotherapy*, 83, 179–192.

Forjaz, M. J., Martinez-Martin, P., Dujardin, K., et al. (2013). Rasch analysis of anxiety scales in Parkinson's disease. *Journal of Psychosomatic Research*, 74, 414–419.

Gallagher, D. A., Goetz, C. G., Stebbins, G., Lees, A. J. and Schrag, A. (2012). Validation of the MDS-UPDRS Part I for nonmotor symptoms in Parkinson's disease. *Movement Disorders*, 27, 79–83.

George, S., Van Den Buuse, M., San Mok, S., Masters, C. L., Li, Q. X. and Culvenor, J. G. (2008). Alpha-synuclein transgenic mice exhibit reduced anxiety-like behaviour. *Experimental Neurology*, 210, 788–792.

Graham, D. R. and Sidhu, A. (2010). Mice expressing the A53T mutant form of human alpha-synuclein exhibit hyperactivity and reduced anxiety-like behavior. *Journal of Neuroscience Research*, 88, 1777–1783.

Harding, A. J., Stimson, E., Henderson, J. M. and Halliday, G. M. (2002). Clinical correlates of selective pathology in the amygdala of patients with Parkinson's disease. *Brain*, 125, 2431–2445.

Heinrichs, N., Hoffman, E. C. and Hofmann, S. G. (2001). Cognitive–behavioral treatment for social phobia in Parkinson's disease: a single-case study. *Cognitive and Behavioral Practice*, 8, 328–335.

Hu, M., Cooper, J., Beamish, R., et al. (2011). How well do we recognise non-motor symptoms in a British Parkinson's disease population? *Journal of Neurology*, 258, 1513–1517.

Huang, C., Ravdin, L. D., Nirenberg, M. J., et al. (2013). Neuroimaging markers of motor and nonmotor features of Parkinson's disease: an ^{18}F fluorodeoxyglucose positron emission computed tomography study. *Dementia and Geriatric Cognitive Disorders*, 35, 183–196.

Hyman, C., Hofer, M., Barde, Y. A., et al. (1991). BDNF is a neurotrophic factor for dopaminergic neurons of the substantia nigra. *Nature*, 350, 230–232.

Jacob, E. L., Gatto, N. M., Thompson, A., Bordelon, Y. and Ritz, B. (2010). Occurrence of depression and anxiety prior to Parkinson's disease. *Parkinsonism & Related Disorders*, 16, 576–81.

Khedr, E. M., El Fetoh, N. A., Khalifa, H., Ahmed, M. A. and El Beh, K. M. A. (2012). Prevalence of depression, anxiety, dementia and other non motor features of a large cohort of Egyptian Parkinson's disease patients. *Life Science Journal*, 9, 509–518.

Kim, S., Park, J. M., Moon, J. and Choi, H. J. (2014). Alpha-synuclein interferes with cAMP/PKA-dependent upregulation of dopamine beta-hydroxylase and is associated with abnormal adaptive responses to immobilization stress. *Experimental Neurology*, 252, 63–74.

Kraepelien, M., Svenningsson, P., Lindefors, N. and Kaldo, V. (2015). Internet-based cognitive behavioral therapy for depression and anxiety in Parkinson's disease – a pilot study. *Internet Interventions*, 2, 1–6.

Kulisevsky, J., Pagonabarraga, J., Pascual-Sedano, B., Garcia-Sanchez, C. and Gironell, A. (2008). Prevalence and correlates of neuropsychiatric symptoms in Parkinson's disease without dementia. *Movement Disorders*, 23, 1889–1896.

Kulisevsky, J., Pascual-Sedano, B., Barbanoj, M., Gironell, A., Pagonabarraga, J. and Garcia-Sanchez, C. (2007). Acute effects of immediate and controlled-release levodopa on mood in Parkinson's disease: a double-blind study. *Movement Disorders*, 22, 62–67.

Kummer, A., Cardoso, F. and Teixeira, A. L. (2008). Frequency of social phobia and psychometric properties of the Liebowitz social anxiety scale in Parkinson's disease. *Movement Disorders*, 23, 1739–1743.

Kummer, A., Cardoso, F. and Teixeira, A. L. (2010). Generalized anxiety disorder and the Hamilton Anxiety Rating Scale in Parkinson's disease. *Arquivos de Neuro-Psiquiatria*, 68, 495–501.

Lauterbach, E. C., Freeman, A. and Vogel, R. L. (2003). Correlates of generalized anxiety and panic attacks in dystonia and Parkinson disease. *Cognitive and Behavioral Neurology*, 16, 225–233.

Lauterbach, E. C., Freeman, A. and Vogel, R. L. (2004). Differential DSM-III psychiatric disorder prevalence profiles in dystonia and Parkinson's disease. *Journal of Neuropsychiatry and Clinical Neurosciences*, 16, 29–36.

Leentjens, A. F., Dujardin, K., Marsh, L., Martinez-Martin, P., Richard, I. H. and Starkstein, S. E. (2012). Anxiety and motor fluctuations in Parkinson's disease: a cross-sectional observational study. *Parkinsonism & Related Disorders*, 18, 1084–1088.

Leentjens, A. F., Dujardin, K., Marsh, L., Richard, I. H., Starkstein, S. E. and Martinez-Martin, P. (2011). Anxiety rating scales in Parkinson's disease: a validation study of the Hamilton Anxiety Rating Scale, the Beck Anxiety Inventory, and the Hospital Anxiety and Depression Scale. *Movement Disorders*, 26, 407–415.

Leentjens, A. F., Dujardin, K., Pontone, G. M., Starkstein, S. E., Weintraub, D. and Martinez-Martin, P. (2014). The Parkinson Anxiety Scale (PAS): development and validation of a new anxiety scale. *Movement Disorders*, 29, 1035–1043.

Leentjens, A. F., Dujardin, K., Marsh, L., et al. (2008). Anxiety rating scales in Parkinson's disease: critique and recommendations. *Movement Disorders*, 23, 2015–2025.

Macht, M., Schwarz, R. and Ellgring, H. (2005). Patterns of psychological problems in Parkinson's disease. *Acta Neurologica Scandinavica*, 111, 95–101.

Manor, Y., Balas, M., Giladi, N., Mootanah, R. and Cohen, J. T. (2009). Anxiety, depression and swallowing disorders in patients with Parkinson's disease. *Parkinsonism & Related Disorders*, 15, 453–456.

Marinus, J., Leentjens, A. F., Visser, M., Stiggelbout, A. M. and Van Hilten, J. J. (2002). Evaluation of the hospital anxiety and depression scale in patients with Parkinson's disease. *Clinical Neuropharmacology*, 25, 318–324.

Marxreiter, F., Ettle, B., May, V. E., et al. (2013). Glial A30P alpha-synuclein pathology segregates neurogenesis from anxiety-related behavior in conditional transgenic mice. *Neurobiology of Disease*, 59, 38–51.

Matheson, S. F., Byrne, G. J., Dissanayaka, N. N., et al. (2012). Validity and reliability of the Geriatric Anxiety Inventory in Parkinson's disease. *Australasian Journal on Ageing*, 31, 13–16.

Matsui, H., Nishinaka, K., Oda, M., et al. (2007). Depression in Parkinson's disease. diffusion tensor imaging study. *Journal of Neurology*, 254, 1170–1173.

McLean, G., Lawrence, M., Simpson, R. and Mercer, S. W. (2017). Mindfulness-based stress reduction in Parkinson's disease: a systematic review. *BMC Neurology*, 17, 92.

Menza, M., Marin, H., Kaufman, K., Mark, M. and Lauritano, M. (2004). Citalopram treatment of depression in Parkinson's disease: the impact on anxiety, disability, and cognition. *Journal of Neuropsychiatry and Clinical Neurosciences*, 16, 315–319.

Menza, M. A., Palermo, B., Dipaola, R., Sage, J. I. and Ricketts, M. H. (1999). Depression and anxiety in Parkinson's disease: possible effect of genetic variation in the serotonin transporter. *Journal of Geriatric Psychiatry and Neurology*, 12, 49–52.

Menza, M. A., Robertson-Hoffman, D. E. and Bonapace, A. S. (1993). Parkinson's disease and anxiety: comorbidity with depression. *Biological Psychiatry*, 34, 465–470.

Mohlman, J., Reel, D. H., Chazin, D., et al. (2010). A novel approach to treating anxiety and enhancing executive skills in an older adult with Parkinson's disease. *Clinical Case Studies*, **9**, 74–90.

Mondolo, F., Jahanshahi, M., Granà, A., Biasutti, E., Cacciatori, E. and Di Benedetto, P. (2007). Evaluation of anxiety in Parkinson's disease with some commonly used rating scales. *Neurological Sciences*, **28**, 270–275.

Moonen, A. J., Wijers, A., Leentjens, A. F., et al. (2014). Severity of depression and anxiety are predictors of response to antidepressant treatment in Parkinson's disease. *Parkinsonism & Related Disorders*, **20**, 644–646.

Moriyama, T. S., Felicio, A. C., Chagas, M. H., et al. (2011). Increased dopamine transporter density in Parkinson's disease patients with social anxiety disorder. *Journal of the Neurological Sciences*, **310**, 53–57.

Negre-Pages, L., Grandjean, H., Lapeyre-Mestre, M., et al. (2010). Anxious and depressive symptoms in Parkinson's disease: the French cross-sectional DoPaMiP study. *Movement Disorders*, **25**, 157–166.

Okai, D., Askey-Jones, S., Samuel, M., et al. (2013). Trial of CBT for impulse control behaviors affecting Parkinson patients and their caregivers. *Neurology*, **80**, 792–799.

Ozdilek, B. and Gunal, D. I. (2012). Motor and non-motor symptoms in Turkish patients with Parkinson's disease affecting family caregiver burden and quality of life. *Journal of Neuropsychiatry and Clinical Neurosciences*, **24**, 478–483.

Pachana, N. A., Byrne, G. J., Siddle, H., Koloski, N., Harley, E. and Arnold, E. (2007). Development and validation of the Geriatric Anxiety Inventory. *International Psychogeriatrics*, **19**, 103–114.

Pachana, N. A., Egan, S. J., Laidlaw, K., et al. (2013). Clinical issues in the treatment of anxiety and depression in older adults with Parkinson's disease. *Movement Disorders*, **28**, 1930–1934.

Pena-Oliver, Y., Buchman, V. L. and Stephens, D. N. (2010). Lack of involvement of alpha-synuclein in unconditioned anxiety in mice. *Behavioural Brain Research*, **209**, 234–240.

Peron, J., Dondaine, T., Le Jeune, F., Grandjean, D. and Verin, M. (2012). Emotional processing in Parkinson's disease: a systematic review. *Movement Disorders*, **27**, 186–199.

Picillo, M., Amboni, M., Erro, R., et al. (2013). Gender differences in non-motor symptoms in early, drug naive Parkinson's disease. *Journal of Neurology*, **260**, 2849–2855.

Pickut, B. and Vanneste, S. (2015). Mindfulness training among individuals with Parkinson's disease: neurobehavioral effects. *Hindawi*, **2015**, 816404.

Pickut, B., Vanneste, S., Hirsch, M. A., et al. (2015). Mindfulness training among individuals with Parkinson's disease: neurobehavioral effects. *Parkinson's Disease*, **2015**, 816404.

Pontone, G. M., Williams, J. R., Anderson, K. E., et al. (2009). Prevalence of anxiety disorders and anxiety subtypes in patients with Parkinson's disease. *Movement Disorders*, **24**, 1333–1338.

Prediger, R. D., Matheus, F. C., Schwarzbold, M. L., Lima, M. M. and Vital, M. A. (2012). Anxiety in Parkinson's disease: a critical review of experimental and clinical studies. *Neuropharmacology*, **62**, 115–124.

Qureshi, S. U., Amspoker, A. B., Calleo, J. S., Kunik, M. E. and Marsh, L. (2012). Anxiety disorders, physical illnesses, and health care utilization in older male veterans with Parkinson disease and comorbid depression. *Journal of Geriatric Psychiatry and Neurology*, **25**, 233–239.

Rahman, S., Griffin, H. J., Quinn, N. P. and Jahanshahi, M. (2011). On the nature of fear of falling in Parkinson's disease. *Behavioural Neurology*, **24**, 219–228.

Remy, P., Doder, M., Lees, A., Turjanski, N. and Brooks, D. (2005). Depression in Parkinson's disease: loss of dopamine and noradrenaline innervation in the limbic system. *Brain*, **128**, 1314–1322.

Richard, I. H., Frank, S., McDermott, M. P., et al. (2004). The ups and downs of Parkinson disease: a prospective study of mood and anxiety fluctuations. *Cognitive and Behavioral Neurology*, **17**, 201–207.

Richard, I. H., McDermott, M. P., Kurlan, R., et al. (2012). A randomized, double-blind, placebo-controlled trial of antidepressants in Parkinson disease. *Neurology*, **78**, 1229–1236.

Rodriguez-Blazquez, C., Frades-Payo, B., Forjaz, M. J., De Pedro-Cuesta, J. and Martinez-Martin, P. (2009). Psychometric attributes of the Hospital Anxiety and Depression Scale in Parkinson's disease. *Movement Disorders*, **24**, 519–525.

Rodriguez-Violante, M., Cervantes-Arriaga, A., Corona, T., Martinez-Ramirez, D., Morales-Briceno, H. and Martinez-Martin, P. (2013). Clinical determinants of health-related quality of life in Mexican patients with Parkinson's disease. *Archives of Medical Research*, **44**, 110–114.

Rothman, S. M., Griffioen, K. J., Vranis, N., et al. (2013). Neuronal expression of familial Parkinson's disease A53T alpha-synuclein causes early motor impairment, reduced anxiety and potential sleep disturbances in mice. *Journal of Parkinson's Disease*, **3**, 215–229.

Schrag, A., Jahanshahi, M. and Quinn, N. (2000). How does Parkinson's disease affect quality of life? A comparison with quality of life in the general population. *Movement Disorders*, **15**, 1112–1118.

Shiba, M., Bower, J. H., Maraganore, D. M., et al. (2000). Anxiety disorders and depressive disorders preceding Parkinson's disease: a case–control study. *Movement Disorders*, **15**, 669–677.

Shulman, L. M., Singer, C., Bean, J., et al. (1996). Therapeutic effects of sertraline in patients with Parkinson's disease [abstract]. *Movement Disorders*, **11**, 12.

Shulman, L. M., Taback, R. L., Bean, J. and Weiner, W. J. (2001). Comorbidity of the nonmotor symptoms of Parkinson's disease. *Movement Disorders*, **16**, 507–510.

Siemers, E. R., Shekhar, A., Quaid, K. and Dickson, H. (1993). Anxiety and motor performance in Parkinson's disease. *Movement Disorders*, **8**, 501–506.

Solla, P., Cannas, A., Floris, G. L., et al. (2011). Behavioral, neuropsychiatric and cognitive disorders in Parkinson's disease patients with and without motor complications. *Progress in Neuro-Psychopharmacology & Biological Psychiatry*, **35**, 1009–1013.

Solla, P., Cannas, A., Ibba, F. C., et al. (2012). Gender differences in motor and non-motor symptoms among Sardinian patients with Parkinson's disease. *Journal of the Neurological Sciences*, **323**, 33–39.

Sproesser, E., Viana, M. A., Quagliato, E. M. and De Souza, E. A. (2010). The effect of psychotherapy in patients with PD: a controlled study. *Parkinsonism & Related Disorders*, **16**, 298–300.

Stefanova, E., Ziropadja, L., Petrović, M., Stojković, T. and Kostić, V. (2013). Screening for anxiety symptoms in Parkinson disease: a cross-sectional study. *Journal of Geriatric Psychiatry and Neurology*, **26**, 34–40.

Stein, M. B., Heuser, I. J., Juncos, J. L. and Uhde, T. W. (1990). Anxiety disorders in patients with Parkinson's disease. *American Journal of Psychiatry*, **147**, 217–220.

Svetel, M., Pekmezovic, T., Markovic, V., et al. (2013). No association between brain-derived neurotrophic factor G196A polymorphism and clinical features of Parkinson's disease. *European Neurology*, **70**, 257–262.

Sylvester, C. M., Corbetta, M., Raichle, M. E., et al. (2012). Functional network dysfunction in anxiety and anxiety disorders. *Trends in Neurosciences*, **35**, 527–535.

Tarczy, M. and Szombathelyi, E. (1998). Depression in Parkinson's disease with special regard to anxiety: experiences with paroxetine treatment [abstract]. *Movement Disorders*, **13**, 275.

Tessitore, A., Hariri, A. R., Fera, F., et al. (2002). Dopamine modulates the response of the human amygdala: a study in Parkinson's disease. *Journal of Neuroscience*, **22**, 9099–9103.

Tinaz, S., Courtney, M. G. and Stern, C. E. (2011). Focal cortical and subcortical atrophy in early Parkinson's disease. *Movement Disorders*, **26**, 436–441.

Trend, P., Kaye, J., Gage, H., Owen, C. and Wade, D. (2002). Short-term effectiveness of intensive multidisciplinary rehabilitation for people with Parkinson's disease and their carers. *Clinical Rehabilitation*, 16, 717–725.

Troeung, L., Egan, S. J. and Gasson, N. (2014). A waitlist-controlled trial of group cognitive behavioural therapy for depression and anxiety in Parkinson's disease. *BMC Psychiatry*, 14, 19.

Veazey, C., Cook, K. F., Stanley, M., Lai, E. C. and Kunik, M. E. (2009). Telephone-administered cognitive behavioral therapy: a case study of anxiety and depression in Parkinson's disease. *Journal of Clinical Psychology in Medical Settings*, 16, 243–253.

Vriend, C., Boedhoe, P. S., Rutten, S., et al. (2016). A smaller amygdala is associated with anxiety in Parkinson's disease: a combined FreeSurfer-VBM study. *Journal of Neurology, Neurosurgery, and Psychiatry*, 87, 493–500.

Wade, D. T., Gage, H., Owen, C., Trend, P., Grossmith, C. and Kaye, J. (2003). Multidisciplinary rehabilitation for people with Parkinson's disease: a randomised controlled study. *Journal of Neurology, Neurosurgery, and Psychiatry*, 74, 158–162.

Weintraub, D., Moberg, P. J., Duda, J. E., Katz, I. R. and Stern, M. B. (2004). Effect of psychiatric and other nonmotor symptoms on disability in Parkinson's disease. *Journal of the American Geriatrics Society*, 52, 784–788.

Weintraub, D., Newberg, A. B., Cary, M. S., et al. (2005). Striatal dopamine transporter imaging correlates with anxiety and depression symptoms in Parkinson's disease. *Journal of Nuclear Medicine*, 46, 227–232.

Weisskopf, M. G., Chen, H., Schwarzschild, M. A., Kawachi, I. and Ascherio, A. (2003). Prospective study of phobic anxiety and risk of Parkinson's disease. *Movement Disorders*, 18, 646–651.

Wen, M. C., Chan, L. L., Tan, L. C. and Tan, E. K. (2016). Depression, anxiety, and apathy in Parkinson's disease: insights from neuroimaging studies. *European Journal of Neurology*, 23, 1001–1019.

Yamakado, H., Moriwaki, Y., Yamasaki, N., et al. (2012). Alpha-synuclein BAC transgenic mice as a model for Parkinson's disease manifested decreased anxiety-like behavior and hyperlocomotion. *Neuroscience Research*, 73, 173–177.

Yang, S., Sajatovic, M. and Walter, B. L. (2012). Psychosocial interventions for depression and anxiety in Parkinson's disease. *Journal of Geriatric Psychiatry and Neurology*, 25, 113–121.

Chapter 1

Anxiety in Older Adults across Care Settings

Veronica L. Shead, Rachel L. Rodriguez, Samuel J. Dreeben, and Shalagh A. McBride

The presentation of anxiety in older adults can differ across treatment and care settings. Therefore, providers must be mindful of these differences in order to adjust assessment and identify appropriate interventions to address the impact of anxiety on the patient and, in many cases, their overall health. This chapter aims to provide a brief description of anxiety across settings for older adults. The chapter will address anxiety in subacute treatment settings, home-based care, long-term care, and palliative/hospice care environments. It is important to remember that in these settings anxiety is often a secondary issue that accompanies acute, chronic, and terminal disease processes. Therefore, in addition to assessment and intervention, the impact of anxiety on the disease and treatment processes is also discussed in relation to overall health and treatment outcomes.

Anxiety in Subacute Settings

Subacute care can be defined as integrative medical care for patients no longer requiring acute medical treatment yet still needing a higher level of care than is typically available at long-term facilities or with home-based care. Subacute inpatient care is often the best option for rehabilitation following a serious medical crisis. Patients in a subacute care setting have a range of medical needs including physical and functional rehabilitation, pain management, postsurgical care, wound care, intravenous antibiotic treatment, oncology care, cardiac care, and pulmonary care. Due to the transitional and time-limited nature of subacute care, mental health interventions are often best accomplished using a coordinated interdisciplinary approach targeting specific, short-term behavioral, cognitive, and functional goals. While a certain degree of anxiety is to be expected given the context, older patients' ability to adjust to change and cope with anxiety can profoundly influence prospects for physical rehabilitation, long-term mental health, and further medical complications.

Research has identified anxiety as a major risk factor for a number of populations in subacute settings and as a predictive factor for various geriatric syndromes including falling, incontinence, and functional dependence (Keister, 2006; Tinetti et al., 1995). Older adult patients with premorbid anxiety issues are at even higher risk for reduced physical functioning and comorbid mental health disorders (Le Roux et al., 2005). Common sources of anxiety for subacute patients, such as fear of falling, have also been correlated with avoidance of activities, loss of confidence, and greater dependence (Watanabe, 2005).

Astrom (1996) found that 28% of stroke patients met criteria for generalized anxiety in the acute stage post-stroke and that there was no significant decrease at a 3-year follow-up. Generalized anxiety symptoms were further associated with social isolation, dysphasia, and functional dependence.

A study (Singh et al., 2007) examining amputees in subacute rehabilitative settings found that anxiety symptoms peaked shortly after surgery and subsequently decreased over time. However, a follow-up study (Singh et al., 2009) revealed a rebound effect for anxiety symptoms after patients returned home. The authors speculate that patients experience a decrease in anxiety in a subacute setting due to the high level of support received. This short-term reduction in anxiety does not appear to last, however, unless the individual can maintain high levels of functional independence living away from the subacute setting. This underscores the importance of prioritizing increased self-efficacy and functional ability in subacute care, even when rehabilitation is itself anxiety-provoking.

Some anxiety can be beneficial in a subacute setting, as learning typically occurs best with mid-level arousal (Yerkes & Dodson, 1908); however, too much anxiety can have profoundly detrimental effects. Striking the appropriate balance between being supportive of patients and challenging patients is particularly critical as patients slowly regain confidence and functional abilities. Even for patients who regain most or nearly all functional independence, the anxiety associated with discharge and functioning outside of the subacute unit still needs to be anticipated and addressed. Maintaining a focus on the reality of discharge both serves as a motivator and allows the patient to prepare for the mental transition of reduced levels of care.

The subacute model of care can encourage patients to face their fears and develop positive coping strategies during the rehabilitation process. Subacute patients will frequently use avoidance strategies for immediate distress reduction in lieu of fully engaging with therapy. In a study of chronic obstructive pulmonary disease (COPD) patients in a subacute setting (Ninot et al., 2006), patients were found to use fewer avoidance and emotional coping strategies and more problem-solving strategies after 4 weeks of intensive physical rehabilitation with supplementary psychoeducation regarding COPD.

For older adults in subacute settings, the perception of limited control over oneself and/or external events increases the expected probability of danger, resulting in heightened anticipatory anxiety (Chorpita & Barlow, 1998). Control can be reasserted by subacute patients via improved strength and functioning related to physical rehabilitation; however, it can also be developed via cognitive strategies that allow the individual to maximize functional ability within imposed physical limitations. One important example is nonpharmacological pain management strategies, whereby patients learn to reframe the meaning of chronic pain, use relaxation strategies, and focus on engaging in value-based behavior to increase functional activation and reduce emotional reactivity to pain. Psychoeducation regarding the etiology of pain and the rehabilitative process can shift the patient from perceiving rehabilitation and pain as something to fear into challenges to overcome.

Although rehabilitation suggests a return to greater levels of functional ability and self-efficacy, there is the real possibility that losses of function and independence could be permanent for older adults in subacute settings. The anxiety related to this perceived loss of control may evoke particularly powerful fear, anger, and resentment from individuals accustomed to having significant independence and control over their lives. Being suddenly unable to dictate one's life and becoming reliant on others can be a tremendous threat to self-perception and self-worth. Older adults who are already coping with societal prejudices against the elderly are now faced with the additional judgment of being viewed as disabled (Hartke, 1991, p. 3). These negative appraisals of self can be compounded by eager young and healthy team members who push the residents to work harder and struggle to empathize with their debilitated states (Gans, 1987, p. 186).

For patients who are anxious about rehabilitation and/or mourning the loss of functional ability, focusing on personal values and goals of care can help reassert a degree of autonomy and a sense of self-efficacy. By explicitly identifying the personal values and options available to the patient, patients frequently become more willing to make difficult decisions about rehabilitation. For instance, the promise of improving functional ability enough to play with grandchildren may be just the motivation needed for a patient to persevere through difficult rehabilitation. Identifying values can also be the gateway to creating meaningful experiences within the subacute setting, as the older adult might begin to invest more in the people or causes he or she cares about most.

Providers sometimes attempt to protect patients from experiencing anxiety by presenting information in broad, nonthreatening terms or in coded medical jargon that is difficult to understand. In reality, clearly communicated information is typically far less threatening to a patient. By shielding patients from information about their own medical conditions, providers inadvertently can create the impression they do not respect the patient's autonomy and/or that they are withholding the information for self-serving reasons. A trust deficit can develop, resulting in patients experiencing anxiety when new medical procedures are suggested, decreasing medical adherence, and sometimes causing greater agitation, anger, and acting out. The prophylactic approach to preventing medical anxiety is to develop a nonjudgmental interest in the patient. Asking one or two questions about the patient's day, interests, or family can quickly build a reserve of trust. This communicates caring and provides space for patients to process unspoken fears while offering providers valuable clinical information (Greif & Matarazzo, 1982, p. 43).

Subacute patients frequently experience anxiety related to the unpredictability of a new environment. Many patients have developed a careful routine at home that compensates for reduced functional ability and provides maximum comfort given physical, financial, cognitive, and social limitations. Patients may experience anxiety as they work to decode how a patient is supposed to act within an inpatient rehabilitative context. Patients worry that they will be perceived as overly demanding if they are frequently asking for nursing staff's assistance and that they will be treated differently depending on their expressed level of need. If patients' medications, meals, or treatments occur at irregular time intervals or if the patient struggles to remember his or her new schedule, anxiety about coping with daily living in a subacute setting can become overwhelming. Having predictable, positively anticipated activities or social interactions included in the schedule can also have profound effects on the emotional adjustment of older adults (Schulz, 1976).

Preadmission or early admission orientation to the unit is particularly important for addressing anxiety related to uncertainty in the new environment (Hartke, 1991, p. 84). This can include formal orientation classes, printed materials, or Q&A's with staff and current residents. Developing a sense of community within the subacute setting can have a strong protective influence on feelings of anxiety and isolation. Other patients can be useful in providing empathy about the transition and offering advice validating overlooked sources of anxiety without the perceived agenda of medical providers. For instance, peers can be a valuable resource for asking questions perceived as too embarrassing or trivial to ask medical staff. Peers within the subacute setting also establish new social norms for incoming patients, destigmatizing potential sources of shame that often accompany reduced functional abilities. These temporary friendships and communities can provide meaningful contributions of encouragement, instrumental aid, information, humor, and perspective-taking.

Anxiety in Home-Based Care

Defining Need for and Types of Home-Based Care Services

Homebound older adults are an often-overlooked subpopulation of the larger community of older adults aged 65 and over. Homebound older adults suffer from higher rates of chronic illness, disability, cognitive impairment, and psychiatric conditions than their community-dwelling counterparts (Qiu et al., 2010). Recent studies indicate that 40.8% of homebound elders have two to three comorbid medical/psychiatric conditions, while 31.9% suffer from four or more comorbid conditions (Beck et al., 2009). These medical conditions often render the individual dependent in at least one activity of daily living (ADLs), such as feeding, dressing, medication management, financial management, mobility/transportation, bathing, or toileting. With this increased need for assistance and homebound status, it is clear that traditional office-based primary medical care does not meet the needs of this medically complex, physically frail population.

There are several variations of home health care programs that better meet the needs of the medically complex, physically frail homebound patient. One such program in the USA is the Medicare Skilled Home Care Program (www.medicare.gov/coverage/home-health-services.html). This program offer patients with short-term conditions focused, skilled health care such as intermittent skilled nursing care, physical therapy, speech-language pathology therapy, and/or occupational therapy. In the UK and Europe, there are similar outreach programs that provide multidimensional, home-based, geriatric assessments aimed at defining needs and developing care plans for the homebound elderly (Stall et al., 2013). While these programs may provide some level of assistance to homebound, ill older adults, they often utilize multiple providers who often do not work together to coordinate or integrate care. Furthermore, neither type of program is designed to provide ongoing primary care services to address acute and/or changing care needs. Without regular access to primary care services, these medically frail individuals must utilize alternative programs in times of health crises, such as emergency room visits and/or hospitalization (Stall et al., 2014). While these solutions may address the acute need, there is still no coordination of care responsibilities, often resulting in a disjointed post-discharge care plan with little chance of success. Medically frail individuals who do not receive adequate follow-up services then are further at risk for continued decline, readmission, or admission to a long-term care facility.

Home-based primary care (HBPC) programs have developed as an answer to this call for coordinated care services to meet the needs of the medically complex, homebound patient. HBPC programs provide comprehensive, longitudinal primary care services in the homes of individuals with complex, chronic disabling disease using an interprofessional team of skilled practitioners. HBPC interprofessional teams utilize practitioners from a wide range of disciplines, often including geriatricians, nurse practitioners, registered nurses, social workers, pharmacists, dieticians, occupational therapists, physical therapists, mental health providers (psychologists or psychiatrists), and dental assistants. A recent review found that HBPC programs can reduce both hospitalizations and long-term care admissions while improving care recipient and caregiver quality of life and satisfaction with care (Edes et al., 2014; Stall et al., 2014).

As discussed previously, the need for transition to home-based medical care usually arises when, due to increased medical burden and loss of function, the patient is no longer able to regularly attend medical appointments without assistance or transportation. This transition can elicit a number of emotions for patients from relief and happiness to anxiety and feeling overwhelmed. Many patients may express relief that they are receiving medical assistance in their home and happiness that they are having the opportunity for increased social interaction on a regular basis. However, the introduction of new individuals into the home can be overwhelming and distressing for some patients, especially those with dementia, cognitive impairment, or other psychiatric concerns. From a non-pathological standpoint, patients may feel shy about having new individuals enter their home, concerned about invasions of privacy, or even embarrassed about the state of their home. Moreover, some patients may feel as though they are losing connections with long-standing medical providers or the clinical community. Despite the emotional ups and downs that may arise from the transition to home care, research has consistently shown that homebound medical care not only improves patient access to care, but patients also report high levels of satisfaction with the care provided (Beck et al., 2009; Edes et al., 2014).

Assessment of Anxiety in Home Care Settings

While HBPC services may first seek to treat the chronic medical concerns of the patients enrolled, the psychiatric concerns do not go unnoticed. Although exact prevalence rates are not known, it has been estimated that 40.5% of homebound elders suffer from at least one psychiatric disorder, with depression and dementia being among the most common (Qui et al., 2010). However, given that it is well documented that anxiety disorders are common in older adults with medical illnesses, including cardiovascular disease, pain conditions (migraine, arthritis), lung diseases, and gastrointestinal problems (El-Gabalawy et al., 2011; Tolin et al., 2005; Wolitzky-Taylor et al., 2010), and that anxiety symptoms appear to be associated with increased levels of disability among older adults with medical comorbidities (Brenes et al., 2005, 2008; Kessler et al., 1999; Wetherell et al., 2004, 2005), it can be deduced that anxiety symptoms may in fact be high among the group of medically compromised, physically limited patients receiving home care services.

Recognizing and treating anxiety symptoms in homebound patients requires that the treatment team and the patient work together to overcome several barriers. For the treatment providers, it will be important to recognize that older adults may use different language to describe anxiety symptoms ("concerns" or "on edge," not "worry" or "nervous") (Bryant et al., 2013; El-Gabalawy et al., 2011). Relatedly, subsyndromal presentation of anxiety often also results in clinically significant distress that interferes with health and well-being (Teachman, 2006; Wolitzky-Taylor et al., 2010) and the patient's ability to engage in treatment. Therefore, the treatment team must pay special attention to the language that the patient uses to describe possible anxiety symptoms, as well as provide intervention even if the full criteria for diagnosis are not met.

From the patient perspective, homebound older adults with physical limitations and social isolation may expect to feel distressed and therefore not recognize their psychological symptoms as abnormal (Gum et al., 2009). Similarly, they may misinterpret symptoms as resulting from chronic illness and not related to anxiety. With proper psychoeducation from treatment providers, the patient may be open to interventions to treat previously undiagnosed anxiety symptoms.

Notably, providers working with homebound elders are in the unique position to witness behaviors during home visits that might be unreported in the traditional clinical setting. One such set of behaviors includes those related to compulsive hoarding. These behaviors include persistent difficulty and distress associated with discarding possessions, regardless of actual value. Now a distinct disorder in itself in Diagnostic and Statistical Manual of Mental Disorders, 5th Edition (DSM-5) (American Psychiatric Association, 2013), hoarding disorder has high comorbidity with other anxiety and mood disorders. Hoarding is a chronic and progressive condition that increases in severity with age (Ayers et al., 2010), and in late life is associated with significant functional impairment and health risk (Ayers et al., 2010; Diefenbach et al., 2013). Hoarding is particularly dangerous for older persons because of increased risk of physical and cognitive limitations. Possible consequences include increased fall risk, fire hazard, food contamination, social isolation, and medication mismanagement (Ayers et al., 2010; Kim et al., 2001).

Mental Health Treatment/Intervention in Home Care Settings

While the specific pharmacotherapy and psychotherapeutic interventions used to address symptoms of anxiety in home care settings do not differ from those in traditional clinical and other settings, there are several factors to keep in mind when providing care in the home. A distinct advantage is that patients may feel more comfortable and in control in their own homes versus an office or clinical setting, and thus more willing to accept and actively engage in psychotherapy with a mental health provider in their own home (Hicken & Plowhead, 2010). Additionally, providing care in the home not only allows for more detailed assessment of patient's current functioning in light of the anxiety symptoms, but also allows for enhanced treatment planning and intervention (Hicken & Plowhead, 2010; Yang, 2009). For example, when teaching relaxation techniques, the patient can practice *in vivo* and potential environmental problems can be resolved. In addition, with the permission of the patient, other individuals living in the home can potentially be brought into treatment planning and intervention phases to assist the patient with carrying out the intervention. One disadvantage, particularly as it applies to the treatment and management of anxiety disorders, is the reduced opportunity for exposure among homebound patients. Patients who are unable to leave the home for medical reasons or due to physical limitations are unlikely to be able to engage in interventions utilizing exposure to anxiety triggers outside of the home. This eliminates a critical treatment option in the management of anxiety disorders.

Anxiety in Long-Term Care

Defining Long-Term Care

Long-term care is a broad range of services and supports designed to address the needs of older individuals whose capacity for self-care is limited due to chronic illness, injury, physical, cognitive, or mental disability, or other health-related conditions. This includes assistance with personal and health care needs, often referred to as basic and instrumental ADLs (Harris-Kojetin et al., 2013). Overall, the purpose of long-term care services is to promote the maintenance of or improvements toward an individual's ability to operate at an optimal level of physical functioning and with the highest quality of life possible.

Levels of long-term care occur on a continuum. The lowest level of care along the continuum can be classified as residence within a retirement or independent living community, which typically only offers aid with room and meals. The next step along the continuum consists of assisted living communities. These are for individuals who are ambulatory but require some assistance with ADLs. The concept of assisted living is grounded in a social model emphasizing choice, dignity, independence, privacy, and autonomy in a minimally restrictive environment (Hawes et al., 1999; Reinardy & Kane, 2003). The highest level of care along this continuum consists of nursing facilities, which operate within a medical model context as they are suited for individuals who require daily nursing care or monitoring and aid with most ADLs (Applebaum et al., 2000; Hawes et al., 1999).

Characteristics of Individuals Living in Long-Term Care

According to the World Health Organization, there is considerable variability in the prevalence rates of older adults residing in long-term care across countries. Higher prevalence is noted in low- and middle-income countries than in high-income countries. This can be accounted for by differences in supporting infrastructure available to meet this need. For example, high-income countries, such as Germany, Japan, The Netherlands, Sweden, and the USA, are shifting the emphasis away from long-term care services to residential and community-based care. In general, international prevalence rates for long-term care services increase among adults aged 74 years and older (World Health Organization, 2015). According to the 2010 US Census, approximately 3.1% or 1.3 million adults aged 65 years or older utilize long-term care services in the form of a skilled nursing facility (US Census Bureau, 2010). The number of US individuals using long-term care facilities is projected to increase from 15 million in 2000 to 27 million by 2050 (HHS, 2003). In addition to age, a number of factors increase the possibility that an individual may need to utilize long-term care services. For example, gender is such a factor, as older women are more likely to require long-term care services, experience disability or chronic illness, live alone, and face a change in health status (Harris-Kojetin et al., 2013; World Health Organization, 2015). Furthermore, the majority of assisted living residents are likely to move in directly from their homes or retirement apartments, and very few are admitted after a stay in the hospital (Reinardy & Kane, 2003).

Patient Experience of Long-Term Care

General research on the impact of relocation on mental health reveals that relocation is considered a significant stressor and potential source of anxiety for individuals of all ages and is characterized by loss of social support systems and fear of the unknown (Drummet et al., 2003). For older adults, a move to a community where one's peers are physically or cognitively impaired might be unpleasant, distressing, and possibly threatening to individuals who fear that their own health may consequently become impaired, particularly if their own move occurred in association with health challenges or a change in functional status (Lee et al., 2002). Relocation for older adults also seems to be associated with loss of independence or autonomy, loss of agency, loss of valued possessions, loss of self-sufficiency, and feelings of powerlessness and frustration about the care setting system/environment (Jungers, 2010). Individuals who experience increased loneliness and encounter negative stereotypes about older adults appear to endorse adjustment difficulties to long-term care settings (Jungers, 2010). Positive transition experiences seem to be characterized by the individual's active involvement in the relocation decision, feelings of social relatedness, and resistance to the culturally constructed worldview that aging represents a period of decline (Jungers, 2010). Social support also appears to mediate positive physical and mental health outcomes for older adults (Cook, 2006; Cummings, 2002).

Anxiety in Long-Term Care

Very little research has been conducted on the presence of anxiety in older adults in long-term care settings. However, the research available suggests that high anxiety symptoms in clinical hospitalized settings implicate anxiety as both a source of significant distress for older adults with physical illnesses and as a risk factor for poor outcomes (Bryant et al., 2008). Furthermore, preexisting anxiety is the best predictor for anxiety in older adulthood. Premorbid anxiety can be exacerbated or maintained by stressors unique to older adulthood, such as changes in physical and cognitive status, chronic illness, and functional limitations (Hess, 2012; Le Roux et al., 2005; Schoevers et al., 2003). Mental health diagnoses are prevalent in geriatric and rehabilitation settings, which are ideal settings for detecting and treating mental health issues in older adults (Lichtenberg & MacNeill, 2003).

Dementia and Anxiety in Long-Term Care

Anxiety has been shown to be common in older adults with dementia (Ballard et al., 1996; Ferretti et al., 2001; Mack et al., 1999; Neville & Teri, 2011; Porter et al., 2003). The symptoms of anxiety most frequently reported in older adults with dementia include tension, worry, apprehension, fear, situational anxiety, physiological anxiety, irritability that centers on concerns about and implications of cognitive impairments, and panic attacks (Ballard et al., 1996; Reisberg et al., 1990). Individuals with dementia are more likely to experience more frequent and severe symptoms of anxiety as their cognitive abilities become more and more impaired (Starkstein et al., 2007; Teri et al., 1998). Furthermore, research suggests that older adults with dementia who experience anxiety symptoms frequently also experience symptoms of depression (Ballard et al., 1996; Ferretti et al., 2001; Teri et al., 1998). Some research suggests that a mixed presentation of anxiety and depression symptoms may actually represent a generalized distress experience rather than a specific psychopathology (Meeks et al., 2003). Other research seems to suggest that anxiety and depression are actually separate but related symptom presentations in that they are both forms of negative affect but present with different physiological symptoms (Hess, 2012).

Notably, agitation in individuals with dementia has been conceptualized by some as a behavioral manifestation of anxiety that can occur in cognitively impaired adults (Logsdon et al., 1999; Mintzer & Brawnman-Mintz, 1996; Shankar & Orrell, 2000). Within such a framework, some behavioral manifestations might include increased disruptive behaviors, aggression, verbal agitation, aberrant motor behavior, and disinhibition (Cohen-Mansfield & Bilig, 1986; Ferretti et al., 2001; Mega et al., 1996; Porter et al., 2003). Managing individuals experiencing agitation in a nursing home facility can be challenging for caregivers and staff; thus, identifying ways to prevent and manage these behaviors is very important in an institutional setting. In a long-term care environment, this requires a proactive collaborative approach between health care providers and caregivers to recognize and manage the symptoms and to treat the underlying cause. Historically, pharmacological interventions have been utilized, but with moderate effectiveness and a greater potential risk for side effects. Nonpharmacological interventions, on the other hand, can be effective in decreasing agitation without the risk of potential medication side effects, as well as attempting to address the underlying cause of the agitation (Cohen-Mansfield et al., 2011). Increasing evidence supports the use of nonpharmacological approaches, including behavioral methods, to reduce agitation and anxiety in patients with dementia, and they are found to be most helpful for wandering behaviors, hoarding or hiding objects, repetitive questioning, withdrawal, and social inappropriateness.

Several systematic reviews of nonpharmacological interventions for agitation in dementia found several effective interventions that included the implementation of activities such as exercise training, occupational activities, music therapy, sensory interventions such as massage or aromatherapy, and person-centered communication skills training for caregivers. However, the benefits tended to be short term (Livingston et al., 2014;; Martini de Oliveira et al., 2015; O'Neil et al., 2011). Most behavioral interventions for the management of agitation include identifying whether or not there is a preceding event that generates agitation, determining whether or not the patient has an unmet need that can be anticipated or alleviated, and avoiding or controlling for triggers in the environment. One of the postulated mechanisms underlying the effectiveness of behavioral interventions involves a reduction in the insistent, task-focused, impersonal, and often intrusive typical care that is administered in a long-term care setting. Thus, symptoms of agitation in individuals with dementia are often best managed by educating staff and caregivers in strategies that may reduce environmental triggers, identify unmet needs, and reduce preceding events. This might involve learning strategies for distraction and redirection, implementing structured routines, and addressing patients calmly and with reassurance when patients seem anxious. At times, pharmacological interventions can also be beneficial, but generally, behavioral, environmental, and other nonpharmacological interventions are the preferred therapies for agitation in dementia.

Assessment of Anxiety in Long-Term Care

Despite its importance, very little psychometric research exists concerning the assessment of anxiety in long-term care. Furthermore, assessing anxiety in a long-term care setting may be problematic because individuals are often experiencing coexisting medical conditions or cognitive impairments. The Geriatric Anxiety Inventory (GAI), the GAI – Short Form (GAI-SF), and the Geriatric Anxiety Scale (GAS) are referenced in the literature as appropriate for use in long-term care residents, particularly nursing home residents with psychological disorders (Boddice et al., 2008; Gerolimatos et al., 2013; Gould et al., 2014; Segal et al., 2010).

Anxiety in Palliative Care Settings

The World Health Organization defines palliative care as "an approach that improves the quality of life of patients and their families facing the problem associated with life-threatening illness, through the prevention and relief of suffering by means of early identification and impeccable assessment and treatment of pain and other problems, physical, psychosocial and spiritual" (www.who.int/cancer/palliative/definition/en). Palliative care can be provided across settings, from primary care, acute care, long-term care, and inpatient hospice care, as well as in the home. Palliative care is provided by an interdisciplinary team inclusive of physicians, nurses, chaplains, social workers, and other specialists who work together to provide symptom management and comfort measures in combination with or in lieu of curative treatments. The patients with chronic and/or life-limiting disease are treated in keeping with their values and goals of care. Palliative care can be practiced at any point from the time of diagnosis as an additional service or as the primary focus of care, as is the case in hospices, when a patient's life expectancy is estimated to be less than 6 months and no further curative interventions have been elected.

Although palliative care can be elected at any age due to the nature of the service, it has been estimated that 85% of hospice services were provided to adults over the age of 65 years. Of these older adults, there were estimates that 70% would experience symptoms of anxiety in comparison to 50% experiencing depression, 11% experiencing dementia, and almost 100% experiencing delirium at some point in the end-of-life process (Irwin, 2012). These numbers are indicative of a need to assess and provide interventions to address anxiety symptoms and distress in those receiving palliative and especially hospice care. In addition, these numbers are inclusive of persons who may have had preexisting psychiatric diagnoses including generalized anxiety disorder (GAD), depression, post-traumatic stress disorder (PTSD), and other disorders, which can be exacerbated during the treatment of chronic and life-limiting disease. This, however, is also inclusive of many other patients who develop symptoms of anxiety without necessarily reaching diagnostic criteria (Miovic & Block, 2007). Anxiety in the context of palliative care likely has multiple causes and may present differently than in other settings.

Anxiety as a Symptom

Palliative care is integrated care, as it works to address the biological, psychological, social, and spiritual needs of patients as well as their families. This model of care acknowledges the influences of each area on the other. It is understood that psychological distress can influence biological, social, and spiritual manifestations and vice versa. Therefore, a patient with a history of anxiety may have greater perceived pain, which would influence pain and other symptom management. In another instance, a terminal diagnosis may elicit fear of death and anxiety surrounding the unknown, resulting in insomnia perpetuated by a patient ruminating over thoughts of being a burden and failing to prepare and provide financially and otherwise for their family. In palliative care, the challenge lies in making distinctions between anxiety as a symptom, psychiatric disorder, or normal reaction.

It is important to document and treat anxiety because it has been shown to decrease quality of life, increase insomnia, impact communication with physicians by decreasing trust, and result in poor compliance (Anderson et al., 2014; Kolva et al., 2011). In addition, anxiety has been associated with poor prognosis, a reaction to the treatment process, accelerated disease progression, uncontrolled pain, dying, and the uncertainty of the afterlife (Anderson et al., 2014; Irwin & Hirst, 2015; Kolva et al., 2011). Anxiety may also result from substance abuse, medication side effects, delirium, or undertreated symptoms. With medications, some may contribute to anxiety, such as antipsychotics and antiemetics. With other medications, such as opioids, corticosteroids, anticonvulsants, benzodiazepines, nicotine, and clonidine, the effects of rapid withdrawal of the drug may cause anxiety (Miovic & Block, 2007)

Exacerbation of Anxiety-Related Diagnoses at End of Life

Although most patients exhibiting symptoms of anxiety in palliative care do not meet criteria for an anxiety or related disorders, it is possible that end-of-life issues and treatments may exacerbate symptoms for those with a history of those disorders. For instance, for many patients with PTSD, pain can be a stimulus that may heighten or reinitiate PTSD symptoms. The same can be true of patients with GAD and panic attacks. Providers must be aware of the patient's psychological/psychiatric history and attend to any past anxiety-related diagnoses. Most patients who will meet criteria for an anxiety disorder diagnosis will have a history that occurred prior to diagnosis of their life-limiting condition. For patients without a history but with significant anxiety symptoms that impact their functioning and treatment, they may develop an adjustment disorder with anxious mood. In the case of patients in palliative care with life-limiting illness, the illness is an identifiable stressor for which the patient develops clinically significant emotional and/or behavioral symptoms as a result (Kangas et al., 2002; Roth et al., 2006). This diagnosis is often more accurate for those in the palliative care and hospice settings.

Recommendations for Evaluating and Treating Anxiety in Cancer/Palliative Care

The American Society of Clinical Oncology (ASCO) recommends that all patients with cancer and cancer survivors be evaluated for symptoms of depression and anxiety periodically across the trajectory of the disease process using validated assessment measures. Evidence suggests that untreated anxiety and depression in the context of cancer increases the risk for poor outcomes, decreased quality of life, and increased disease-related morbidity and mortality (Anderson et al., 2014).

Palliative care teams should attend to patients who demonstrate limited ability to understand clinical information, are less comfortable answering questions related to their health, and are more distrustful regarding treatments offered, as these may be due to anxiety (Irwin & Hirst, 2015). Anxiety has many manifestations across a number of domains of symptoms: emotional, cognitive, and behavioral problems, autonomic symptoms, fears, spiritual duress, and worries about death. Therefore, the assessment of and intervention in anxiety symptoms should be standard of care.

Intervention for Anxiety

Treatments for anxiety within palliative care should be individualized and integrated into the overall treatment plan. Since the symptoms of anxiety can vary widely, input from the interdisciplinary team is necessary to assist with diagnosis and management. If a mental health provider is not included on the team, consultation may be useful. When providing treatment, the team must consider the life-limiting illness and prognosis, comorbidities, the patient's present functional condition, and, importantly, the patient's and family's wishes (Irwin et al., 2012). Many may simply need supportive care and services provided by the team. Other patients whose symptoms are impactful may require multiple interventions consisting of a combination of supportive therapy, psychotherapy, pharmacotherapy, and complementary therapies (Irwin, 2012). Brief psychotherapies have been shown to have empirical validity, including meaning-centered therapy and dignity therapy (Breitbart, 2002; Chochinov et al., 2011).

Caregivers/Families and Anxiety

Notably, when working in palliative care, one must also consider the caregivers and family members. They may also demonstrate symptoms of anxiety surrounding the end-of-life process and be coping with anticipatory grief. As with patients, this may influence communication, decision-making, and patient treatment outcomes. In addition, this may influence bereavement and complicate the grief process.

References

American Psychiatric Association (2013). *Diagnostic and Statistical Manual of Mental Disorders*, 5th ed. Washington, DC: American Psychiatric Association.

Andersen, B. L., DeRubeis, R. J., Berman, B. S., et al. (2014). Screening, assessment, and care of anxiety and depressive symptoms in adults with cancer: an American Society of Clinical Oncology guideline adaptation. *Journal of Clinical Oncology*, 32, 1605–1619.

Applebaum, R. A., Straker, J. K. and Geron, S. M. (2000). *Assessing Satisfaction in Health and Long-Term Care*. New York: Springer.

Åström, M. (1996). Generalized anxiety disorder in stroke patients a 3-year longitudinal study. *Stroke*, 27(2), 270–275.

Ayers, C. R., Saxena, S., Golshan, S. and Wetherell, J. L. (2010). Age at onset and clinical features of late life compulsive hoarding. *International Journal of Geriatric Psychiatry*, 25, 142–149.

Ayers, C. R., Wetherell, J. L., Golshan, S. and Saxena, S. (2011). Cognitive–behavioral therapy for geriatric compulsive hoarding. *Behaviour Research and Therapy*, 49, 689–694.

Ballard, C., Boyle, A., Bowler, C. and Linedesay, J. (1996). Anxiety disorders in dementia sufferers. *International Journal of Geriatric Psychiatry*, 11, 987–990.

Beck, R. A., Arizmendi, A., Purnell, C., Fultz, B. A. and Callahan, C. M. (2009). House calls for seniors: Building and sustaining a model of care for homebound seniors. *Journal of the American Geriatrics Society*, 57(6), 1103–1109.

Block, S. D. (2006). Psychological issues in end-of-life care. *Journal of Palliative Medicine*, 9, 751–772.

Boddice, G., Pachana, N. A. and Byrne, G. J. (2008). The clinical utility of the geriatric anxiety inventory in older adults with cognitive impairment. *Nursing Older People*, 20(8), 36–39.

Breitbart, W. (2002). Spirituality and meaning in supportive care: spirituality- and meaning-centered group psychotherapy interventions in advanced cancer. *Support Care Cancer*, 10, 272–280.

Breitbart, W., Chochinov, H. M. and Passik, S. (2005). Psychiatric symptoms in palliative medicine. In D. Doyle, G. W. C. Hanks, N. I. Cherny, and K. Calman, eds., *Oxford Textbook of Palliative Medicine*, 3rd ed. New York: Oxford University Press, p. 747.

Brenes, G. A., Guralink, J. M., Williamson, J. D., et al. (2005). The influence of anxiety on the progression of disability. *Journal of the American Geriatrics Society*, 53, 34–39.

Brenes, G. A., Pennix, B. W. J. H., Judd, P. H., Rockwell, E., Sewell, D. D. and Wetherell, J. L. (2008). Anxiety, depression, and disability across the lifespan. *Aging and Mental Health*, 12(1), 158–163.

Bryant, C., Jackson, H. and Ames, D. (2008). The prevalence of anxiety in older adults: methodological issues and a review of the literature. *Journal of Affective Disorders*, 109 (3), 223–250.

Bryant, C., Mohlman, J., Gum, A., et al. (2013). Anxiety disorders in older adults: Looking to DSM-5 and beyond. *American Journal of Geriatric Psychiatry*, 21, 872–876.

Chochinov, H. M., Kristjanson, L. J., Breitbart, W., et al. (2011). Effect of dignity therapy on distress and end-of-life experience in terminally ill patients: a randomised controlled trial. *Lancet Oncology*, 12(8), 753–762.

Chorpita, B. F. and Barlow, D. H. (1998). The development of anxiety: the role of control in the early environment. *Psychological Bulletin*, 124(1), 3–21.

Cohen-Mansfield, J. and Bilig, N. (1986). Agitated behaviors in the elderly: a conceptual review. *Journal of the American Geriatric Society*, 34(10), 711–721.

Cohen-Mansfield, J., Marx, M. S., Freedman, L. S., Murad, H., Regier, N. G., Thein, K. and Dakheel-Ali, M. (2011). The comprehensive process model of engagement. *American Journal of Geriatric Psychiatry*, 19(10), 859–870.

Cook, G. (2006). The risk to enduring relationships following the move to a care home. *International Journal of Older People Nursing*, **1**(3), 182–185.

Cummings, S. M. (2002). Predictors of psychological well-being among assisted-living residents. *Health and Social Work*, **27**(4), 293–313.

Diefenbach, G. J., Dimauro, J., Frost, R., Steketee, G. and Tolin, D. F. (2013). Characteristics of hoarding in older adults. *American Journal of Geriatric Psychiatry*, **21** (10), 1043–1047.

Drummet, A. R., Coleman, M. and Cable, S. (2003). Military families under stress: implications for family life education. *Family Relations*, **52**, 279–287.

Edes, T., Kinosian, B., Vuckovic, N. H., Nichols, L. O., Becker, M. M. and Hossain, M. (2014). Better access, quality, and cost for clinically complex veterans with home-based, primary care. *Journal of the American Geriatrics Society*, **62**, 1954–1961.

El-Gabalawy, R., Mackenzie, C. S., Shooshtari, S. and Sareen, J. (2011). Comorbid physical health conditions and anxiety disorders: a population-based exploration of prevalence and health outcomes among older adults. *General Hospital Psychiatry*, **33**, 556–564.

Fairman, N. and Irwin, S. A. (2013). Palliative care psychiatry: update on an emerging dimension of psychiatric practice. *Current Psychiatry Report*, **15**(7), 374.

Ferretti, L., McCurry, S. M., Logsdon, R., Gibbons, L. and Teri, L. (2001). Anxiety and Alzheimer's disease. *Journal of Geriatric Psychiatry and Neurology*, **14**(1), 52–58.

Gans, J. S. (1987). Facilitating staff/patient interaction in rehabilitation. In B. Caplan, ed., *Rehabilitation Psychology Desk Reference*. New York: Aspen Publishers, pp. 185–218.

Garuti, G., Cilione, C., Dell Orso, D., et al. (2003). Impact of comprehensive pulmonary rehabilitation on anxiety and depression in hospitalized COPD patients. *Monaldi Archives for Chest Disease*, **59**(1), 56–61.

Gerolimatos, L. A., Gregg, J. J. and Edlestein, B. A. (2013). Assessment of anxiety in long-term care: examination of the Geriatric Anxiety Inventory (GAI) and its short form. *International Psychogeriatrics*, **25** (9), 1533–1542.

Gould, C., Segal., D. L., Yochim, B. P., Pachana, N.A., Byrne, G. J. and Beaudreau, S. A. (2014). Measuring anxiety in late life: a psychometric examination of the Geriatric Anxiety Inventory and Geriatric Anxiety Scale. *Journal of Anxiety Disorders*, **28**, 804–811.

Greif, E. and Matarazzo, R. G. (1982). *Behavioral Approaches to Rehabilitation: Coping with Change*, Vol. **3**. New York: Springer Publishing Company.

Gum, A. M., Petkus, A., McDougal, S. J., Present, M., King-Kallimanis, B. and Schonfield, L. (2009). Behavioral health needs and problem recognition by older adults receiving home-based aging services. *International Journal of Geriatric Psychiatry*, **24**, 400–408.

Harris-Kojetin, L., Sengupta, M., Park-Lee, E. and Valverde, R. (2013). Long-term care services in the United States: 2013 overview. *National Center for Health Statistics: Vital Health Statistics*, 3(37), 1–107.

Hartke, R. (1991). Introduction. In R. Hartke, ed., *Psychological Aspects of Geriatric Rehabilitation*. New York: Aspen Publishers, pp. 1–8.

Hartke, R. (1991). The older adult's adjustment to the rehabilitation setting. In R. Hartke, ed., *Psychological Aspects of Geriatric Rehabilitation*. New York: Aspen Publishers, pp. 73–96.

Hawes, C., Phillips, C. D. and Rose, M. (1999). A national study of assisted living for the frail elderly: final summary report. U.S. Department of Health and Human Services Office of Disability, Aging, and Long-Term Care Policy Office of the Assistance Secretary for Planning and Evaluation. http://aspe .hhs.gov/daltcp/reports/finales.pdf

Hess, L. S. (2012). *Anxiety in Older Adults with Dementia Residing in Long-term Care Facilities*. Doctoral dissertation, University of Louisville.

HHS (2003). The future supply of long-term care workers in relation to the aging baby boom generation: report to Congress.

Washington, DC: HHS. Retrieved from http://aspe.hhs.gov/daltcp/reports/ltcwork.pdf

Hicken, B. L. and Plowhead, A. (2010). A model for home-based psychology from the Veterans Health Administration. *Professional Psychology: Research and Practice*, **41**, 340–346.

Irwin, S. A. (2012). Palliative care, geriatric psychiatry, and you. *American Journal of Geriatric Psychiatry*, **20**(4), 281–283.

Irwin, S. A. and Hirst, J. M. (2015). Overview of anxiety in palliative care. In S. D. Block, ed., UptoDate. www.uptodate.com/contents/overview-of-anxiety-in-palliative-care/abstract/37

Irwin, S. A., Montross, L. P. and Chochinov, H. M. (2012). What treatments are effective for anxiety in patients with serious illness? In R. S. Morrison, and N. Goldstein, eds., *Evidence-Based Practice of Palliative Medicine*. Philadelphia, PA: Elsevier Saunders, pp. 191–197.

Jungers, C. M. (2010). Leaving home: an examination of late-life relocation among older adults. *Journal of Counseling and Development*, **88**, 416–423.

Kales, H. C., Gitlin, L. N. and Lyketsos, C. G. (2014). Management of neuropsychiatric symptoms of dementia in clinical settings: recommendations from a multidisciplinary expert panel. *Journal of the American Geriatric Society*, **62**, 762–769.

Kangas, M., Henry, J.L. and Bryant, R. A. (2002). Posttraumatic stress disorder following cancer. A conceptual and empirical review. *Clinical Psychological Review*, **22**, 499–524.

Keister, K. J. (2006). Predictors of self-assessed health, anxiety, and depressive symptoms in nursing home residents at week 1 post-relocation. *Journal of Aging and Health*, **18**(5), 722–742.

Kessler, R. C., DuPont, R. L., Berglund, P. and Wittchen, H. U. (1999). Impairment in pure and comorbid generalized anxiety disorder and major depression at 12 months in two national surveys. *American Journal of Psychiatry*, **156**, 1915–1923.

Kim, H., Stektee, G. and Frost, R. O. (2001). Hoarding by elderly people. *Health and Social Work*, **26**, 176–184.

Kolva, E., Rossenfield, B., Pessin, H., Breitbart, W. and Brescia, R. (2011), Anxiety in terminally ill cancer patients. *Journal of Pain and Symptom Management*, **42**(5), 691–701.

Le Roux, H., Gatz, M. and Wetherell, J. L. (2005). Age at onset of generalized anxiety disorder in older adults. *American Journal of Geriatric Psychiatry*, **13**, 23–30.

Lee, D., Woo, J. and Mackenzie, A. E. (2002). The cultural context of adjusting to nursing home life: Chinese elders' perspectives. *Gerontologist*, **42**, 667–675.

Lichtenberg, P. A. and MacNeill, S. E. (2003). Streamlining assessments and treatments for geriatric mental health in medical rehabilitation. *Rehabilitation Psychology*, **48**(1), 56–60.

Livingston, G., Kelly, L., Lewis-Holmes, E. and Cooper, C. (2014). Non-pharmacological interventions for agitation in dementia: systematic review of randomized controlled trials. *British Journal of Psychiatry*, **205**, 436–442.

Logsdon, R. G., Gibbons, L. E., McCurry, S. M. and Teri, L. (1999). Quality of life in Alzheimer's disease: patient and caregiver reports. *Journal of Mental Health and Aging*, **5**, 21–32.

Mack, J. L., Patterson, M. B. and Tariot, P. N. (1999). Behavior rating scale for dementia: development of test scales and presentation of data for 555 individuals with Alzheimer's disease. *Journal of Geriatric Psychiatry and Neurology*, **12**(4), 211–223.

Martini de Oliveira, A., Radanovic, M. and Cotting Homem de Mello, P., et al. (2015). Non-pharmacological interventions to reduce behavioral and psychological symptoms of dementia: a systematic review. *BioMed Research International*, **2015**, 218980.

Meeks, S., Woodruff-Borden, J. and Depp, C. (2003). Structural differentiation of self-reported depression and anxiety in late life. *Journal of Anxiety Disorders*, **17**, 627–646.

Mega, M. S., Cummings, J. L., Fiorello, T. and Gornbein, J. (1996). The spectrum of behavioral changes in Alzheimer's disease. *Neurology*, **46**(1), 130–135.

Mintzer, J. E. and Brawman-Mintzer, O. (1996). Agitation as possible expression of generalized anxiety disorder in demented elderly patients: toward a treatment approach. *Journal of Clinical Psychiatry*, **57**, 55–63.

Miovic, M. and Block, S. (2007). Psychiatric disorders in advanced cancer. *Cancer*, **110**(8), 1665–1676.

Neville, C. and Teri, L. (2011). Anxiety, anxiety symptoms, and associations among older people with dementia in assisted-living facilities. *International Journal of Mental Health Nursing*, **20**(3), 195–201.

Ninot, G., Fortes, M., Poulain, M., et al. (2006). Gender difference in coping strategies among patients enrolled in an inpatient rehabilitation program. *Heart & Lung*, **35**(2), 130–136.

O'Neil, M., Freeman., M., Christensen, V., Telerant, A., Addleman, A. and Kansagara, D. (2011). *Non-pharmacological Interventions for Behavioral Symptoms of Dementia: A Systematic Review of the Evidence*. VA-ESP Project #05-225. Washington, DC: US Department of Veterans Affairs.

Porter, R. J., Gallagher, P., Thompson, J. M. and Young, A. H. (2003). Neurocognitive impairment in drug-free patients with major depressive disorder. *British Journal of Psychiatry*, **182**, 214–220.

Qiu, W. Q., Dean, M., Liu, T., et al. (2010). Physical and mental health of the homebound elderly: an overlooked population. *Journal of the American Geriatrics Society*, **58**(12), 2423–2428.

Reinardy, J. R. and Kane, R. A. (2003). Anatomy of a choice: deciding on assisted living or nursing home care in Oregon. *Journal of Applied Gerontology*, **22**, 152–174.

Reisberg, B., Franssen, E., Kluger, A., et al. (1990). The clinical course of Alzheimer's patients. *Neurobiology of Aging*, **11**, 253.

Roth, A. Nelson, C.J., Rosenfeld B., et al. (2006). Assessing anxiety in men with prostate cancer: further data on the reliability and validity of the Memorial Anxiety Scale for Prostate Cancer (MAX-PC). *Psychosomatics*, **47**, 340–347.

Schoevers, R. A., Beekman, A. T. F., Deeg, D. J. H., et al. 2003. The natural history of late-life depression: results from the Amsterdam Study of the Elderly (AMSTEL). *Journal of Affective Disorders*, **76**, 5–14.

Schulz, R. (1976). Effects of control and predictability on the physical and psychological well-being of the institutionalized aged. *Journal of Personality and Social Psychology*, **33**(5), 563–573.

Segal, D. L., June, A., Payne, M., Coolidge, F., L. and Yochim, B. (2010). Development and initial validation of a self-report assessment tool for anxiety among older adults: the Geriatric Anxiety Scale. *Journal of Anxiety Disorders*, **24**, 709–214.

Shankar, K. K. and Orrell, M. W. (2000). Detecting and managing anxiety in people with dementia. *Current Opinion in Psychiatry*, **13**, 55–59.

Singh, R., Hunter, J. and Philip, A. (2007). The rapid resolution of depression and anxiety symptoms after lower limb amputation. *Clinical Rehabilitation*, **21**(8), 754–759.

Singh, R., Ripley, D., Pentland, B., et al. (2009). Depression and anxiety symptoms after lower limb amputation: the rise and fall. *Clinical Rehabilitation*, **23**(3), 281–286.

Stall, N, Nowaczynski, M. and Sinha, S. K. (2013). Back to the future: home-based primary care for older homebound Canadians: part 2: where we are going. *Canadian Family Physician*, **59**, 243–245.

Stall, N, Nowaczynski, M. and Sinha, S. K. (2014). Systematic review of outcomes from home-based primary care programs for homebound older adults. *Journal of the American Geriatrics Society*, **62**, 2243–2251.

Starkstein, S. E., Jorge, R., Mizrahi, R., Adrian, J. and Robinson, R. G. (2007). Insight and danger in Alzheimer's disease. *European Journal of Neurology*, **14**(4), 455–460.

Teachman, B. A. (2006). Aging and negative affect: the rise and fall and rise of anxiety and depression symptoms. *Psychology and Aging*, **21**, 201–207.

Teri, L. E., McCurry, S. M., Logsdon, R. G., et al. (1998). Exercise and activity level in Alzheimer's disease: a potential treatment focus. *Journal of Rehabilitation Research and Development*, 35(4), 411–419.

Tinetti, M. E., Inouye, S. K., Gill, T. M. and Doucette, J. T. (1995). Shared risk factors for falls, incontinence, and functional dependence: unifying the approach to geriatric syndromes. *JAMA*, 273(17), 1348–1353.

Tolin, D. F., Robison, J. T., Gaztambide, S. and Blank, K. (2005). Anxiety disorders in older Puerto Rican primary care patients. *American Journal of Geriatric Psychiatry*, 13, 150–156.

US Census Bureau (2010). National population projections: summary. www.census.gov/population/www/cen2010/glance/

Watanabe, Y. (2005). Fear of falling among stroke survivors after discharge from inpatient rehabilitation. *International Journal of Rehabilitation Research*, 28(2), 149–152.

Wetherell, J. L., Sorrell, J. T., Thorp, S. R. and Patterson, T. L. (2005). Psychological interventions for late-life anxiety: a review and early lessons from the CALM study. *Journal of Geriatric Psychiatry and Neurology*, 18, 72–82.

Wetherell, J. L., Thorp, S. R., Patterson, T. L., Golshan, S., Jeste, D. V. and Gatz, M. (2004). Quality of life in geriatric generalized anxiety disorder: a preliminary investigation. *Journal of Psychiatric Research*, 38, 305–312.

Wolitzky-Taylor, K. B., Castriotta, N., Lenze, E. J., Stanley, M. A. and Craske, M. G. (2010). Anxiety disorders in older adults: a comprehensive review. *Depression and Anxiety*, 27, 190–211.

World Health Organization (2015). World report on ageing and health. http://apps.who.int/iris/bitstream/10665/186463/1/9789240694811_eng.pdf

Yang, J. A., Garis, J., Jackson, C. and McClure, R. (2009). Providing psychotherapy to older adults in home: benefits, challenges, and decision-making guidelines. *Clinical Gerontologist*, 32, 333–346.

Yerkes, R. M. and Dodson, J. (1908). The relation of strength of stimulus to rapidity of habit-formation. *Journal of Comparative Neurology and Psychology*, 18, 459–482.

Psychosocial Treatment of Anxiety in Later Life

Katherine Ramos and Melinda A. Stanley

Anxiety disorders are common in older adulthood, with 12-month and lifetime prevalence rates of 11.6% and 15.3%, respectively, in the USA (Kessler et al., 2005). International prevalence ranges from 1% to 15% (Prina et al., 2011). Anxiety disorders and/or subsyndromal anxiety are associated with decreased quality of life (Porensky et al., 2009), increased disability (Tampi & Tampi, 2014), cognitive impairment (Beaudreau & O'Hara, 2008), decreased physical activity (Norton et al., 2012), sleep disturbance (Brenes et al., 2009), and increased dependence in activities of daily living (Lenze et al., 2001). Those suffering from clinically impairing anxiety symptoms or a diagnosable anxiety disorder are also less likely to access mental health services (Bower & Wetherell, 2015) than their counterparts without these problems, underscoring the importance of improving access to treatment delivery.

Evidence-based psychosocial treatments for late-life anxiety are promising. However, over half of older adults with anxiety do not seek treatment (Byers et al., 2012), and age differences in treatment response suggest that older adults with anxiety may not benefit from evidence-based treatments as much as their younger counterparts (Wetherell et al., 2013b). More work is needed to improve access and outcomes for this underserved population. This chapter provides an overview of available late-life anxiety psychosocial treatments with attention to both traditional efficacy trials and the development and testing of new models of care designed to improve reach, access, and outcomes.

Overview of Traditional Efficacy Trials

Initial efficacy trials of psychosocial treatments for late-life anxiety disorders focused on cognitive behavioral therapy (CBT), given the success of this approach in younger adults. Within the past 8 years, meta-analytic research and independent studies support the efficacy of CBT for older adults in the treatment of anxiety disorders, with particular attention being paid to generalized anxiety disorder (GAD) and panic disorder (PD) with or without agoraphobia.

Meta-analytic evaluation of late-life anxiety interventions across a range of anxiety disorders (GAD, PD, mixed anxiety samples) supports the efficacy of behavioral and pharmacological treatments (Pinquart & Duberstein, 2007). Both treatment approaches demonstrate significant reductions in anxiety symptoms, with equivalent effects across the two modalities when analyses control for nonspecific changes. However, because the influence of medication placebo is more robust than control conditions for behavioral treatments (e.g., wait list, treatment as usual (TAU)), the effects of pharmacological interventions without consideration of nonspecific effects are greater relative to behavioral treatment.

In two meta-analyses focused only on cognitive behavioral treatments for a range of anxiety problems (GAD, PD, mixed anxiety disorders, and anxiety symptoms; Gould et al., 2012; Thorp et al., 2009), outcomes following CBT were effective relative to control conditions, although effects were larger relative to wait-list control conditions and TAU than in comparison with alternative active treatments. Moreover, outcomes following relaxation therapy alone were comparable to effects of more comprehensive CBT models (Thorp et al., 2009).

Because most late-life anxiety efficacy work has focused on GAD, one recent meta-analysis examined the effects of both medication and psychosocial interventions (mostly CBT) for the treatment of this disorder (Gonçalves & Byrne, 2012). Positive effects occurred for both benzodiazepines and antidepressant medication, and CBT was effective for late-life GAD compared with wait-list controls, minimal contact, or TAU. Effects for CBT were not significant, however, when comparison conditions involved active treatments, suggesting the need for modifications to enhance outcomes. In a more recent small-scale randomized controlled trial (RCT) examining CBT as an augmentation strategy for antidepressant medication in the treatment for GAD, results suggested sustained remission without the aid of long-term pharmacotherapy (i.e., three-quarters of participants receiving CBT were able to discontinue their medication) (Wetherell et al., 2013c).

CBT has also been effective in the reduction of PD symptoms with or without agoraphobia in a direct comparison with pharmacotherapy (i.e., paroxetine) and wait-list control (Hendriks et al., 2012). Late-life PD onset and shorter duration of PD symptoms were predictors of stronger outcomes following CBT treatment. In a more recent study comparing panic symptom reduction following CBT among younger versus older adults, results suggested similar symptom reduction (with moderate to large effect sizes) in both groups, although avoidance behavior improved more in older adults (Hendriks et al., 2014). Less is known about the efficacy of CBT for other anxiety disorders due to a lack of RCTs. However, CBT has also been efficacious for late-life specific phobia (Pachana et al., 2007) and obsessive–compulsive disorders according to uncontrolled case reports (Calamari et al., 2012).

Evidence supports the efficacy of CBT for late-life anxiety, although effects are not as robust in older adults as in younger populations (Ayers et al., 2007; Wetherell et al., 2013b). Older adults are at higher risk for cognitive impairment and memory decline than younger adults, which may limit the benefits of the cognitive components of CBT (Mohlman & Gorman, 2005). Thus, relaxation training and other behavioral approaches may be preferable to complex cognitive skills, and data support the comparable effects of relaxation training relative to a full course of CBT (Thorp et al., 2009). Additionally, changes in visual acuity and scanning and processing speeds in the aging may suggest that simplification of CBT materials and assignments is necessary to improve adherence and to demonstrate greater reductions in psychologically impairing symptoms.

Notably, when CBT was enhanced via provision of weekly reading assignments, learning aids, reminder calls, and weekly reviews, homework compliance improved, and significant reductions in anxiety symptoms were found compared with standard CBT delivery (Mohlman et al., 2003). Additional suggestions for modifying CBT to meet the unique needs of older adults include prioritizing individual above group treatment, decreasing the duration of treatment sessions, simplifying practice skills, providing learning and memory aids, increasing psychoeducation, having a greater focus on behavioral components and skills acquisition, and including caretakers or family in treatment planning (Ayers et al., 2007; Mohlman, 2008).

Limitations of Efficacy Studies and the Need for New Models of Care

Most CBT efficacy studies focus primarily on samples that are homogeneous with regard to both diagnosis (i.e., GAD or PD) and demographic characteristics (e.g., participants are predominantly Caucasian, of middle to high socioeconomic status, and mostly in the young-old age category (60–69 years of age)). Additionally, most studies have been conducted in academic clinical settings, where older adults do not typically present for care. Recent work has demonstrated positive effects of CBT for late-life anxiety in primary care settings (Stanley et al., 2009; Wetherell et al., 2009), but these studies still reflect homogeneity of clinical and demographic characteristics, as well as a number of practice procedures (e.g., expert providers, long in-person sessions) that do not adequately reflect what is feasible in real-world care.

There is an ongoing need to examine unique constellations of anxiety symptoms in older adults to improve models of care and service delivery. For example, older adults with late-life anxiety present with trauma (Thorp et al., 2012), unique anxiety symptoms (e.g., hoarding, fear of falling), cognitive deficits (e.g., poor concentration and memory impairment) (Beaudreau & O'Hara, 2008), and frequent coexistent physical health issues (e.g., chronic illness, disability). Psychosocial stressors, including changes in marital status (e.g., divorce, separation, or being single), cultural stigmas/taboos, limited finances, retirement, and concerns of becoming a burden to family, are additional areas necessitating attention in clinical care.

The Institute of Medicine (2012) further highlights the complexity of mental health issues in older adults (e.g., medication treatment worsening physical and mental health problems), suggesting that effective delivery will consist of systematic outreach, diagnosis, and further inclusion of a larger, more diverse interdisciplinary workforce with adequate geriatric training to improve service delivery. Within the last decade, there has been an increase in service delivery models to improve care in the aging (e.g., the Improving Mood – Promoting Access to Collaborative Treatment program model (IMPACT; Unützer et al., 2001) and the Geriatric Resources for Assessment and Care of Elders model (GRACE; Counsell et al., 2007)).

The IMPACT model, originally conceived to treat late-life depression, provides participants with education materials, including a relapse-prevention plan and psychiatry services (if there is no response to treatment). In addition, interdisciplinary teams consisting of nurses, social workers, and psychologists work alongside the participant's primary care provider to develop and implement a treatment plan. Similarly, the GRACE model, a home-based geriatric care program, also uses an interdisciplinary team that together develops an initial assessment plan, followed by weekly care plan meetings for patient progress and monthly visits to the participant's home. Such programming and treatment show promise. However, these models were specifically developed solely for the treatment of late-life depression, and programming for treating late-life anxiety is also needed. In brief, effective mental health services for late-life anxiety will require novel delivery models that are patient-centered and use the expertise of care managers within an interdisciplinary team to personalize care and increase access.

Novel Approaches to Address Anxiety Symptoms Unique to Older Adults

To address current limitations of efficacy trials, recent programs of research have begun to develop and pilot-test treatment models that address heterogeneity in clinical samples with late-life anxiety. Additionally, more attention has been given to treating elders from diverse backgrounds (e.g., across ethnicity, Veteran versus non-Veteran status, and nonacademic clinical settings with interdisciplinary teams) to more sensitively address the unique needs in older adults. Below is a summary of current and novel psychosocial treatments addressing post-traumatic stress disorder (PTSD), hoarding, fear of falling, cognitive impairment, and chronic illness.

PTSD

Per the Diagnostic and Statistical Manual of Mental Disorders, Fifth Edition (DSM-5; American Psychiatric Association, 2013), PTSD is characterized by exposure to a traumatic event, with the presence of intrusive symptoms, avoidance, negative alterations in cognitions and mood, and alterations in arousal and reactivity. Symptoms cause significant impairment in social and occupational functioning and last longer than 1 month or may have a 6-month delayed onset.

Among the general population, about 70–90% of adults aged 65 and over are exposed to at least one traumatic event in their lifetime (Frans et al., 2005). In large epidemiological studies, prevalence rates of PTSD vary in older adults and by gender (e.g., more men report higher rates of lifetime exposure to trauma than women). Within the USA, the lifetime prevalence rate in adults aged 60 and older was 2.5% (Kessler et al., 2005); internationally rates range from 1.5% to 6.5% (Frans et al., 2005). Among older US Veterans, in particular, lifetime exposure to trauma is as high as 85% (Hankin et al., 1999), suggesting a significant need to research appropriate evidence-based mental health services to address these types of symptoms in older adults.

Current treatments for PTSD among the general population include pharmacotherapy, exposure therapies (typically the preferred treatment of choice), and CBT (the most widely tested in RCTs) (Thorp et al., 2011). The utility of these evidence-based treatments for older adults with PTSD has been questioned given potential age-associated cognitive limitations (Schuitevoerder et al., 2013) and concerns about possible adverse outcomes of intensive exposure. Until recently, treatment of older adults with PTSD had been examined only in case studies, with interventions including eye movement desensitization and reprocessing (Thomas & Gafner, 1993), imaginal exposure (Knaevelsrud et al., 2009), life review (Maercker, 2002), and general cognitive behavioral treatment (Snell & Padin-Rivera, 1997).

In a quasi-experimental pilot study of prolonged exposure (PE) for older-adult Veterans with PTSD, significant reduction in PTSD symptoms was evident via clinician rating and self-report compared with TAU (Thorp et al., 2012). In this study, exposure-based treatment was provided for Veterans whose traumas had occurred four to five decades prior to study enrollment. The study findings supported the potential viability of PE for older Veterans. In a subsequent RCT of this intervention with 87 older-adult male combat Veterans, significantly greater PTSD symptom reduction was reported following PE than following relaxation training (Thorp & Sones, 2013). Veterans also self-reported improved symptoms of depression. These data support the value of Veterans Health Administration efforts to disseminate PE. Further work in standardizing PTSD screening procedures for older adults outside PTSD clinics (e.g., during primary-care visits to the Veterans Health Administration) and consistent use of clinical reminders via electronic health records can help further identify and refer older adults who need trauma-focused treatment. Though the literature addressing PTSD treatment in older adults remains nascent, current findings and continuing efforts in addressing treatment efficacy remain promising.

Hoarding

The diagnostic features of hoarding disorder include persistent difficulty discarding possessions, regardless of value, with a strong need to save belongings and clutter that prohibits the use of living spaces (American Psychiatric Association, 2013). Hoarding causes clinically significant distress in important areas of functioning (e.g., social and occupational) that lead to poor maintenance in keeping a safe environment. Based on community samples, general population prevalence in the USA and Europe ranges from 2% to 6%, (Mueller et al., 2009; Samuels et al., 2008).

Hoarding is more common in men than women (Samuels et al., 2008) and more prevalent in older than in younger adults, with severity increasing with age if untreated in early life (Ayers et al., 2013a). Hoarding behavior in late life has been linked with functional impairment and disability (Ayers et al., 2013a), poor quality of life (Saxena et al., 2011), poor executive functioning (Ayers et al., 2013b), and chronic illness (e.g., diabetes, cardiovascular disease, and sleep apnea; Ayers et al., 2014b).

A cognitive behavioral approach for compulsive hoarding that includes education, motivational interviewing, exposure, cognitive restructuring, problem-solving, and skill training across 12 weeks (26 sessions) has demonstrated efficacy relative to a wait-list control among younger adults (Steketee et al., 2010). Use of this same treatment in geriatric populations, however, failed to produce similar positive outcomes (Ayers et al., 2011). Of the 12 participants who completed treatment, only 3 were considered treatment responders, with reductions in depression symptoms and hoarding severity, and the treatment gains for these 3 individuals were not maintained at the 6-month follow-up. Given the possible impact of associated neurocognitive deficits (Ayers et al., 2013b) and pervasive behavioral and experiential avoidance in geriatric hoarders (Ayers et al., 2014a), a modified treatment protocol was developed for older adults. This approach de-emphasizes cognitive therapy techniques, increases focus on behavioral treatment components (i.e., exposure), and adds a cognitive rehabilitation component. A recent open trial of this treatment showed promise, with clinically significant symptom reduction in hoarding severity among 8 of 11 older-adult participants (Ayers et al., 2014c). Further follow-up studies that include a control group and have a larger sample size with more ethnically diverse participants are needed.

Fear of Falling

Fear of falling (regardless whether a fall has been sustained) is a common concern in older persons, one that poses risks for increased physical instability, poor health, functional impairment, and diminished quality of life (Li et al., 2003). Rates of having at least one fall per year range from 30% to 40% in community-dwelling older adults (Ambrose et al., 2013). Home-based exercise programs, tai chi, and treatments, including multifactorial assessment (e.g., fall risk assessment and home safety assessment, cognition and visual acuity testing), have proven effective in reducing the symptoms of fear of falling (Gillespie et al., 2012).

Wetherell and colleagues (2013a) are currently conducting a program of research to examine the feasibility and outcomes of the Activity, Balance, Learning, and Exposure (ABLE) intervention, a home-based integrated intervention to address fears of falling. ABLE includes exposure exercises, medical and home assessments, elements of CBT, and delivery by a physical therapist. The treatment protocol consists of eight sessions that begin with a medication review, followed by three sessions involving exercise, home safety evaluations, and development of an exposure hierarchy. The four remaining sessions include exposure-based CBT and cognitive restructuring, with a last session focused on exercise and relapse prevention. Preliminary results suggest decreased symptoms of fear of falling and a reduction in avoidance following treatment (Wetherell et al., 2013a). To date, this study is the first to target exposure exercises to minimize feared anticipation of falling.

Cognitive Limitations

Executive Dysfunction

As previously mentioned, late-life anxiety is sometimes associated with cognitive impairment and impaired function (Beaudreau & O'Hara, 2008). Of particular importance to the impact of psychosocial interventions is the potential presence of executive dysfunction, which is associated with impaired inhibition, difficulty sustaining attention (Mohlman & Gorman, 2005), and decreased performance in verbal memory, categorization, and set switching among older adults (Yochim et al., 2013). Deficits in executive skills decrease an older adult's ability to organize and integrate new information imperative in learning. These types of deficits carry serious clinical implications regarding the appropriateness of the cognitive components of CBT that rely heavily on the use of "top-down" executive abilities (e.g., logic and reasoning, daily monitoring, cognitive restructuring) for successful treatment outcomes. Recent work, however, has examined the role that executive dysfunction plays in late-life anxiety (Yochim et al., 2013) and, more specifically, how it affects treatment and treatment modifications (Mohlman, 2008).

In a pilot study testing standard CBT versus CBT augmented with executive skills modules from the Attention Process Training II (APT) program for late-life GAD, the CBT/APT intervention resulted in greater improvement in executive skills and lowered levels of worry severity relative to standard CBT (Mohlman, 2008). Patients in CBT/APT received executive skills training in areas that strengthened cognitive control and attention across an 8-week period. Overall, twice the number of CBT/APT participants (i.e., $n = 4$; 100% of the sample) relative to CBT participants (i.e., $n = 2$; 50% of the sample) responded to treatment at post-treatment and at the 6-month follow-up. Subsequently, CBT/APT was used effectively to reduce anxiety symptoms in an older adult with Parkinson's disease (Mohlman et al., 2010).

Dementia

Anxiety is common among people with dementia, with prevalence as high as 70% in community-dwelling patients with Alzheimer's disease and prevalence of anxiety disorders ranging from 5% to 21% (Ferretti et al., 2001; Seignourel et al., 2008). Anxiety in dementia is associated with reduced quality of life (Hoe et al., 2006), and it is positively associated with challenging dementia-related behaviors (Ferretti et al., 2001).

CBT for anxiety has been adapted to meet the needs of persons with dementia. In an open trial of "Peaceful Mind," an intervention targeting anxiety in persons with dementia, favorable outcomes included treatment satisfaction and reduction of anxiety and depression symptoms among persons with dementia and reductions in caregiver distress (Paukert et al., 2010). In a follow-up pilot RCT, results among 32 patients with either mild or moderate dementia showed significant post-treatment (3 months) reductions in anxiety symptoms and caregiver distress ratings, in addition to higher self-reported quality of life by participants, relative to usual care (Stanley et al., 2013). Improvements, however, were not maintained at the 6-month follow-up, suggesting the need for more sustained involvement in the intervention. The Peaceful Mind treatment (Paukert et al., 2013) includes elements of home-based treatment delivery, caregiving coaching, and a greater focus on behavioral skills (e.g., diaphragmatic breathing and calming statements) than regular CBT.

In another pilot RCT, 50 participants with mild to moderate dementia and anxiety experienced reductions in anxiety and depression at 15 weeks following a 10-session CBT treatment protocol compared to TAU (Spector et al., 2015). However, after adjusting for baseline anxiety and cognition, group differences in anxiety symptoms were no longer statistically significant. At the 6-month follow-up, anxiety scores were lower in the CBT group compared to the TAU group, although these findings failed to reach statistical significance. Qualitative analyses from this work suggested improved interpersonal relationships among patients and their caregivers. Improved overall well-being and acceptance of dementia were also reported.

Chronic Illness

Given that a large part of the aging population faces chronic health difficulties, psychosocial interventions that target both chronic illness self-management and mental health conditions become imperative. Cully and colleagues (2009, 2010) used a time-limited CBT intervention, known as Adjusting to Chronic Conditions Using Education, Support, and Skills (ACCESS), which concurrently focuses on psychological and physical concerns associated with managing chronic illness. ACCESS is a patient-centered treatment that provides services in person or via phone. The CBT protocol consists of six treatment sessions with brief follow-up booster sessions. Content from the manual includes psychoeducation about chronic illness (in this case, congestive heart failure and chronic obstructive pulmonary disease) with elective modules teaching skills related to managing physical health (exercise, nutrition, provider communication, managing medications and flare-ups, sleep hygiene), relaxation strategies, changing thoughts, increasing pleasant activities, and problem-solving. Results from a series of case studies (Cully et al., 2009) showed a significant reduction in anxiety symptoms at the end of 8 weeks and at the 3-month follow-up. A larger study recently tested the ACCESS intervention in a hybrid effectiveness/implementation design within primary care settings. The results demonstrated significant improvements in anxiety, depression, and physical health outcomes (Cully et al., 2015).

Similarly, an integrated CBT intervention for anxiety, depression, and chronic illness resulted in large effect sizes (range = 0.73–1.49) at post-treatment and at the 1-month follow-up among patients with Parkinson's disease (Calleo et al., 2015), although sample sizes were small and changes were not consistently different across CBT and enhanced usual care. As in the ACCESS protocol, session content focused on both chronic disease self-management (healthy diet and exercise, improving sleep, communication) and traditional skills training to manage anxiety and depression (exposure, relaxation, behavioral activation, managing negative thoughts). Adaptations to CBT interventions that offer brief, patient-centered, and flexible care with special attention to concurrent emotional and physical difficulties may prove fruitful in treating late-life anxiety comorbid with other chronic health conditions.

Novel Approaches to Personalizing Care and Expanding Reach

In addition to addressing the unique and heterogeneous symptoms characteristic of older adults, changes in treatment delivery models are also needed to improve care for late-life anxiety and associated symptoms. Here, we review data related to innovative treatment models and delivery options that seek to enhance access and improve outcomes of evidence-based care.

Novel Treatment Models

Treatment models that diverge from traditional CBT may serve as alternatives to improve outcomes and better meet the needs of older adults. In particular, two approaches anchored in mindfulness theory and practice – acceptance and commitment therapy (ACT) and mindfulness-based stress reduction (MBSR) – have been suggested as potentially useful approaches for older adults with significant worry and anxiety (Lenze et al., 2014; Wetherell et al., 2011). Although seen as alternatives to traditional CBT, both approaches include components that align with behavioral models (i.e., breathing retraining in MBSR, behavioral activation in ACT). The enhanced benefits of these approaches for older people may result from their alignment with the need to adapt to life events that, in themselves, are not always modifiable (e.g., declining health, loss of family or friends, functional impairment). Recent open trials of ACT and MBSR have demonstrated the feasibility of these models and benefits in symptom reduction among older adults with GAD (Wetherell et al., 2011) and with significant worry accompanied by subjective cognitive difficulties (Lenze et al., 2014). Larger clinical trials are needed to establish the effectiveness and relative benefits of these approaches.

Another potentially important treatment model for older adults with anxiety relies on modular approaches that represent more "real-world" care than typical standardized CBT. These models are similar to those described earlier that address coexistent anxiety/depression and chronic illness, but this approach also may be useful for targeting anxiety more specifically. Modular treatments facilitate a person-centered approach wherein patients and providers work together to determine which treatment components best match the patient's primary symptoms and preferences. An initial test of modular treatment for late-life GAD allowed patients to choose from a range of coping modules, some of which represented traditional CBT skills (e.g., relaxation, thought stopping, behavioral activation) and others were anchored in alternative approaches (e.g., life review, acceptance and commitment) (Wetherell et al., 2009). Outcome data indicated the feasibility and acceptability of this approach, although symptoms did not improve relative to an enhanced community treatment comparison group, in which most patients received pharmacological treatment and other services. In a more recent and larger clinical trial, a modular approach anchored primarily in a CBT model demonstrated improvements in GAD severity, anxiety, depression, and mental health quality of life among older adults with GAD (Stanley et al., 2014).

Other innovations in treatment models for late-life anxiety include the integration of religion and/or spirituality (R/S) and additional treatment components to meet the unique needs of older adults, particularly those in underserved, low-income communities. Older adults and minority populations (African Americans, Hispanics) endorse particularly high levels of religious involvement and spirituality (Newport, 2006), and some forms of R/S coping (e.g., prayer, attending church) are associated with physical and mental health benefits (Chatters et al., 2008; Schnall et al., 2010). Furthermore, over 75% of older adults who received psychosocial treatment for anxiety/depression reported a preference for integrating R/S into a skills-based approach (Stanley et al., 2011). Along these lines, Calmer Life, an innovative model of modular skills-based treatment for late-life anxiety, includes the opportunity for participants to incorporate R/S. In this person-centered approach, participants may choose to incorporate R/S into some or all coping skills or may elect to omit R/S completely. In an initial open trial of Calmer Life in a sample of older adults from low-income, mostly minority communities (Shrestha et al., 2012), 78% of participants ($n = 7$) chose to incorporate R/S. Other data indicated the feasibility and potential positive outcomes of this approach.

Participant-expressed needs during the open trial, however, made it increasingly clear that a skills-based intervention alone was insufficient to allow adequate attention to worry in this population. In line with late-life depression work in low-income communities (Areán et al., 2010), worry content often represented participants' significant unmet service needs (e.g., chronic illness, personal care needs, financial difficulties) that limited the potential value of a worry-focused, skills-based approach. In addition, the pilot work revealed significant need for enhancing communication with health care providers, who frequently are unaware of anxiety symptoms and non-medication treatment approaches. Thus, Calmer Life was modified further to incorporate resource counseling that addresses basic unmet needs and to facilitate communication with an identified health care provider. An initial pilot randomized trial of this modified version of Calmer Life revealed positive outcomes in worry, anxiety, depression, sleep, and mental health quality of life relative to Enhanced Community Care (ECC), an intervention anchored in standard community-based information and referral (Stanley et al., 2016). A larger trial is ongoing (Shrestha et al., 2015), and a Spanish-language version of the intervention, Vida Calma, was created and piloted with one participant who experienced meaningful improvements in worry, depression, and satisfaction with life (Ramos et al., 2017).

Novel Delivery Options

To address limitations in access and other barriers to mental health care for older adults (e.g., limited availability of providers, stigma, transportation), recent models of care for late-life anxiety have included telephone and Internet-based treatment, delivery of care in nontraditional settings (primary care, home, community settings), and training of nontraditional providers.

Telephone-based treatment has been incorporated into the modular approaches that have already been discussed, in which participants are given the option to receive care either in person or by telephone after an initial session or two (Shrestha et al., 2012; Stanley et al., 2014, 2016). In these studies, approximately 40–60% of sessions were conducted by telephone. Skills-based treatment for late-life anxiety delivered entirely by phone also is effective. In one clinical trial (Brenes et al., 2012), telephone-based cognitive behavioral treatment (CBT-T) for late-life GAD was more effective than an information-only control condition in reducing general anxiety, worry, anxiety sensitivity, and insomnia, although only reductions in worry were maintained at the 6-month follow-up. In a more recent study (Brenes et al., 2015), CBT-T was more effective than nondirective, supportive therapy in reducing worry, GAD symptoms, and depressive symptoms in a sample of rural older adults with GAD. Reductions in worry severity and greater declines in GAD symptoms were evidenced at the 4-month and 15-month follow-ups (Brenes et al., 2017); the improvements in both trials were equivalent to those seen when similar treatments are delivered face-to-face.

In the last 5 years, there has been a growing interest in the potential effectiveness of Internet-delivered CBT (iCBT) to increase access to evidence-based care for late-life anxiety. While, to date, few studies directly address the use of iCBT for older adults with GAD, preliminary results are promising. For example, in two open trials, large within-group effect sizes were found among older adults with clinical-level symptoms of depression and anxiety (Dear et al., 2015b; Zou et al., 2012). In one RCT with a small sample size, clinical-guided iCBT improved symptoms of anxiety and depression, with symptom reduction maintained at the 3- and 12- month follow-ups (Dear et al., 2015a). The results also supported iCBT as a cost-effective treatment compared to a control comparison. Self-guided iCBT has shown sustained improvements in anxiety and depression at the 12-month follow-up (Titov et al., 2014). Despite promising results, most participants across current iCBT studies are relatively young (e.g., between 50 and 65 years of age), and treatment effectiveness for older adults with cognitive impairments remains mixed (Silfvernagel et al., 2018).

Other innovative delivery options for the treatment of late-life anxiety, some of which are modeled after strategies already tested in the late-life depression literature, include delivery in nontraditional settings, such as primary care (Stanley et al., 2009, 2014; Wetherell et al., 2009) and home-based care. As noted earlier, home-based delivery has been used successfully in the treatment of anxiety among patients with dementia (Stanley et al., 2013), and case reports document the value of home-based care for older adults receiving community care management (Diefenbach et al., 2008) and Veterans receiving home-based primary care (Cummings et al., 2013). Another option for the nontraditional delivery of late-life anxiety care derives from community–academic partnership models that allow participants to be seen in community settings (community service settings, churches, residential settings). In the Calmer Life model of care, described earlier, participants have the option of meeting with providers by telephone or in person at their homes or in a community partner setting (Shrestha et al., 2012, 2015; Stanley et al., 2016). This type of flexibility in delivery options facilitates person-centered care and meets Institute of Medicine (2012) guidelines for novel treatment models that can extend the reach and access to mental health care for older adults.

The Institute of Medicine recommendations also emphasize the need to develop a broader workforce, including nontraditional health care providers. In a recent clinical trial of modular CBT for late-life anxiety (Stanley et al., 2014), bachelor-level lay providers (BLPs) were trained to deliver care. Outcomes following CBT delivered by BLPs and PhD-level providers (PLPs) were equivalent and improved relative to usual care. Treatment characteristics and participant expectations and satisfaction were equivalent across BLP and PLP groups (Kraus-Schuman et al., 2015). In the Calmer Life treatment model, community providers (community health workers, case managers) are trained to deliver care (Shrestha et al., 2015). A larger study currently in progress will examine the effectiveness of this intervention relative to ECC when care is delivered by these providers.

Summary

Older adults are a rapidly growing population, and given the commonality of anxiety disorders prevalent in this age group, increasing the reach and access to mental health service delivery becomes paramount. Current evidence-based psychosocial treatments (e.g., mostly CBT-based) for late-life anxiety show promise. However, continued research is needed to improve outcomes. Such improvements underscore meeting the unique needs of older adults by directly addressing the heterogeneity in clinical samples and developing novel treatment models that pay closer attention to diversity in the aging. Of late, innovative treatment models (e.g., inclusion of mindfulness-based techniques, modular-based treatments, or R/S) and delivery options (e.g., service delivery via telephone or in nontraditional settings) have been proposed and pilot tested. This is a budding and societally important area of research. Further work in this domain will carry significant implications in improving clinical care and overall well-being in the lives of elders.

References

Ambrose, A. F., Paul, G. and Hausdorff, J. M. (2013). Risk factors for falls among older adults: a review of the literature. *Maturitas*, 75(1), 51–61.

American Psychiatric Association (2013). *Diagnostic and Statistical Manual of Mental Disorders*, 5th ed. Washington, DC: American Psychiatric Association.

Areán, P., Mackin, S., Vargas-Dwyer, E., et al. (2010). Treating depression in disabled, low-income elderly: a conceptual model and recommendations for care. *International Journal of Geriatric Psychiatry*, 25(8), 765–769.

Ayers, C., Castriotta, N., Dozier, M., Espejo, E. and Porter, B. (2014a). Behavioral and experiential avoidance in patients with hoarding disorder. *Journal of Behavior Therapy and Experimental Psychiatry*, 45(3), 408–414.

Ayers, C., Iqbal, Y. and Strickland, K. (2014b). Medical conditions in geriatric hoarding disorder patients. *Aging & Mental Health*, 18 (2), 148–151.

Ayers, C., Ly, P., Howard, I., Mayes, T., Porter, B. and Iqbal, Y. (2013a). Hoarding severity predicts functional disability in late-life hoarding disorder patients. *International Journal of Geriatric Psychiatry*, 29(7), 741–746.

Ayers, C., Saxena, S., Espejo, E., Twamley, E., Granholm, E. and Wetherell, J. (2014c). Novel treatment for geriatric hoarding disorder: an open trial of cognitive rehabilitation paired with behavior therapy. *American Journal of Geriatric Psychiatry*, 22 (3), 248–252.

Ayers, C., Sorrell, J., Thorp, S. and Wetherell, J. (2007). Evidence-based psychological treatments for late-life anxiety. *Psychology and Aging*, 22(1), 8–17.

Ayers, C., Wetherell, J., Golshan, S. and Saxena, S. (2011). Cognitive–behavioral therapy for geriatric compulsive hoarding. *Behaviour Research and Therapy*, 49(10), 689–694.

Ayers, C., Wetherell, J., Schiehser, D., Almklov, E., Golshan, S. and Saxena, S. (2013b). Executive functioning in older adults with hoarding disorder. *International Journal of Geriatric Psychiatry*, 28(11), 1175–1181.

Beaudreau, S. and O'Hara, R. (2008). Late-life anxiety and cognitive impairment: a review. *American Journal of Geriatric Psychiatry*, 16 (10), 790–803.

Bower, E. and Wetherell, J. (2015). Late life anxiety disorders. In P. A. Lichtenberg, B. T. Mast, B. D. Carpenter and J. L. Wetherell, eds., *APA Handbook of Clinical Geropsychology, Vol. 2: Assessment, Treatment, and Issues of Later Life*. Washington, D.C.: American Psychological Association, pp. 49–77.

Brenes, G. A., Danhauer, S. C., Lyles, M. F., Anderson, A. and Miller, M. E. (2017). Long-term effects of telephone-delivered psychotherapy for late-life GAD. *American Journal of Geriatric Psychiatry*, 25(11), 1249–1257.

Brenes, G., Danhauer, S., Lyles, M., Hogan, P. and Miller, M. (2015). Telephone-delivered cognitive behavioral therapy and telephone-delivered nondirective supportive therapy for rural older adults with generalized anxiety disorder. *JAMA Psychiatry*, 72(10), 1012–1020.

Brenes, G., Miller, M., Stanley, M., Williamson, J., Knudson, M. and McCall, W. (2009). Insomnia in older adults with generalized anxiety disorder. *American Journal of Geriatric Psychiatry*, **17**(6), 465–472.

Brenes, G., Miller, M., Williamson, J., McCall, W., Knudson, M. and Stanley, M. (2012). A randomized controlled trial of telephone-delivered cognitive–behavioral therapy for late-life anxiety disorders. *American Journal of Geriatric Psychiatry*, **20**(8), 707–716.

Byers, A. L., Arean, P. A. and Yaffe, K. (2012). Low use of mental health services among older Americans with mood and anxiety disorders. *Psychiatric Services*, **63**(1), 66–72.

Calamari, J., Pontarelli, N., Armstrong, K. and Salstrom, S. (2012). Obsessive-compulsive disorder in late life. *Cognitive and Behavioral Practice*, **19**(1), 136–150.

Calleo, J., Amspoker, A., Sarwar, A., et al. (2015). A pilot study of a cognitive–behavioral treatment for anxiety and depression in patients with Parkinson disease. *Journal of Geriatric Psychiatry and Neurology*, **28**(3), 210–217.

Chatters, L., Bullard, K., Taylor, R., Woodward, A., Neighbors, H. and Jackson, J. (2008). Religious participation and DSM-IV disorders among older African Americans: findings from the National Survey of American Life. *American Journal of Geriatric Psychiatry*, **16**(12), 957–965.

Counsell, S., Callahan, C., Clark, D., et al. (2007). Geriatric care management for low-income seniors. *JAMA*, **298**(22), 2623–2633.

Cully, J., Armento, M., Mott, J., et al. (2012). Brief cognitive behavioral therapy in primary care: a hybrid type 2 patient-randomized effectiveness-implementation design. *Implementation Science*, **7**(1), 1–12.

Cully, J., Paukert, A., Falco, J. and Stanley, M. (2009). Cognitive–behavioral therapy: innovations for cardiopulmonary patients with depression and anxiety. *Cognitive and Behavioral Practice*, **16**(4), 394–407.

Cully, J., Stanley, M., Deswal, A., Hanania, N., Phillips, L. and Kunik, M. (2010). Cognitive–behavioral therapy for chronic cardiopulmonary conditions. *Primary Care Companion to the Journal of Clinical Psychiatry*, **12**(4), e1–e6.

Cully, J., Stanley, M. A., Kauth, M.R., et al. (2015). Effectiveness and implementation of brief cognitive behavioral therapy in VA primary care settings. Unpublished poster presentation at the annual Health Services Research and Development/QUERI National Conference, July 8–10, 2015, Philadelphia, PA.

Cummings, J.P., Armento, M.E., Kunik, M.E., et al. (2013). A brief intervention for home-bound veterans with anxiety and/or depressive symptoms. Unpublished poster presentation at The Association for Behavioral and Cognitive Therapies, November 21–24, 2013, Nashville, TN.

Dear, B. F., Zou, J. B., Ali, S., et al. (2015a). Clinical and cost-effectiveness of therapist-guided Internet-delivered cognitive behavior therapy for older adults with symptoms of anxiety: a randomized controlled trial. *Behavior Therapy*, **46**(2), 206–217.

Dear, B. F., Zou, J. B., Ali, S., et al. (2015b). Examining self-guided Internet-delivered cognitive behavior therapy for older adults with symptoms of anxiety and depression: two feasibility open trials. *Internet Interventions*, **2**(1), 17–23.

Diefenbach, G., Tolin, D., Gilliam, C. and Meunier, S. (2008). Extending cognitive–behavioral therapy for late-life anxiety to home care: program development and case examples. *Behavior Modification*, **32**(5), 595–610.

Ferretti, L., McCurry, S., Logsdon, R., Gibbons, L. and Teri, L. (2001). Anxiety and Alzheimer's disease. *Journal of Geriatric Psychiatry and Neurology*, **14**(1), 52–58.

Frans, O., Rimmo, P., Aberg, L. and Fredrikson, M. (2005). Trauma exposure and post-traumatic stress disorder in the general population. *Acta Psychiatrica Scandinavica*, **111**(4), 291–290.

Gillespie, L.D., Robertson, M. C., Gillespie, W.J., et al. (2012). Interventions for preventing falls in older people in the community. *Cochrane Database Systematic Review*, **9**, CD007146.

Gonçalves, D. and Byrne, G. (2012). Interventions for generalized anxiety disorder in older adults: systematic review and meta-analysis. *Journal of Anxiety Disorders*, **26**(1), 1–11.

Gould, R., Coulson, M. and Howard, R. (2012). Efficacy of cognitive behavioral therapy for anxiety disorders in older people: a meta-analysis and meta-regression of randomized controlled trials. *Journal of the American Geriatrics Society*, **60**(2), 218–229.

Hankin, C. S., Spiro, A., Miller, D. R., and Kazis, L. (1999). Mental disorders and mental health treatment among U.S. Department of Veterans Affairs outpatients: the Veterans Health Study. *American Journal of Psychiatry*, **156**(12), 1924–1930.

Hendriks, G., Kampman, M., Keijsers, G., Hoogduin, C. and Voshaar, R. (2014). Cognitive–behavioral therapy for panic disorder with agoraphobia in older people: a comparison with younger patients. *Depression and Anxiety*, **31**(8), 669–677.

Hendriks, G., Keijsers, G., Kampman, M., Hoogduin, C. and Oude Voshaar, R. (2012). Predictors of outcome of pharmacological and psychological treatment of late-life panic disorder with agoraphobia. *International Journal of Geriatric Psychiatry*, **27**(2), 146–150.

Hoe, J., Hancock, G., Livingston, G. and Orrell, M. (2006). Quality of life of people with dementia in residential care homes. *British Journal of Psychiatry*, **188**(5), 460–464.

Institute of Medicine (2012). *Mental Health and Substance Use Workforce for Older Adults. In Whose Hands?* Washington, DC: National Academy Press.

Kessler, R., Berglund, P., Demler, O., Jin, R., Merikangas, K. and Walters, E. (2005). Lifetime prevalence and age-of-onset distributions of DSM-IV disorders in the National Comorbidity Survey Replication. *Archives of General Psychiatry*, **62**(6), 593–602.

Knaevelsrud C, Böttche M, and Kuwert P. (2009). Long-term effects of civilian war trauma: epidemiological, sociological and psychotherapeutic aspects. Presented at: 11th European Conference on Traumatic Stress, June 15–18, 2009, Oslo, Norway.

Kraus-Schuman, C., Wilson, N., Amspoker, A., et al. (2015). Enabling lay providers to conduct CBT for older adults: key steps for expanding treatment capacity. *Translational Behavioral Medicine*, **5**(3), 247–253.

Lenze, E., Hickman, S., Hershey, T., et al. (2014). Mindfulness-based stress reduction for older adults with worry symptoms and co-occurring cognitive dysfunction. *International Journal of Geriatric Psychiatry*, **29**(10), 991–1000.

Lenze, E., Rogers, J., Martire, L., et al. (2001). The association of late-life depression and anxiety with physical disability: a review of the literature and prospectus for future research. *American Journal of Geriatric Psychiatry*, **9**(2), 113–135.

Li, F., Fisher, K. J., Harmer, P., McAuley, E. and Wilson, N. L. (2003). Fear of falling in elderly persons: association with falls, functional ability, and quality of life. *Journals of Gerontology Series B: Psychological Sciences and Social Sciences*, **58**(5), P283–P290.

Maercker, A. (2002). Life-review technique in the treatment of PTSD in elderly patients: Rationale and three single case studies. *Journal of Clinical Geropsychology*, **8**(3), 239–249.

Mohlman, J. (2008). More power to the executive? A preliminary test of CBT plus executive skills training for treatment of late-life GAD. *Cognitive and Behavioral Practice*, **15**(3), 306–316.

Mohlman, J. and Gorman, J. (2005). The role of executive functioning in CBT: a pilot study with anxious older adults. *Behaviour Research and Therapy*, **43**(4), 447–465.

Mohlman, J., Gorenstein, E. E., Kleber, M., deJesus, M., Gorman, J. M., and Papp, L. A. (2003). Standard and enhanced cognitive behavior therapy for late life generalized anxiety disorder: two pilot investigations. *American Journal of Geriatric Psychiatry*, **11**(1), 24–32.

Mohlman, J., Reel, D., Chazin, D., et al. (2010). A novel approach to treating anxiety and enhancing executive skills in an older adult with Parkinson's disease. *Clinical Case Studies*, **9**(1), 74–90.

Mueller, A., Mitchell, J., Crosby, R., Glaesmer, H. and de Zwaan, M. (2009). The prevalence of compulsive hoarding and its association with compulsive buying in a German population-based sample. *Behaviour Research and Therapy*, **47**(8), 705–709.

Newport, F. (2006). Religion Most Important to Blacks, Women, and Older Americans. Gallup.com. www.gallup.com/poll/25585/Religion-Most-Important-Blacks-Women-Older-Americans.aspx (accessed July 27, 2015).

Norton, J., Ancelin, M., Stewart, R., Berr, C., Ritchie, K. and Carrière, I. (2012). Anxiety symptoms and disorder predict activity limitations in the elderly. *Journal of Affective Disorders*, **141**(2–3), 276–285.

Pachana, N. A., Woodward, R. M., and Byrne, G. J. (2007). Treatment of specific phobia in older adults. *Clinical Interventions in Aging*, **2**(3), 469–476.

Paukert, A. L., Calleo, J., Kraus-Schuman, C., et al. (2010). Peaceful mind: an open trial of cognitive–behavioral therapy for anxiety in persons with dementia. *International Psychogeriatrics*, **22**(06), 1012–1021.

Paukert, A. L., Kraus-Schuman, C., Wilson, N., et al. (2013). The Peaceful Mind manual: a protocol for treating anxiety in persons with dementia. *Behavior Modification*, **37**(5), 631–664.

Pinquart, M. and Duberstein, P. (2007). Treatment of anxiety disorders in older adults: a meta-analytic comparison of behavioral and pharmacological interventions. *American Journal of Geriatric Psychiatry*, **15**(8), 639–651.

Porensky, E., Dew, M., Karp, J., et al. (2009). The burden of late-life generalized anxiety disorder: effects on disability, health-related quality of life, and healthcare utilization. *American Journal of Geriatric Psychiatry*, **17**(6), 473–482.

Prina, A., Ferri, C., Guerra, M., Brayne, C. and Prince, M. (2011). Prevalence of anxiety and its correlates among older adults in Latin America, India and China: cross-cultural study. *British Journal of Psychiatry*, **199**(6), 485–491.

Ramos, K., Cortes, J., Wilson, N., Kunik, M. E. and Stanley, M. A. (2017). Vida Calma: CBT for anxiety with a Spanish-speaking Hispanic adult. *Clinical Gerontologist*, **40**(3), 213–219.

Samuels, J., Bienvenu, O., Grados, M., et al. (2008). Prevalence and correlates of hoarding behavior in a community-based sample. *Behaviour Research and Therapy*, **46**(7), 836–844.

Saxena, S., Ayers, C., Maidment, K., Vapnik, T., Wetherell, J. and Bystritsky, A. (2011). Quality of life and functional impairment in compulsive hoarding. *Journal of Psychiatric Research*, **45**(4), 475–480.

Schnall, E., Wassertheil-Smoller, S., Swencionis, C., et al. (2010). The relationship between religion and cardiovascular outcomes and all-cause mortality in the women's health initiative observational study. *Psychology & Health*, **25**(2), 249–263.

Schuitevoerder, S., Rosen, J., Twamley, E., et al. (2013). A meta-analysis of cognitive functioning in older adults with PTSD. *Journal of Anxiety Disorders*, **27**(6), 550–558.

Seignourel, P., Kunik, M., Snow, L., Wilson, N. and Stanley, M. (2008). Anxiety in dementia: A critical review. *Clinical Psychology Review*, **28**(7), 1071–1082.

Shrestha, S., Armento, M. E. A., Bush, A. L., et al. (2012). Pilot findings from a community-based treatment program for late-life anxiety. *International Journal of Person Centered Medicine*, **2**(3), 400–409.

Shrestha, S., Wilson, N. L., Amspoker, A. B., et al. (2015). Calmer Life: a hybrid effectiveness-implementation trial for late-life anxiety. Poster presented at the 68th Annual Scientific Meeting of the Gerontological Society of America Conference, November 18–22, 2015, Orlando, FL.

Silfvernagel, K., Westlinder, A., Andersson, S., et al. (2018). Individually tailored internet-based cognitive behaviour therapy for older adults with anxiety and depression: a randomised controlled trial. *Cognitive Behaviour Therapy*, **47**(4), 286–300.

Snell, F. I., and Padin-Rivera, E. (1997). Group treatment for older Veterans with posttraumatic stress disorders. *Journal*

Psychosocial Nursing Mental Health Services, **35**(2), 10–16.

Spector, A., Charlesworth, G., King, M., et al. (2015). Cognitive-behavioural therapy for anxiety in dementia: pilot randomised controlled trial. *British Journal of Psychiatry*, **206**(6), 509–516.

Stanley, M. A., Bush, A., Camp, M., et al. (2011). Older adults' preferences for religion/spirituality in treatment for anxiety and depression. *Aging & Mental Health*, **15**(3), 334–343.

Stanley, M. A., Calleo, J., Bush, A. L., et al. (2013). The peaceful mind program: a pilot test of a CBT-based intervention for anxious patients with dementia. *American Journal of Geriatric Psychiatry*, **21**(7), 696–708.

Stanley, M., Wilson, N., Amspoker, A., et al. (2014). Lay providers can deliver effective cognitive behavior therapy for older adults with generalized anxiety disorder: a randomized trial. *Depression and Anxiety*, **31**(5), 391–401.

Stanley, M., Wilson, N., Novy, D., et al. (2009). Cognitive behavior therapy for generalized anxiety disorder among older adults in primary care. *JAMA*, **301**(14), 1460–1467.

Stanley, M. A., Wilson, N., Shrestha, S., et al. (2016). Calmer Life: a culturally tailored intervention for anxiety in underserved older adults. *American Journal of Geriatric Psychiatry*, **24**(8), 648–658.

Steketee, G., Frost, R., Tolin, D., Rasmussen, J. and Brown, T. (2010). Waitlist-controlled trial of cognitive behavior therapy for hoarding disorder. *Depression and Anxiety*, **27**(5), 476–484.

Tampi, R. and Tampi, D. (2014). Anxiety disorders in late life: a comprehensive review. *Healthy Aging Research*, **14**(3), 1–9.

Thomas, R. and Gafner, G. (1993). PTSD in an elderly male: treatment with eye movement desensitization and reprocessing. *Clinical Gerontologist*, **14**(2), 57–59.

Thorp, S. R. and Sones, H. M. (2013). Prolonged exposure vs. relaxation for older Veterans with PTSD. Paper presented at the 33rd Annual Meeting of the Anxiety Disorders Association of America (ADAA), La Jolla, CA.

Thorp, S. R., Ayers, C., Nuevo, R., Sorrell, J. and Wetherell, J. (2009). Meta-analysis comparing different behavioral treatments for late-life anxiety. *American Journal of Geriatric Psychiatry*, **17**(2), 105–115.

Thorp, S. R., Sones, H. M., and Cook, J. M. (2011). Post-traumatic stress disorder among older adults. In K. Sorroco and S. Lauderdale, eds., *Cognitive Behavior Therapy with Older Adults*, 1st ed. New York: Springer, pp. 291–316.

Thorp, S., Stein, M., Jeste, D., Patterson, T. and Wetherell, J. (2012). Prolonged exposure therapy for older Veteran with post-traumatic stress disorder: a pilot study. *American Journal of Geriatric Psychiatry*, **20**(3), 276–280.

Titov, N., Dear, B. F., Johnston, L., et al. (2014). Improving adherence and clinical outcomes in self-guided internet treatment for anxiety and depression: a 12-month follow-up of a randomised controlled trial. *PLoS ONE*, **9**(2), e89591.

Unützer, J., Katon, W., Williams, J., et al. (2001). Improving primary care for depression in late life: the design of a multicenter randomized trial. *Medical Care*, **39**(8), 785–799.

Wetherell, J. L., Afari, N., Ayers, C., et al. (2011). Acceptance and commitment therapy for generalized anxiety disorder in older adults: a preliminary report. *Behavior Therapy*, **42**(1), 127–134.

Wetherell, J., Ayers, C., Sorrell, J., et al. (2009). Modular psychotherapy for anxiety in older primary care patients. *American Journal of Geriatric Psychiatry*, **17**(6), 483–492.

Wetherell, J. L., Johnson, K., Chnag, D. G., et al. (2013a). Activity, Balance, Learning and Exposure (ABLE): a new intervention for excessive fear of falling. Poster presented at the annual meeting of the American Association for Geriatric Psychiatry, March 14–17, 2013, Los Angeles, CA.

Wetherell, J., Petkus, A., Thorp, S., et al. (2013b). Age differences in treatment response to a collaborative care intervention for anxiety disorders. *British Journal of Psychiatry*, **203**(1), 65–72.

Wetherell, J., Petkus, A., White, K., et al. (2013c). Antidepressant medication augmented with cognitive–behavioral therapy for generalized anxiety disorder in older adults. *American Journal of Psychiatry*, **170**(7), 782–789.

Wetherell, J. L., Thorp, S. R., Patterson, T. L., Golshan, S., Jeste, D. V. and Gatz, M. (2004). Quality of life in geriatric generalized anxiety disorder: a preliminary investigation. *Journal of Psychiatric Research*, **38**(3), 305–312.

Yochim, B., Mueller, A. and Segal, D. (2013). Late life anxiety is associated with decreased memory and executive functioning in community dwelling older adults. *Journal of Anxiety Disorders*, **27**(6), 567–575.

Zou, J. B., Dear, B. F., Titov, N., et al. (2012). Brief internet-delivered cognitive behavioral therapy for anxiety in older adults: a feasibility trial. *Journal of Anxiety Disorders*, **26**(6), 650–655.

Chapter 12

Pharmacological Treatment of Anxiety in Later Life

Gerard J. Byrne

Introduction

Although behavioural and psychological interventions are considered first-line treatments for anxiety disorders in older people (National Institute for Health and Care Excellence, 2014), psychotropic medications are also widely prescribed (Hollingworth & Siskind, 2010). Drugs from a range of psychotropic classes have been used to treat anxiety disorders, including benzodiazepines, antidepressants, anticonvulsants, and antipsychotics (Reinhold et al., 2011). While there is clinical trial evidence for the short-term efficacy of drugs from each of these classes, particularly for generalized anxiety disorder (GAD), there is scant evidence for long-term effectiveness. Psychotropic drugs exhibit a wide range of adverse effects, including some that pose particular hazards in later life.

This chapter will first summarize the pharmacodynamic and pharmacokinetic changes associated with ageing and the clinical challenges posed by prescribing psychotropic drugs in older people. It will then consider the evidence for the use of the main classes of psychotropic medication for older people with anxiety disorders.

General Considerations

Rationale for Drug Use

Anxiety symptoms and disorders develop as a result of interactions between complex polygenetic and epigenetic factors and environmental exposures throughout life. In some older people, there are additional factors of relevance, including cerebrovascular disease and neurodegenerative conditions such as Parkinson's disease and Alzheimer's disease. A further layer of complexity is provided by the co-morbidity of anxiety disorders with other mental disorders and with substance use disorders.

Studies in laboratory animals and in humans have shown that anxiety is mediated by complex brain circuitry involving the medial prefrontal cortex, amygdaloid and hypothalamic nuclei, hippocampal formation, and midbrain central grey matter. This circuitry is susceptible to certain types of pharmacological interventions, particularly by drugs with effects on the γ-aminobutyric acid (GABA) and monoamine systems. The goals of judicious use of psychotropic medication in older people are to reduce emotional distress and improve everyday function. Treatment with psychotropic medication for anxiety disorders is considered symptomatic rather than disease-modifying.

Access to behavioural and psychological treatments for anxiety disorders varies considerably by location, whereas most older people have access to primary care physicians or general practitioners. Pharmacological interventions are often less expensive than psychological treatments. While some older people express a preference for drug treatment over psychological treatment, particularly when symptoms are severe (Landreville et al., 2001), others express a preference for nonpharmacological approaches for anxiety (e.g., Woodward & Pachana, 2009).

Although older people may express a preference for either pharmacological or psychological treatment, a systematic review and meta-analysis (Gonçalves & Byrne, 2012) found that both psychotherapy and pharmacotherapy were effective in the short-term management of GAD in older people and that each was associated with a moderate effect size.

Clinical Context of Drug Treatment

Most older people with anxiety disorders will be seen in primary care settings, and prescribers of psychotropic medication will most often be primary care physicians, although in some places nurse practitioners and other health workers may be licensed to prescribe. For a variety of reasons, consultations with primary care physicians may be of short duration and allow little time for detailed exploration of psychological issues and the application of behavioural or psychological interventions.

In addition, accessible and affordable psychological therapy is not available everywhere. In such situations, prescription of a psychotropic medication is often seen as preferable to no intervention at all. However, some older people are already taking multiple prescribed medications for general medical problems (e.g., cardiovascular disease, Parkinson's disease) and are reluctant to take additional medications.

Older people entering long-term care (nursing homes or skilled nursing facilities) are sometimes commenced on psychotropic medication upon admission to the facility, although this medication is now less likely to be a benzodiazepine than previously.

Psychotropic medication, especially benzodiazepines or related drugs, may sometimes be commenced in hospital for anxiety or insomnia and not ceased upon discharge. This can lead to continuing treatment with a psychotropic medication that was originally intended to be only for short-term use.

Psychiatrists, including those specializing in the treatment of older people, see only a minority of those with anxiety disorders. However, they are more likely to see those older people with severe, treatment-resistant anxiety or those in whom anxiety occurs in co-morbid relation to other general medical and mental disorders. These patients are more likely to be prescribed psychotropic medication.

Geriatric psychiatrists may undertake home visits to see older people who are unable to get to the clinic. In this setting, they may encounter older people with diverse organic and functional mental disorders. Some of these patients have anxiety as a manifestation of their psychotic disorder and some have anxiety as a complication of their mood disorder. Still other older patients will have anxiety as a manifestation of their neurocognitive disorder.

Most of the evidence for the use of psychotropic medication to treat anxiety disorders in older people comes from clinical trials conducted in academic clinics attached to large university teaching hospitals. It is unclear how well this evidence is likely to generalize to the diverse settings in which older people may present with anxiety.

Pharmacokinetic and Pharmacodynamic Considerations

Ageing is associated with both pharmacokinetic and pharmacodynamic changes, although age-related pharmacokinetic changes have been better studied. Put simply, pharmacokinetics refers to how the body deals with medications, and in particular with how medications move within the body. In contrast, pharmacodynamics refers to the effects of medications on the body and their mechanisms of action.

As humans age, there is reduced metabolism of ingested medications both within the gut wall and the liver. In addition, older people have reduced lean body mass and an increased fat to muscle ratio. Older people also have reduced renal excretion. The net effect of these changes is to allow medications to achieve higher serum levels for any given dose and to more readily accumulate within the body. When medications are ceased, they may take longer to be eliminated from the body.

In older people, organ systems, including the brain, become more susceptible to adverse effects from medications. The threshold for sedation, ataxia, and delirium as adverse effects of prescribed medications is reduced in the ageing brain.

The combined effect of these pharmacokinetic and pharmacodynamic changes is such that prescribers should give preference to psychotropic medications with more favourable properties when treating older people. In many instances, this is likely to mean drugs with shorter half-lives and drugs with fewer anticholinergic and antihistaminic side effects. Prescribers should also start older people on lower doses of psychotropic medication than they would use in young and middle-aged individuals. Finally, the rate of dose escalation should be slower to allow time for biological adaptation to the drug. Despite these cautions, some older people may ultimately require the same final dose of psychotropic medication as younger people.

There are two additional factors to be borne in mind when prescribing to older people: multiple physical co-morbidities and polypharmacy. Many older people suffer from a range of general medical conditions, including disorders such as hypertension, ischaemic heart disease, cerebrovascular disease, osteoarthritis, osteoporosis, chronic obstructive pulmonary disease, chronic kidney disease, constipation, and Parkinson's disease. Co-morbid medical conditions sometimes complicate psychotropic prescribing and must be taken into account when prescribing psychotropic medication. In particular, older people with liver or kidney disease may be particularly susceptible to the adverse effects of psychotropic medication. Polypharmacy is the prescription of multiple medications, which may be involved in drug–drug interactions and may lead to an increased adverse effect burden. For instance, the co-prescription of benzodiazepines, anticonvulsants, and opioid analgesics might produce dangerous levels of respiratory depression, sedation, and ataxia.

Measurement of Treatment Effect

Parallel-group, double-blind, placebo-controlled clinical trials remain the gold standard for assessing the efficacy of psychotropic medication in older people. In pharmaceutical trials, a washout period is used to wean participants off existing psychotropic medication. It is preferable also to have a run-in period to establish which participants have a stable diagnosis, although this is much less often a feature of clinical trials involving older people.

Ideally, clinical trials should be independently funded to avoid the suggestion that the study design or outcome reporting may have been influenced by the pharmaceutical industry. In practice, most clinical trials are industry sponsored. Regardless of the funding source, clinical trials should be prospectively registered, with standardized diagnoses and pre-specified hypotheses, power analyses, and data analysis plans. It is generally considered appropriate for investigators to report intention-to-treat analyses using the last observation carried forward method. Secondary hypotheses should also be pre-specified to minimize the temptation for data dredging.

There are a variety of ways of measuring treatment effect. These include assessing the proportion of study participants whose illness resolves. Resolution is generally considered to mean that the participant no longer meets diagnostic criteria for the condition. Another approach involves assessing the proportion of study participants who exhibit clinically significant improvement, preferably defined as a 50% or greater reduction in score on an appropriately valid and reliable clinical scale. Unfortunately, many clinical trials involving drug treatment for anxiety in older people have used either a 25% or a 20% reduction in score on the outcome measure. Some clinical trials have employed dimensional measures of anxiety in samples recruited by advertising in the media rather than formal diagnoses in patients presenting for treatment, calling into question the clinical significance of the anxiety being treated.

There are now several dimensional scales that have been developed specifically for the assessment of anxiety in older people that could be used as outcome measures in clinical trials, such as the Geriatric Anxiety Inventory and the Geriatric Anxiety Scale (Gould et al., 2014; Balsamo et al., 2018). Despite this, many clinical trials have used scales not specifically designed for use in older people. The Hamilton Anxiety Rating Scale (HAM-A; Hamilton, 1959) has been commonly used in pharmaceutical trials in people with anxiety disorders. However, the HAM-A relies heavily on the assessment of somatic symptoms, and its use in older people is likely to be confounded by the presence of co-morbid general medical problems.

Another limitation to the assessment of treatment effects in older people is sample selection. Clinical trials purporting to generate findings relevant to older people sometimes include people as young as 50 or 55 years of age. The number of published clinical trials in people aged 65 years and over is quite small.

Most clinical trials in older people have assessed short-term efficacy rather than longer-term efficacy or effectiveness. This is problematic because most anxiety disorders in older people run a chronic course and have often been present for many years prior to the patient presenting for treatment.

As-Required Medication

Although most medications are prescribed for regular use, some medications are prescribed *pro re nata* (PRN; as needed). This is particularly true for conditions that vary in severity or for conditions where symptoms are only occasionally present. As anxiety disorders often fluctuate in severity, targeted or PRN medications are sometimes used.

Psychological Impact of Drug Treatment

The prescription of psychotropic medication is usually accompanied by a variety of psychological effects, even in the absence of a formal psychotherapeutic intervention. The patient is likely to have fears and expectations in relation to the medication, particularly when it is first prescribed.

For many patients, the prescription of medication validates their reason for attendance at the clinic and provides them with evidence that the prescriber has taken their concerns seriously. Some patients have a high degree of faith in psychotropic medication and believe it to be a powerful and effective intervention.

Other patients fear the 'mind-altering' properties of psychotropic medication or fear the risk of 'drug addiction', and so strongly prefer behavioural and psychological interventions.

Still others seek to please the prescriber by agreeing to the prescription of psychotropic medication without any real intent to have it dispensed at the pharmacy or to actually take it.

In addition, there are some patients who conceal from their prescriber that they are consulting other prescribers and are taking multiple psychotropic medications.

Assessment Prior to Drug Treatment

Standard clinical practice prior to prescribing psychotropic medication for any indication is to make a formal diagnosis using one of the major nosological systems, such as the Diagnostic and Statistical Manual of Mental Disorders (DSM) or International Classification of Diseases (ICD). This is good clinical practice because diagnosis should generally precede treatment, and most of the available evidence comes from clinical trials in which formal diagnoses were made. Diagnostic assessment relies upon detailed history-taking from the patient and suitable informants together with mental state examination. In many cases, physical examination, laboratory investigations, electrocardiograms (ECGs), and neuroimaging studies will supplement the history and mental state examination. In some patients with a long-standing anxiety disorder, comprehensive medical work-up may have been completed previously and there would be little purpose in repeating it. However, in anxiety disorders arising for the first time in later life, more detailed medical work-up is warranted to exclude anxiety due to another medical problem.

Prior to prescribing psychotropic medication, it is prudent to review the past history of treatment for the condition, including behavioural and psychological interventions, and past pharmacological interventions. The efficacy and adverse effects of such interventions should be identified.

Selection of a suitable pharmacological agent should be informed by knowledge of psychiatric and general medical co-morbidities, including substance use disorder. Special consideration should be given to patients with likely liver or kidney diseases, as these may affect dose selection and dose interval. Consideration of the patient's current medication and the likelihood of drug–drug interactions is also important.

Adverse Effects

All psychotropic medications have adverse effects. Just as there are individual differences in response to psychotropic drug treatment, there are also substantial individual differences in the propensity to experience and report adverse effects. Some of these individual differences are due to genetic variations and are referred to as pharmacogenomic factors.

Common adverse effects of psychotropic medication include nausea, constipation, postural hypotension, blurred vision, urinary hesitancy, impaired attention, sedation, amnesia, slurred speech, impaired balance, gait ataxia, falls, altered sleep architecture, reduced respiratory drive, tremor, anxiety, sexual side effects, serotonin syndrome, and headache. In some older people, sedating medication has a paradoxical disinhibiting effect. The use of psychotropic medication may combine with general medical problems to impair driving ability.

Some adverse effects, including Parkinsonism, may take many weeks to manifest and many weeks to resolve once the offending agent is ceased.

The prescriber must monitor the patient's response to treatment or arrange for another clinician to do this. The dose will often need adjustment, and not infrequently one drug will need to be ceased and replaced by another. Many psychotropic drugs will need to be tapered before ceasing to minimize discontinuation symptoms.

Most centrally acting drugs have some propensity to cause hyponatraemia, so this should be checked for, particularly in older patients on diuretics or who have cerebrovascular disease.

Some psychotropic agents are associated with prolongation of the QTc interval on the ECG and increased risk of sudden cardiac death, so it is often prudent to order ECGs before and after initiation of psychotropic drug treatment.

Use of Psychotropic Medication in the Presence of Cognitive Impairment

A general principle of prescribing in older people is to prescribe as few medications as needed, with each medication being given at the lowest effective dose for the shortest period feasible. Regular medication reviews should be undertaken and unnecessary medications tapered and ceased.

Older people are often commenced on temporary medication while in hospital (e.g., hypnotics), which is inadvertently continued upon discharge. It is worthwhile undertaking a careful review of medication changes initiated in hospital to establish which are required in the post-hospital phase.

Drug treatment of anxiety is complicated by the presence of mild cognitive impairment (mild neurocognitive disorder) or dementia (major neurocognitive disorder). Psychotropic medication may further impair cognitive function in older people through anticholinergic (e.g., olanzapine, paroxetine), antihistaminic (e.g., quetiapine, mirtazapine), or $GABA_A$ augmentation (e.g., oxazepam, lorazepam) effects.

Not only may medication further impair cognition, but adherence may be a problem in patients with cognitive impairment. If cognitive impairment is relatively mild, medication can be dispensed by the pharmacist into a blister pack (e.g., Webster-pak™) or a roll of plastic sachets (e.g., DoseAid™) to improve ease of administration, including self-administration. Another method is the use of a Dosette™ box, which has subdivisions for each day of the week and for several times of the day. Dosette boxes are usually filled by the patient or their caregiver once a week. However, if cognitive impairment is more severe, a co-resident spouse, partner, other family member (e.g., adult child), or friend may need to administer medication to the older person. Alternatively, a domiciliary nurse could visit daily or twice daily to administer medication. To ensure safety, medication can be stored in a locked box (e.g., Lockmed™), accessible only by the visiting nurse.

As cognitive function often deteriorates over the day in people with cognitive impairment (the so-called sundowning effect), there may be utility in arranging for medication to be administered in the morning when the patient is likely to be most alert. However, this is not always practicable for sedating medications.

Use of Psychotropic Medication in the Nursing Home Setting

There are additional challenges when employing psychotropic medication to treat anxiety disorders in the nursing home setting.

Historically, sedative and hypnotic drugs, particularly from the benzodiazepine class, have been used excessively in residential aged care settings. However, in many places (e.g., in the USA following Omnibus Budget Reconciliation Act (OBRA) 1987), the use of sedatives and hypnotics has fallen.

Another challenge that may arise is due to relatively infrequent visits from prescribing medical practitioners. In this situation, it may be difficult to rapidly modify prescribed medication in response to changes in the patient.

The provision of individualized patient-centred care may allow for a reduction in dose or the cessation of psychotropic medication in many anxious nursing home residents.

Ceasing Psychotropic Medication

Ceasing psychotropic medication, particularly where it has been used at high doses for long periods, requires a degree of caution. In ambulatory patients and in non-urgent situations, most psychotropic medication, including benzodiazepines and antidepressants, should be tapered over an extended period before being ceased. Rapid discontinuation may lead to cholinergic rebound (e.g., paroxetine) or benzodiazepine withdrawal symptoms (e.g., oxazepam). It may be difficult to distinguish the symptoms of medication discontinuation from the symptoms of the underlying anxiety disorder.

There are some older patients with severe anxiety disorders who have been taking benzodiazepines for decades. In these circumstances, a specialist geriatric psychiatry opinion is likely to be warranted before embarking on discontinuation. In some individuals, it can be prudent to continue such medication if it does not appear to be causing significant adverse effects.

Limitations of the Available Evidence

Patients participating in double-blind placebo-controlled pharmacological trials are likely to believe that they are receiving an active intervention. This is different to the situation in most psychotherapeutic trials in which the patients cannot be blinded to the intervention they are receiving. For this reason, findings from clinical trials of psychotropic medication cannot be directly compared with clinical trials of non-pharmacological interventions.

The absence of discontinuation trials makes it difficult to judge how long a drug treatment should be continued.

The paucity of clinical trials in older people with anxiety disorders in which psychotropic medication is combined with either specific (e.g., cognitive behaviour therapy (CBT)) or non-specific (e.g., psychoeducation) psychosocial interventions is a gap in existing knowledge.

Most of the available clinical trials involve older people with GAD. More work is needed on the treatment of other anxiety disorders in older people.

Most of the available clinical trials have involved short-term treatment only (4–12 weeks). Even for GAD with its minimum duration of 6 months, clinical trials of psychotropic medications have typically been of 4 weeks' duration. Little is known about long-term outcomes of the treatment of anxiety disorders with psychotropic medication. However, the beneficial effects of psychotropic medication tend not to persist for long following cessation of the drug.

Specific Drugs

Antidepressants

Antidepressants are recommended as first-line drug treatments for anxiety disorders other than specific phobia. They also have efficacy as adjunctive treatment in people treated initially with behavioural and psychological interventions. Although antidepressant medications are the preferred drug treatment for anxiety disorders, they are not without their challenges. Modern antidepressants are commonly associated with nausea and reduced appetite, which may lead to weight loss in older people.

Antidepressants prescribed to treat anxiety disorders include drugs from a variety of biochemical classes, including selective serotonin reuptake inhibitors (SSRIs) and serotonin and noradrenaline (norepinephrine) reuptake inhibitors (SNRIs). Older drugs, including tricyclic antidepressants and irreversible monoamine oxidase inhibitors, are much less commonly used because of their adverse effect profiles. Importantly, the SSRIs and SNRIs are safer in overdose.

The SSRIs and SNRIs often cause an initial increase in anxiety and insomnia that sometimes needs to be treated with a low-dose benzodiazepine for a short period (1–2 weeks).

In older people taking antidepressants, particularly older women who have pre-existing cerebrovascular disease or who are also taking diuretics, there is a risk of hyponatraemia (low serum sodium concentration). Hyponatraemia may lead to apparent worsening of anxiety and depression and to confusion. In severe cases, it may be life-threatening.

While antidepressant use in children and youth is associated with an increased risk of completed suicide, this is not the case in older people. In older people, antidepressant use is associated with a reduced risk of suicide (Barbui et al., 2009).

Sertraline

In a 10-week randomized, double-blind, placebo-controlled trial of sertraline (50–200 mg/day) in 326 adult out-patients with GAD, sertraline was modestly superior to placebo (Brawman-Mintzer et al., 2006). The response rate in the sertraline group was significantly higher than in the placebo group (59.2% vs 48.2%; $p = 0.05$). No similar study in older adults has been reported, although two small studies in older adults with anxiety disorders compared sertraline with other interventions.

Schuurmans et al. (2006) randomized 84 patients aged 60 years and over with GAD, panic disorder, agoraphobia, or social phobia to either: (1) 15 sessions of CBT; (2) sertraline to a maximum dose of 150 mg/day; or (3) a wait-list control condition. A completers analysis used data from 52 participants. Both CBT and sertraline led to significant improvements in anxiety and worry. Sertraline showed superior results on worry symptoms and was associated with a larger effect size than CBT at the 3-month follow-up ($d = 1.02$ vs 0.35).

An 8-week single-blind clinical trial (Mokhber et al., 2010) comparing sertraline with buspirone in 46 patients aged 60 years and over with GAD on the HAM-A found that buspirone was superior following 2 and 4 weeks of treatment, but that there was no significant difference between the two drugs at 8 weeks. Both drugs were associated with clinically meaningful improvements in anxiety.

Citalopram

In an 8-week randomized, double-blind trial in 34 patients aged 60 years and over with a DSM-IV anxiety disorder, citalopram was compared with placebo (Lenze et al., 2005). Eleven (65%) of 17 citalopram-treated patients had responded by 8 weeks versus 4 (24%) of 17 placebo-treated patients. There were a number of methodological limitations to this study, challenging interpretation of its findings (Kruszewski, 2005).

Escitalopram

In a 12-week out-patient trial conducted in primary care and specialty clinics, 177 participants aged 60 years and over with GAD were randomized to either escitalopram (10–20 mg/day) or placebo (Lenze et al., 2009). In an intention-to-treat analysis, there was no significant difference between the cumulative response rate between the escitalopram and placebo arms (57% vs 45%; $p = 0.11$). In an analysis based on completers, the response rate in the escitalopram arm was better than the response rate in the placebo arm (69% vs 51%; $p = 0.03$).

Venlafaxine

There appear to be no published placebo-controlled trials of extended-release venlafaxine in older patients with anxiety disorders. However, one pooled analysis of five placebo-controlled trials of venlafaxine in GAD extracted data from patients aged 60 years and over (Katz et al., 2002). Two of the studies were of 12 weeks' duration and three of the studies were of 8 weeks' duration. The dose of extended-release venlafaxine varied between 37.5 and 225 mg/day. The older patients included in the analyses represented 10% of the 1,839 adult out-patients with GAD who participated in the studies. Extended-release venlafaxine was found to have similar efficacy in older and younger adults.

Duloxetine

In a 10-week study conducted in adults aged 65 years and over with GAD, 291 patients were randomized to either duloxetine (30–120 mg/day) or placebo (Alaka et al., 2014). At 10 weeks, duloxetine was found to be superior to placebo, with the mean change in HAM-A score from baseline favouring duloxetine (–15.9 vs –11.7; $p < 0.001$). Treatment-emergent adverse effects, including constipation, dry mouth, and somnolence, were reported more frequently in the duloxetine arm.

Mirtazapine

Mirtazapine is a modern antidepressant with less propensity to cause anxiety and insomnia. It is structurally a tetracyclic and similar biochemically to the older tetracyclic mianserin. Mirtazapine is not an SSRI or SNRI, but has a novel mode of action and strong antihistaminic effects. It is more commonly associated with sedation and increased appetite than the SSRI and SNRI antidepressants. There is evidence in adults of efficacy in major depressive disorder with co-morbid anxiety or agitation (Fawcett & Barkin, 1998), but scant evidence for efficacy in anxiety disorders. There appear to be no published placebo-controlled trials for the efficacy of mirtazapine in late-life anxiety disorders.

Nortriptyline

Similarly, there appear to be no published placebo-controlled trials of the tricyclic antidepressant nortriptyline in older patients with uncomplicated anxiety disorders. However, one small pooled analysis has been reported in which 27 patients with post-stroke depression with co-morbid GAD were randomized to nortriptyline or placebo (Kimura et al., 2003). Those treated with nortriptyline did better, and anxiety symptoms responded earlier than depressive symptoms.

Benzodiazepines and Related Drugs

Beginning in the 1960s, prescribers began substituting the much safer benzodiazepines for barbiturates, which were lethal in overdose in people with anxiety disorders. Benzodiazepines are positive allosteric modulators at the $GABA_A$ receptor. By this mechanism, they amplify the activity of the inhibitory $GABA_A$ receptor. GABA is the main inhibitory neurotransmitter in the central nervous system.

Benzodiazepines vary in their speed of onset and their duration of action. Some benzodiazepines undergo both glucuronidation and oxidation in the liver and have active metabolites with long half-lives (e.g., diazepam, chlordiazepoxide), whereas other benzodiazepines undergo only glucuronidation and have inactive metabolites (e.g., oxazepam, lorazepam). Glucuronidation involves linking a molecule to the drug to make it water soluble and easier to excrete. Oxidation involves increasing the positive valence of the drug molecule by removing a hydrogen ion or an electron. Benzodiazepines that undergo oxidative metabolism can accumulate and lead to excessive sedation and respiratory depression. As a consequence, oxazepam and lorazepam are the preferred benzodiazepines for use in older people and in those with liver disease.

Benzodiazepines are effective at reducing anxiety symptoms in the short term, but there is little evidence of longer-term efficacy in adults or older people with anxiety disorders.

Alprazolam and Ketazolam

There are no published placebo-controlled studies of lorazepam in older people with anxiety disorders. Alprazolam (Cohn, 1984) and ketazolam (Bresolin et al., 1988) have both been studied in relatively small 4-week placebo-controlled clinical trials in older patients with GAD. The alprazolam study did not specify a definition of response, so it is difficult to assess its findings (Gonçalves & Byrne, 2012). The ketazolam study demonstrated an effect size of $d = -0.89$ favouring the active drug (Bresolin et al., 1988). Ketazolam is not available in Australia, the UK, or the USA. Alprazolam has widespread availability, although its abuse potential is increasingly being recognized.

Oxazepam

One study of oxazepam has been reported. In a 4-week double-blind multicentre study, 220 out-patients aged 60 years and over with anxiety neurosis were randomized to either oxazepam or placebo (Koepke et al., 1982). The dose of oxazepam was titrated up to a maximum of 15 mg four times daily, although most participants received 15 mg thrice daily. Although the outcome analyses presented were not sophisticated by contemporary standards, participants in the oxazepam arm improved significantly on the HAM-A.

Z-Drugs

The so-called z-drugs include agents from the imidazopyridine group (e.g., zolpidem), the cyclopyrrolone group (e.g., zopiclone), and the pyrazolopyrimidine group (e.g., zaleplon). All z-drugs are thought to have their primary effects as agonists at the $GABA_A$ receptor and as a consequence have similar properties to the benzodiazepines. It is unclear whether the z-drugs offer any major advantages over the benzodiazepines, although they do have shorter half-lives, so they might be associated with less risk of morning 'hangover' when used as hypnotics.

No z-drugs currently marketed have been tested for efficacy in anxiety disorders in older people. Alpidem, a drug from the imidazopyridine group, was tested in a 3-week placebo-controlled trial in 40 older subjects with GAD (Frattola et al., 1992). It was subsequently marketed briefly in France before being withdrawn.

In summary, despite their documented widespread use in older people (Hollingworth & Siskind, 2010), there is a remarkable paucity of evidence for the use of benzodiazepines and z-drugs in the treatment of anxiety disorders in later life.

Antipsychotics

Over recent decades, prescribers have become increasingly aware of the problems associated with benzodiazepines, and it appears that some may have turned to sedating antipsychotics as a substitute for benzodiazepines. In Australia, women over the age of 80 years have been reported to have the highest utilization of antipsychotic medication (Hollingworth et al., 2010). It is likely that the anxiolytic effects of sedating antipsychotics are mediated principally by antagonism of the histamine 1 (H1) receptor.

Second-generation antipsychotics, including aripiprazole, olanzapine, quetiapine, risperidone, and ziprasidone, have been studied in short-term trials in adults with GAD (Reinhold et al., 2011). However, it appears that only quetiapine has been studied in older adults.

Quetiapine

Quetiapine has become a popular alternative to benzodiazepines and is being prescribed to anxious older people. Quetiapine is a low-potency second-generation antipsychotic medication and a strong H1 receptor antagonist. Through this mechanism it causes sedation and weight gain, although the latter might be less of a problem in older people.

Mezhebovsky et al. (2013) reported an 11-week clinical trial of extended-release quetiapine fumarate monotherapy (50–300 mg/day) or placebo in patients aged 66 years and over with DSM-IV GAD and a HAM-A total score of 20 or more. This study had also been reported in shorter form in 2008 in a subsequently discontinued journal (Eriksson et al., 2008). A total of 450 patients were recruited at 47 sites in the USA and Eastern Europe and were randomized to quetiapine or placebo for 9 weeks with follow-up 2 weeks later. Quetiapine was superior to placebo after 9 weeks on the HAM-A (least mean squares – 14.97 vs –7.21; $p < 0.001$), and this separation was evident after only 1 week of treatment. Adverse effects occurring in more than 5% of patients in either group included somnolence, dry mouth, dizziness, headache, and nausea.

There are several practical and ethical issues raised by the use of antipsychotic medication to treat non-psychotic disorders in older people. In a series of studies conducted mainly in nursing home patients with dementia associated with agitation, aggression, and psychosis, the use of low-dose antipsychotic medication was shown to be associated with increased all-cause mortality. Antipsychotic medications are associated with an increased risk of stroke and cognitive deterioration in older people and are subject to a 'black box' warning in many jurisdictions. Drugs such as quetiapine may also cause orthostatic hypotension leading to falls and may cause excessive sedation leading to hypoventilation and pneumonia. Although this evidence does not come from studies of older people with anxiety disorders, it nevertheless raises issues of potential risk. As a consequence, antipsychotics should not generally be used as first-line medications in the management of anxiety disorders in older people.

Buspirone

Buspirone is a strong 5-HT_{1A} agonist and a weak dopamine D_2 antagonist from the azapirone class. While it is ineffective as an antipsychotic, it has anxiolytic and antidepressant properties. The Sequenced Treatment Alternatives to Relieve Depression (STAR*D) study demonstrated the likely value of buspirone as an augmentation agent in patients treated with SSRIs for severe depression (Appelberg et al., 2001).

In a 4-week double-blind placebo-controlled study, 40 anxious patients aged 65 years and over were randomized to either buspirone 5–30 mg/day (mean 18 mg/day) or placebo

(Böhm et al., 1990). Buspirone treatment was superior to placebo on the HAM-A and on a clinical global assessment scale. However, clinical trial data from younger samples have shown more equivocal findings (e.g., see Lader et al., 1998).

As noted in the 'Sertraline' section, Mokhber et al., (2010) compared buspirone with sertraline in 46 older people with GAD, finding no significant difference between the two drugs after 8 weeks of treatment.

Majercsik and Haller (2004), in their study of 384 older inpatients (mean age approximately 80 years), found interactions between anxiety, social support, health status, and buspirone efficacy. Buspirone was associated with improved anxiety overall, but it worked better in patients with many social contacts and many diseases.

Buspirone has a speed of onset that is similar to antidepressants, and its beneficial effects are generally seen after 2 or more weeks of treatment. There is evidence that buspirone might be more effective in benzodiazepine-naïve patients (DeMartinis et al., 2000). Buspirone is generally well tolerated, although dizziness and nausea can occur, and extrapyramidal side effects have occasionally been reported. Buspirone is metabolized in the liver by the cytochrome P450 3A4 (CYP3A4) enzyme, so drugs that inhibit this enzyme are likely to interact with buspirone. Buspirone is excreted via the liver and the kidneys, so care should be taken in patients with liver or kidney disease.

Anticonvulsants

There is limited evidence for the use of anticonvulsants in patients with anxiety disorders (Mula et al., 2007). In particular, there is some evidence from studies in adults for the use of pregabalin in social anxiety disorder (Feltner et al., 2011) and GAD (Generoso et al., 2017), for lamotrigine in post-traumatic stress disorder (Hertzberg et al., 1999), and for gabapentin in social anxiety disorder (Pande et al., 1999). In older adults, the evidence for the use of anticonvulsants in anxiety disorders appears to be limited to a single trial of pregabalin in GAD (Montgomery et al., 2008).

Pregabalin

Pregabalin is a GABA analogue used mainly as an anticonvulsant and for the treatment of neuropathic pain. A systematic review and meta-analysis that included 2,299 patients of all ages with GAD from eight clinical trials found pregabalin to be superior to placebo with a Hedges' g of 0.37 (Generoso et al., 2017). The reviewers noted that pregabalin had comparable efficacy to the benzodiazepines, but with a lower dropout rate. Montgomery et al. (2008) undertook an 8-week double-blind placebo-controlled trial of pregabalin (150–600 mg/day) in 273 patients aged 65 years and over (mean age 72 years) with GAD and a HAM-A score of 20 or more. The end point was change in HAM-A score between baseline and week 8. Pregabalin was significantly better than placebo from week 2 onwards, with a difference of two points on the HAM-A at week 8. Pregabalin was well tolerated.

Other Drugs

There is very little evidence to support the use of lithium and the cognition-enhancing drugs such as donepezil, galantamine, rivastigmine, and memantine in the management of anxiety disorders in older people.

β-Blockers are sometimes prescribed to manage tremor in musicians with performance anxiety, but the quality and the quantity of the evidence for their use in anxiety disorders is poor (Steenen et al., 2016). The use of β-blockers in older people may exacerbate chronic obstructive pulmonary disease and heart block.

Pharmacotherapy versus Psychotherapy

Hendricks et al. (2010) randomized 49 panic disorder patients aged 60 years and over to 14 weeks of treatment with paroxetine, CBT, or a wait-list condition. Patients randomized to either paroxetine or CBT did better than patients randomized to the wait-list condition. Older age at onset and shorter duration of illness were predictors of better outcomes with CBT.

As noted in the 'Antidepressants' section, Schuurmans et al. (2006) compared sertraline to CBT and a wait-list control condition in 84 older people with anxiety disorder. Using data from 52 completers, sertraline was found to be superior to CBT on worry symptoms at the 3-month follow-up.

Combination Treatment with Pharmacotherapy and Psychotherapy

There is evidence from studies in adults with anxiety disorders that combination treatment with psychotherapy and pharmacotherapy is superior to either treatment alone (Cuijpers et al., 2014), but there is limited evidence in older people.

Wetherell et al. (2013) reported a clinical trial of combination treatment with antidepressant medication and CBT in older people with GAD. In a complex design, outpatients aged 60 years and over ($n = 73$) were treated with open-label escitalopram for 12 weeks and then randomized to either: (1) escitalopram plus CBT followed by maintenance escitalopram; (2) escitalopram plus CBT followed by pill placebo; (3) escitalopram alone followed by maintenance escitalopram; or (4) escitalopram alone followed by pill placebo. At 28 weeks, all three active treatment arms were superior to placebo alone. The relapse rate was lower in the arms that included maintenance escitalopram than in the arms that included pill placebo. Combination treatment was superior to escitalopram alone when the dimensional outcome was measured on the Penn State Worry Questionnaire, but not when measured on the HAM-A.

Complementary Medicine

Older people often use complementary medicine to manage anxiety symptoms and disorders (McIntyre et al., 2016), although the evidence base for such use is limited. So-called phytomedicines, which have effects on the GABA receptor, are reported to include ashwagandha, chamomile, *Ginkgo biloba*, hops, kava, lemon balm, passion flower, pennywort, skullcap, and valerian (Savage et al., 2018). A review of the use of herbal medicines in the treatment of psychiatric disorders (Sarris, 2018) found some evidence for the efficacy of kava (*Piper methysticum*), passion flower (*Passiflora* spp.), and galphimia (*Galphimia glauca*) in anxiety disorders. Clinical trials of these phytomedicines have not been conducted in older people.

St John's wort (*Hypericum perforatum*) is a widely used phytomedicine that is taken mainly to treat depression. Available formulations may vary in the levels of their active ingredients. St John's wort interacts with many prescribed drugs, including psychotropic medications, via both pharmacokinetic and pharmacodynamic mechanisms. Of particular note, St John's wort can lead to increased serotonergic effects when taken by patients on SSRIs and related drugs. Patients considering starting or stopping St John's wort should consult their doctor or pharmacist for advice.

Next Steps

The available evidence for drug treatment of anxiety disorders in older people is limited in its scope. Most of the reported clinical trials have involved older people with GAD and have employed antidepressants. There is scant evidence for pharmacotherapy in older people with anxiety disorders other than GAD, so prescribers must extrapolate from evidence in younger adults. There is a need for clinical trials of longer duration and in settings such as residential aged care. Finally, discontinuation studies in antidepressant-treated older people are needed in order to clarify the appropriate duration of treatment and the extent and severity of discontinuation symptoms.

Summary

Psychotropic medications are often used as adjuncts to the behavioural and psychological treatment of anxiety disorders in older people. They are also used as an alternative to behavioural and psychological treatment when this is inaccessible, unaffordable, or unacceptable to the patient. Antidepressant medications appear to be particularly valuable in this context, but they suffer from a delayed onset of action. Historically, benzodiazepine sedatives have been widely prescribed to anxious older people, but these are no longer recommended except for in short-term use. Antipsychotic medications should not generally be used as first-line drugs in the treatment of anxiety disorders in older people.

References

Alaka, K. J., Noble, W., Montejo, A., et al. (2014). Efficacy and safety of duloxetine in the treatment of older adult patients with generalized anxiety disorder: a randomized, double-blind, placebo-controlled trial. *International Journal of Geriatric Psychiatry*, **29**(9), 978–986.

Appelberg, B. G., Syvälahti, E. K., Koskinen, T. E., Mehtonen, O. P., Muhonen, T. T. and Naukkarinen, H. H. (2001). Patients with severe depression may benefit from buspirone augmentation of selective serotonin reuptake inhibitors: results from a placebo-controlled, randomized, double-blind, placebo wash-in study. *Journal of Clinical Psychiatry*, **62**(6), 448–452.

Balsamo, M., Cataldi, F., Carlucci, L. and Fairfield, B. (2018). Assessment of anxiety in older adults: a review of self-report measures. *Clinical Interventions in Aging*, **13**, 573–593.

Barbui, C., Esposito, E. and Cipriani, A. (2009). Selective serotonin reuptake inhibitors and risk of suicide: a systematic review of observational studies. *Canadian Medical Association Journal*, **180**(3), 291–297.

Böhm, C., Robinson, D. S., Gammans, R. E., et al. (1990). Buspirone therapy in anxious elderly patients: a controlled clinical trial. *Journal of Clinical Psychopharmacology*, **10** (Suppl. 3), 47S–51S.

Brawman-Mintzer, O., Knapp, R. G., Rynn, M., Carter, R. E. and Rickels, K. (2006). Sertraline treatment for generalized anxiety disorder: a randomized, double-blind, placebo-controlled trial. *Journal of Clinical Psychiatry*, **67**(6), 874–881.

Bresolin, N., Monza, G., Scarpini, E., et al. (1988). Treatment of anxiety with ketazolam in elderly patients. *Clinical Therapeutics*, **10** (5), 536–542.

Cohn, J. B. (1984). Double-blind safety and efficacy comparison of alprazolam and placebo in the treatment of anxiety in geriatric-patients. *Current Therapeutic Research: Clinical and Experimental*, **35**(1), 100–112.

Cuijpers, P., Sijbrandij, M., Koole, S. L., Andersson, G., Beekman, A. T. and Reynolds, C. F. (2014). Adding psychotherapy to antidepressant medication in depression and anxiety disorders: a meta-analysis. *World Psychiatry*, **13**(1), 56–67.

DeMartinis, N., Rynn, M., Rickels, K. and Mandos, L. (2000). Prior benzodiazepine use and buspirone response in the treatment of generalized anxiety disorder. *Journal of Clinical Psychiatry*, **61**(2), 91–94.

Eriksson, H., Mezhebovsky, I., Magi, K., She, F. and Datto, C. (2008). Double-blind, randomised study of extended release quetiapine fumarate (quetiapine XR) monotherapy in elderly patients with generalized anxiety disorder (GAD). *International Journal of Psychiatry in Clinical Practice*, **12**(4), 332–333.

Fawcett, J. and Barkin, R. L. (1998). A meta-analysis of eight randomized, double-blind, controlled clinical trials of mirtazapine for the treatment of patients with major depression and symptoms of anxiety. *Journal of Clinical Psychiatry*, **59**(3), 123–127.

Feltner, D. E., Liu-Dumaw, M., Schweizer, E. and Bielski, R. (2011). Efficacy of pregabalin in generalized social anxiety disorder: results of a double-blind, placebo-controlled, fixed-dose study. *International Clinical Psychopharmacology*, **26**(4), 213–220.

Frattola, L., Piolti, R., Bassi, S., et al. (1992). Effects of alpidem in anxious elderly outpatient: a double-blind, placebo-controlled trial. *Clinical Neuropharmacology*, **15**(6), 477–487.

Generoso, M. B., Trevizol, A. P., Kasper, S., Cho, H. J., Cordeiro, Q. and Shiozawa, P. (2017). Pregabaling for generalized anxiety disorder: an updated systematic review and meta-analysis. *International Clinical Psychopharmacology*, **32**(1), 49–55.

Gonçalves, D. A. and Byrne, G. J. (2012). Interventions for generalized anxiety disorder in older adults: systematic review and meta-analysis. *Journal of Anxiety Disorders*, **26**, 1–11.

Gould, C. E., Segal, D. L., Yochim, B. P., Pachana, N. A., Byrne, G. J. and Beaudreau, S. A. (2014). Measuring anxiety in late life: a psychometric examination of the geriatric anxiety inventory and geriatric anxiety scale. *Journal of Anxiety Disorders*, **28**(8), 804–811.

Hamilton, M. (1959). The assessment of anxiety states by rating. *British Journal of Medical Psychology*, **32**, 50–55.

Hendriks, G. J., Keijsers, G. P., Kampman, M., et al. (2010). A randomized controlled study of paroxetine and cognitive–behavioural therapy for late-life panic disorder. *Acta Psychiatrica Scandinavica*, **122**(1), 11–19.

Hertzberg, M. A., Butterfield, M. I., Feldman, M. E., et al. (1999). A preliminary study of lamotrigine for the treatment of posttraumatic stress disorder. *Biological Psychiatry*, **45**(9), 1226–1229.

Hollingworth, S. A. and Siskind, D. J. (2010). Anxiolytic, hypnotic and sedative medication use in Australia. *Pharmacoepidemiology and Drug Safety*, **19**(3), 280–288.

Hollingworth, S. A., Siskind, D. J., Nissen, L. M., Robinson, M. and Hall, W. D. (2010). Patterns of antipsychotic medication use in Australia 2002–2007. *Australian and New Zealand Journal of Psychiatry*, **44**(4), 372–377.

Katz, I. R., Reynolds, C. F., Alexopoulos, G. S. and Hackett, D. (2002). Venlafaxine ER as a treatment for generalized anxiety disorder in older adults: pooled analysis of five randomized placebo-controlled clinical trials. *Journal of the American Geriatrics Society*, **50**(1), 18–25.

Kimura, M., Tateno, A. and Robinson, R. G. (2003). Treatment of post-stroke generalized anxiety disorder comorbid with poststroke depression: merged analysis of nortriptyline trials. *American Journal of Geriatric Psychiatry*, **11**(3), 320–327.

Koepke, H. H., Gold, R. K., Linden, M. E., Lion, J. R. and Kickels, K. (1982). Multicenter controlled study of oxazepam in anxious elderly outpatients. *Psychosomatics*, **23**(6), 641–645.

Kruszewski, S. P. (2005). Conclusions inconsistent with results with citalopram. *American Journal of Psychiatry*, **162**(11), 2195–2196.

Lader, M. and Scotto, J. C. (1998). A multicentre double-blind comparison of hydrozyzine, buspirone and placebo in patients with generalized anxiety disorder. *Psychopharmacology (Berlin)*, **54** (Suppl.), 64–68.

Landreville, P., Landry, J., Baillargeon, L., Guerette, A. and Matteau, E. (2001). Older adults' acceptance of psychological and pharmacological treatments for depression. *Journals of Gerontology Series B: Psychological Sciences and Social Sciences*, **56**(5), P285–P291.

Lenze, E. J., Mulsant, B. H., Shear, M. K., et al. (2005). Efficacy and tolerability of citalopram in the treatment of late-life anxiety disorders: results from an 8-week randomized, placebo-controlled trial. *American Journal of Psychiatry*, **162**(1), 146–150.

Lenze, E. J., Rollman, B. L., Shear, M. K., et al. (2009). Escitalopram for older adults with generalized anxiety disorder: a randomized controlled trial. *Journal of the American Medical Association*, **301**(3), 295–303.

Majercsik, E. and Haller, J. (2004). Interactions between anxiety, social support, health status and buspirone efficacy in elderly patients. *Progress in Neuropsychopharmacology and Biological Psychiatry*, **28**, 1161–1169.

McIntyre, E., Saliba, A. J., Wiener, K. K. and Sarris, J. (2016). Herbal medicine use behaviour in Australian adults who experience anxiety: a descriptive study. *BMC Complementary and Alternative Medicine*, **16**, 60.

Mezhebovsky, I., Magi, K., She, F., Datto, C. and Eriksson, H. (2013). Double-blind, randomized study of extended release quetiapine fumarate (quetiapine XR) monotherapy in older patients with generalized anxiety disorder. *International Journal of Geriatric Psychiatry*, **28**(6), 615–625.

Mokhber, N., Azarpazhooh, M. R., Khajehdaluee, M., Velayati, A. and Hopwood, M. (2010). Randomized, single-blind trial of sertraline and buspirone for treatment of elderly patients with generalized anxiety disorder. *Psychiatry and Clinical Neuroscience*, **64**(2), 128–133.

Montgomery, S., Chatamra, K., Pauer, L., Whalen, E. and Baldinetti, F. (2008). Efficacy and safety of pregabalin in elderly people with generalised anxiety disorder. *British Journal of Psychiatry*, **193**(5), 389–394.

Mula, M., Pini, S. and Cassano, G. B. (2007). The role of anticonvulsant drugs in anxiety disorders: a critical review of the evidence.

Journal of Clinical Psychopharmacology, **27** (3), 263–372.

National Institute for Health and Care Excellence (2014). Anxiety Disorders, Quality Standard QS53, February 2014, NICE, UK. www.nice.org.uk/guidance/qs53/chapter/About-this-quality-standard (accessed 7 May 2018).

Pande, A. C., Davidson, J. R., Jefferson, J. W., et al. (1999). Treatment of social phobia with gabapentin: a placebo-controlled study. *Journal of Clinical Psychopharmacology*, **19** (4), 341–348.

Reinhold, J. A., Mandos, L. A., Rickels, K. and Lohoff, F. W. (2011). Pharmacological treatment of generalized anxiety disorder. *Expert Opinion on Pharmacotherapy*, **12**(16), 2457–2467.

Sarris, J. (2018). Herbal medicines in the treatment of psychiatric disorders: 10-year updated review. *Phytotherapy Research*, **32** (7), 1147–1162.

Savage, K., Firth, J., Stough, C. and Sarris, J. (2018). GABA-modulating phytomedicines for anxiety: A systematic review of preclinical and clinical evidence. *Phytotherapy Research*, **32**(1), 3–18.

Schuurmans, J., Comijs, H., Emmelkamp, P. M., et al. (2006). A randomized, controlled trial of the effectiveness of cognitive–behavioral therapy and sertraline versus a waitlist control group for anxiety disorders in older adults. *American Journal of Geriatric Psychiatry*, **14**(3), 255–263.

Steenen, S. A., van Wijk, A. J., van der Heijden, G. J. M. G., van Westrhenen, R., de Lange, J. and de Jongh, A. (2016). Propranolol for the treatment of anxiety disorders: systematic review and meta-analysis. *Journal of Psychopharmacology*, **30**(2), 128–139.

Wetherell, J. L., Petkus, A. J., White, K. S., et al. (2013). Antidepressant augmented with cognitive–behavioral therapy for generalized anxiety disorder in older adults. *American Journal of Psychiatry*, **170**(7), 782–789.

Woodward, R. and Pachana, N. A. (2009). Attitudes towards psychological treatment among older Australians. *Australian Psychologist*, **44**(2), 86–93.

Chapter 13

Animal Models in Anxiety Research

Madhusoothanan Bhagavathi Perumal and Pankaj Sah

Man is not worried by real problems so much as by his imagined anxieties about real problems.
Epictetus (55–135 CE)

Fear and anxious apprehension are highly evolutionarily conserved responses triggered by a real or perceived imminent threat. These are adaptive responses, classically described as fight or flight responses, which comprise emotional, autonomic, and motor arousal. They are rapidly initiated and diminish as the danger abates. Anxiety states display physiological features that are similar to those evoked by fear, but as defined in the Diagnostic and Statistical Manual of Mental Disorders (DSM) of the American Psychiatric Association, these behavioural disturbances persist beyond the appropriate period. Anxiety disorders are prevalent in all societies, and in 2014 they were the sixth leading cause of disability worldwide in terms of years lived with disability.

Charles Darwin, in his seminal book *The Expression of the Emotions in Man and Animals*, laid the foundation for comparative and systemic investigations of emotional responses and behaviour in animals. A broad definition of an animal model is given by: 'An animal model is a living organism in which normative biology or behavior can be studied, or in which a spontaneous or induced pathological process can be investigated, and in which the phenomenon in one or more respects resembles the same phenomenon in humans or other species of animal' (Held, 1983, p. 13). Understanding human psychiatric disorders using animal models is difficult, firstly, because these conditions are intrinsically subjective with individual-specific spectra of symptoms, and secondly, because of the difficulty in identifying specific behavioural correlates between humans and animals. Although the emotional aspects of threat responses are subjective and cannot be directly studied in animals, certain behavioural correlates and patterns of brain activity triggered by the experience of fear can be investigated in animals. Indeed, both the behavioural outputs and neural circuits involved are highly conserved amongst animals and humans, presumably owing to the necessity of the fear response for an organism's survival. Behavioural responses to fear and anxiety include autonomic arousal as well as defensive coping behaviours like the fight or flight response and freezing, when animals become immobile to avoid detection. The major circuits typically disturbed in anxiety disorders involve brain regions crucial for associative learning and memory (amygdala and hippocampus) and decision-making processes (prefrontal cortex), each of which influences the hypothalamic–pituitary–adrenal (HPA) axis in generating the hormonal and autonomic responses associated with fear and anxiety. Cholinergic, serotonergic, and adrenergic neurotransmission are critical for mediating the arousal associated with these responses, and many current therapeutic strategies for anxiety disorders are aimed at modulating these mechanisms.

The major anxiety disorders include generalized anxiety disorder (GAD), panic disorder, specific phobias, social anxiety disorder, and post-traumatic stress disorder (PTSD). As may be expected, interactions between nature (genetic), nurture (developmental), and environmental influences on intrinsic factors (epigenetic and synaptic mechanisms) underlie the development of disturbances in anxiety and fear responses. This poses challenges for developing efficient treatments of these disorders, as it makes the individual susceptibility, temporal evolution, and symptom spectra of anxiety disorders highly variable. Nevertheless, common behavioural disturbances observed in these conditions suggest that specific, highly conserved neural circuits of the fear response are critical to the underlying pathology. Studies based on experimental animal models are already revealing new mechanisms involved in the generation of fear and anxiety. Here, we discuss the neural circuits that underpin fear responses in animal models and how this understanding provides insight into avenues for treating anxiety-related disorders.

Pavlovian Fear Conditioning

Our understanding of the neural circuits that underpin fear comes largely from the study of Pavlovian fear conditioning. In this paradigm, an emotionally neutral stimulus, such as a tone or light (described as the conditioned stimulus (CS)), is contingently paired with an aversive stimulus (the unconditioned stimulus (US)), typically a footshock. Following a small number of pairings, the CS comes to evoke an evasive response, called the conditioned response (CR). This is manifest as immobility (freezing), autonomic changes in heart rate, and biochemical changes in the hypothalamic–pituitary axis. The behavioural response reflects a rapidly learnt association made between the CS and US, requires a single or at most a few pairings, and is long lasting. However, subsequent presentations of the CS that are not paired with the US loosen this association, leading to a gradual reduction in the CR, a process known as extinction (Pavlov, 1927). While extinction breaks the association between the original CS and US, it does not result from erasure of the previous memory. Rather, it requires new learning that the CS no longer predicts the US.

The neural circuitry for evaluating and storing fear memories has its genesis in the need to learn about and rapidly respond to dangerous situations and to modify this response appropriately when circumstances change. In both fear learning and extinction, the amygdala has emerged as a key structure that plays a central role in the acquisition and expression of learnt fear (Hitchcock & Davis, 1986; LeDoux et al., 1990; Slotnick, 1973). The amygdala is extensively interconnected with cortical and subcortical regions (McDonald, 1998; Sah et al., 2003), and it has become increasingly clear that the hippocampus (Maren, 2001) and the medial prefrontal cortex (mPFC) are two structures that play significant roles in fear conditioning and extinction (Sotres-Bayon & Quirk, 2010). These circuits are largely preserved in humans, with fear conditioning and presentations of fearful stimuli activating the amygdala (LaBar et al., 1998; Morris et al., 1996), and fear extinction resulting in prefrontal activity (Delgado et al., 2008; LaBar et al., 1998).

Fear and anxiety share a remarkable number of features, and anxiety states in humans are thought to be an exaggeration of these normal fear states (Blanchard & Blanchard, 2008). Irrational or overgeneralized fear is one of the most prevalent symptoms in anxiety disorders, particularly phobias, PTSD, and panic disorder, all of which involve a clear dysregulation of fear (Blanchard & Blanchard, 2008).

Understanding the neural circuits engaged during fear learning will therefore provide insight into the neural circuits that underpin anxiety. Moreover, the management of such disorders with procedures like exposure therapy have their roots in fear extinction (McNally, 2007).

Thus, understanding the biology that underpins fear learning and extinction will provide insight into the genesis of anxiety-related disorders and help define the neurons and neurotransmitter systems that drive the activity in these circuits. Together, this understanding will provide the starting point for the development of new therapeutic pharmaceutical and behavioural procedures to treat these disorders.

The Amygdala

The amygdala complex, located in the mid-temporal lobe, is divided into over 20 subnuclei with extensive internuclear and extranuclear connections (Pape & Paré, 2010; Sah et al., 2003). These nuclei are commonly divided into three groups (Price et al., 1987; Sah et al., 2003): a deeper basolateral (BLA) group consisting of the lateral nucleus (LA), the basal nucleus (BA), and the accessory basal nucleus; a more superficial or cortical-like group that includes the cortical amygdalar nuclei and the nucleus of the lateral olfactory tract; and a centromedial group composed of the medial and central nuclei (CeA). The BLA is the primary sensory input zone of the amygdala, receiving afferents from many cortical and subcortical regions, while the CeA is the primary output structure that initiates physiological responses of fear (Pape & Paré, 2010; Sah et al., 2003).

The BLA, a cortical-like structure, contains two types of neuron: glutamatergic principal neurons that form ~80% of the total cell population; and GABAergic interneurons that make up the rest (McDonald, 1982, 1992, McDonald & Mascagni, 2001; Spampanato et al., 2011). Principal neurons resemble cortical pyramidal neurons (Faber et al., 2001; Power & Sah, 2008; Washburn & Moises, 1992). As in other cortical- like areas (Ascoli et al., 2008), several families of interneuron are present within the BLA (McDonald & Mascagni, 2001; Spampanato et al., 2011), providing both feedforward and feedback inhibition within the BLA (Ehrlich et al., 2009; Jasnow et al., 2009; Spampanato et al., 2011; Woodruff & Sah, 2007b). CS and US information from both cortical and subcortical regions is carried by glutamatergic afferents that innervate both types of neuron (Farb & Ledoux, 1999; Lanuza et al., 2008; Sah et al., 2003; Smith et al., 1998, 2000), forming classical dual-component glutamatergic synapses that express two types of receptors: α-amino-3-hydroxy-5-methyl-4-isoxazolepropionic acid (AMPA) receptors and N-methyl-D-aspartate (NMDA) receptors (Hestrin et al., 1990; Mahanty & Sah, 1999; Weisskopf & LeDoux, 1999). At these synapses, AMPA receptors are engaged during normal synaptic transmission, whereas NMDA receptors are engaged during learning (Collingridge & Bliss, 1987). Incoming CS/US information is first processed in the BLA, whose principal neurons then project to the CeA. Connections from the CeA then initiate the physiological responses of fear (Ehrlich et al., 2009; Sah et al., 2003).

Interneurons within the BLA can be divided into distinct populations based on their expression of particular markers and firing properties (Spampanato et al., 2011). Recent studies have begun to reveal the intrinsic organization and roles of some of these interneuron families, showing that different types of interneuron make different types of local connections (Jasnow et al., 2009; Rainnie et al., 1991; Woodruff & Sah, 2007a, 2007b; Woodruff et al., 2006). While they form a relatively small population of cells, local inhibition is potent in the amygdala, controlling the activity of most cells. Recent work has shown that different interneurons are engaged during fear learning, each playing a distinct role (Tovote et al., 2015).

In contrast to the BLA, the CeA is a striatal-like structure that consists entirely of GABAergic neurons (de Olmos et al., 1985), and it is divided into lateral and medial divisions (Cassell et al., 1986). Projections from the BLA innervate the lateral CeA, which in turn projects to the medial CeA (Tovote et al., 2015). Outputs from the medial CeA to hypothalamic and brainstem nuclei then initiate fear responses (Paré & Duvarci, 2012).

Neurons in both divisions of the CeA can also be separated into distinct populations based on their expression of peptides (Cassell et al., 1986) and intrinsic firing properties (Dumont et al., 2002; Lopez de Armentia & Sah, 2004; Martina et al., 1999). Excitatory afferents from the BLA activate lateral division of the central amygdala (CeL) neurons (Lopez de Armentia & Sah, 2004), but also drive feedforward disynaptic inhibitory responses (Amano et al., 2010; Lopez de Armentia & Sah, 2004; Royer et al., 1999). This inhibition is provided by two distinct sources: firstly, a cluster of GABAergic neurons interposed between the BLA and CeA – the intercalated cells (ITCs) (Millhouse, 1986) – that receives inputs from the BLA and projects to the CeA (Delaney & Sah, 2001; Royer et al., 1999). Secondly, neurons within the CeA, which are all GABAergic, are extensively interconnected, providing strong local inhibition upon afferent activation (Haubensak et al., 2010; Lopez de Armentia & Sah, 2004).

The intrinsic organization within the CeA is complex and recordings from the lateral CeA *in vivo* show that following fear conditioning some neurons increases their response to the CS, while others are inhibited (see below), suggesting that different cells within the CeA also receive different types of input. In the medial CeA, neurons that project to different downstream targets and mediate different physiological responses constitute distinct populations of neurons that can be separated on electrophysiological as well as pharmacological grounds (Viviani et al., 2011). Finally, apart from the BLA, the CeA also receives inputs from a variety of cortical and subcortical regions (Sah et al., 2003).

Medial Prefrontal Cortex and Hippocampus

The mPFC, a neocortical structure, is divided into four distinct regions from dorsal to ventral: the medial precentral cortex (PrCm), the anterior cingulate cortex (ACd), the prelimbic (PL), and the infralimbic (IL) prefrontal cortices (Heidbreder & Groenewegen, 2003). Most neocortical regions, particularly sensory areas, are divided into six distinct layers (I–VI), with pyramidal cells confined to layers II/III, V, and VI. Layer IV is largely devoid of pyramidal neurons, but it is the primary target for sensory input from the thalamus (Miller et al., 2001). The rodent prefrontal cortex appears to have well-defined layers I, II/III, and V/VI; however, the existence of a discrete layer IV is not clear (Van De Werd et al., 2010).

Pyramidal cells located in layers II/III and V/VI show a range of firing properties (Wang et al., 2006) that are similar to those described for other neocortical regions (Connors & Gutnick, 1990). The mPFC also contains a variety of types of interneuron (Van De Werd et al., 2010), with the expected distribution of interneuronal markers (Markram et al., 2004).

The hippocampal formation is a very distinctive structure that has historically been considered the gate for the formation of declarative memories (Milner et al., 1998). This view arose from studying the now-famous case of H.M., who lost the ability to form new memories when much of his mid-temporal pole was removed to treat intractable epilepsy. This basic finding has been recapitulated many times in both humans and rodents (Milner et al., 1998). However, there is also a growing literature that implicates septohippocampal activity in depression and anxiety disorders (Gray & McNaughton, 2000). Connections of the hippocampal formation are stereotactically organized with widespread projections to cortical and subcortical areas (Moser & Moser, 1998). In particular, the ventral (temporal) hippocampus is strongly reciprocally connected with the mPFC and amygdala (Fanselow & Dong, 2010). These projections from the hippocampus innervate distinct cell groups in the amygdala and mPFC and gate fear responses (Sotres-Bayon et al., 2012).

Different Circuits Mediate Fear Learning and Extinction

The Amygdala

As described above, CS and US inputs converge on neurons within the amygdala (Pape & Paré, 2010; Sah et al., 2003). Inhibiting synaptic transmission in the BLA during learning using pharmacological agents blocks fear learning and extinction, and post-learning infusions block the expression of learnt fear (Falls et al., 1992; Kim et al., 1993), confirming the key role of the BLA in fear conditioning and extinction. In contrast, infusion of selective NMDA receptor antagonists into the amygdala blocks learning during both fear conditioning and extinction, but has no effect on previously learnt responses (Goosens & Maren, 2004; Miserendino et al., 1990). These results support the idea that learning during both fear conditioning and extinction requires NMDA receptor-mediated synaptic plasticity within the BLA (Mayford et al., 2012). Consistent with this proposal, inputs to BLA principal neurons show NMDA receptor-dependent plasticity (Bissiere et al., 2003; Humeau et al., 2003; McKernan & Shinnick-Gallagher, 1997; Rodrigues et al., 2004; Rogan et al., 1997; Rumpel et al., 2005; Weisskopf et al., 1999). However, how this plasticity is initiated during fear conditioning and extinction is not clear (Sah et al., 2008).

Single -unit recordings *in vivo* have shown that, following fear conditioning, principal neurons in the BLA show enhanced responses to stimuli that were paired with footshock (Goosens et al., 2003; Quirk et al., 1995). These cells have been called 'fear neurons' (Herry et al., 2008). Following extinction, some of these neurons reduce their response to the CS, and a new population of previously silent neurons now begins to respond to the CS – these neurons have been called 'extinction neurons' (Amano et al., 2011; Herry et al., 2008). In the current model, it seems likely that 'fear neurons' arise due to NMDA receptor-dependent plasticity of CS inputs to BLA neurons (Miserendino et al., 1990; Rogan et al., 1997). Similarly, as extinction is blocked by infusion of NMDA receptor antagonists into the BLA, 'extinction neurons' presumably arise as a result of plasticity at inputs to a different set of neurons during extinction training. The reduction in activity of 'fear neurons' with extinction may result from synaptic plasticity of CS input to interneurons and the enhancement of local inhibition (Ehrlich et al., 2009; Mahanty & Sah, 1998; Polepalli et al., 2010).

Fear learning evokes NMDA receptor-mediated plasticity of CS inputs to principal neurons in the BLA, and this plasticity is able to drive the activity of 'fear neurons'.

Subsequent presentation of the CS evokes fear responses by activating these cells. Following fear extinction, CS presentation inhibits the activity of fear neurons but drives the firing of extinction neurons, and together this activity reduces fear responses. While fear and extinction learning require the BLA, physiological responses to fear are driven by outputs from the medial CeA (Pape & Paré, 2010; Paré & Duvarci, 2012). Afferents from the BLA innervate the lateral CeA, and single-unit recordings show that, following auditory cued conditioning, the CS now drives a population of neurons in the lateral CeA, called 'ON neurons'. These 'ON neurons' make local connections that inhibit the activity of a different population of neurons that have been called 'OFF neurons' (Ciocchi et al., 2010; Haubensak et al., 2010). OFF neurons are GABAergic and project to the medial CeA. Thus, inhibiting OFF neurons results in disinhibition of neurons in the medial CeA by the CS (Ciocchi et al., 2010; Haubensak et al., 2010). The resulting activity of medial CeA neurons evokes a fear response (Ciocchi et al., 2010).

In extinction, there is a reduction in the activity of 'fear neurons' and a new population of 'extinction neurons' becomes active (Herry et al., 2008). This inhibition of 'fear neuron' activity is thought to be mediated by enhanced GABAergic activity in the BLA, resulting from plasticity of inputs to local interneurons. What, then, is the role of extinction neurons? In addition to the local GABAergic interneurons within the BLA, clusters of small GABAergic cells also surround the BLA, and are called ITCs (Millhouse, 1986; Pinard et al., 2012). ITCs are divided into the lateral (lITC) and medial (mITC) clusters, located within the external and intermediate capsules of the amygdala, respectively. Of these, the mITC neurons are thought to form an inhibitory interface between the input (BLA) and output (CeA) nuclei of the amygdala (Palomares-Castillo et al., 2012; Paré & Duvarci, 2012; Paré & Smith, 1993). BLA principal neurons provide input to the mITC neurons and drive feedforward inhibition in the CeA (Paré & Smith, 1993; Strobel et al., 2015). The BLA–mITC synapse exhibits NMDA receptor-dependent plasticity (Royer & Paré, 2002), and it has been proposed that, following extinction, plasticity of this input results in an increase in disynaptic inhibition to the CeA, effectively reducing the activity of ON neurons, thus inhibiting the fear response (Amano et al., 2010). However, whether 'extinction neurons' in the BLA are the cells that drive mITC neurons to inhibit CeA output following fear extinction is not known.

The Medial Prefrontal Cortex and Hippocampus

Fear conditioning and extinction both require activity in the amygdala; however, stimulation and inactivation studies indicate that that the mPFC is also involved in both forms of learning (Burgos-Robles et al., 2007; Corcoran & Quirk, 2007; Laurent & Westbrook, 2008, Sotres-Bayon & Quirk, 2010), with the IL and PL having distinct roles (Burgos-Robles et al., 2007). These studies show that while the amygdala is required during the acquisition and expression of learnt fear, PL activity is required for consolidation and recall of fear memory (Maren & Quirk, 2004; Quirk & Mueller, 2008). Thus, inactivation of the PL after fear learning results in reduced fear responses (Corcoran & Quirk, 2007), and microstimulation of the PL enhances freezing to learnt CS's (Vidal-Gonzalez et al., 2006).

Similarly, the IL does not have a significant role in extinction learning, but it is required for consolidation of extinction memory. Thus, extinction memory is significantly blunted when IL activity is silenced (Laurent & Westbrook, 2009), but it is enhanced if the IL is microstimulated during extinction training (Vidal-Gonzalez et al., 2006).

Electrophysiological recordings from neurons in the IL show that, following extinction training, neurons show enhanced responses to the CS (Milad & Quirk, 2002). Moreover, infusion of NMDA receptor antagonists into the IL, either prior to or immediately after extinction training, impaired extinction learning (Burgos-Robles et al., 2007). Together, these results suggest that consolidation of extinction memory engages NMDA receptor-dependent plasticity within the IL. It has long been appreciated that memory consolidation requires gene transcription and protein synthesis (Lubin et al., 2011), and consistent with the role of the mPFC in the consolidation of memory for fear extinction, protein synthesis and gene transcription within the mPFC have been shown to be required during consolidation of fear extinction memories (Mamiya et al., 2009; Santini et al., 2004). Moreover, similarly to learning in other brain regions (Blaze & Roth, 2013), this synaptic plasticity within the IL is under the control of epigenetic mechanisms (Marek et al., 2011; Wei et al., 2012).

Aside from interactions with the mPFC and (ventral?) hippocampus, the BLA and CeA make reciprocal connections with a variety of other cortical and subcortical regions (Sah et al., 2003), and these regions are now being implicated in controlling the behavioural response evoked by amygdala activation. For example, the bed nucleus of the stria terminalis (BNST), often referred to as being part of the extended amygdala and located in the temporal lobe, receives large input from the BLA and CeA. Recent evidence from rodents suggests a distinct role for the BNST in anxiogeneis and anxiolysis (Davis et al., 2010). The BNST sends both excitatory and inhibitory projections to the ventral tegmental area (VTA), a key neuromodulatory structure for learning and memory (see below). Activation of the VTA by BNST glutamatergic projections induces avoidance and enhanced anxiety, whereas activation of BNST GABAergic terminals to the VTA produces rewarding and anxiolytic effects (Jennings et al., 2013).

Neuromodulation of Fear and Anxiety Circuits

In addition to its use of neurotransmitters such as glutamate, GABA, and glycine for point-to-point fast neurotransmission, the mammalian nervous system is endowed with a range of slow transmitter systems that powerfully influence neural network synchronization and plasticity. These transmitter systems arise from nuclei in the midbrain and brainstem that send ascending projections throughout the brain, and many of these have been implicated in anxiety disorders (Nestler et al., 2015).

Neurons expressing serotonin (5-hydroxytryptamine (5-HT)) are localized in the midbrain raphe nuclei comprising the dorsal and median raphe nuclei, and they send projections throughout the brain (Nestler et al., 2015). The amygdala shows dense expression of 5-HT receptors and receives strong projections from the dorsal raphe nucleus (Vertes, 1991). The hippocampus is innervated by the medial raphe nucleus, whereas the prefrontal cortex receives input from both medial and dorsal raphe nuclei (Azmitia & Segal, 1978; Bauer, 2015; McQuade & Sharp, 1997). Midbrain 5-HT neurons are activated during behavioural arousal and by stress during US presentation. During fear conditioning, 5-HT levels increase in the amygdala and prefrontal cortex, modulating network activity and synaptic plasticity in these regions (Kawahara et al., 1993; Yokoyama et al., 2005). In humans, the short allele of the promoter for the 5-HT transporter is presumed to induce increased extracellular 5-HT. Humans with the short allele also exhibit greater amygdala activity in response to fearful stimuli (Lesch et al., 1996).

5-HT mediates its actions through seven distinct families of receptors (5-HT1–7) that have distinct distributions in the brain, suggesting a dynamic role for this neuromodulator (Nestler et al., 2015). Pharmacological investigations in animal models using specific agonists and antagonists suggest region-specific functions for these receptor families in fear and anxiety behaviours. 5-HT1A receptors act as autoreceptors, regulating the tone of serotonergic output, and agonists of these receptors have anxiolytic actions in both humans and animals (Lacivita et al., 2008). 5-HT2A receptor agonists administered immediately following fear learning enhance memory consolidation and increase avoidance behaviour (Zhang et al., 2013). Interestingly, 5-HT2A/C-knockout mice do not show deficits in fear conditioning paradigms, yet they have reduced anxious behaviour (Weisstaub et al., 2006), while 5-HT2AC overexpression in the amygdala induces increased anxiety-like behaviour (Campbell & Merchant, 2003; Gibson et al., 1994). Thus, the serotonergic system plays a complex and dynamic role in regulating fear circuits through distinct synaptic targets. It will be important to dissect these functions at a synaptic level to understand the role of serotonergic systems in anxiety disorders.

The locus coeruleus, a pontine nucleus, is the main noradrenergic system projecting throughout the brain and spinal cord (Nestler et al., 1984). Noradrenergic receptors (α1, α2, and β) are present throughout the fear circuits (Nestler et al., 1984), and noradrenergic transmission strongly influences synaptic plasticity in various regions, including the amygdala and hippocampus. In rodents, activation of the noradrenergic system enhances fear acquisition and consolidation (Tully & Bolshakov, 2010).

Dopaminergic neurotransmission is crucial for learning and memory processes, including fear acquisition and extinction (Abraham et al., 2014). Four major dopaminergic pathways can be described (Beaulieu & Gainetdinov, 2011). The mesocortical (dopaminergic projections from the ventral tegmentum (VT) to cortical regions) and mesolimbic (VT to the nucleus accumbens, amygdala, and hippocampus) pathways are important for both fear- and reward-associated behavioural responses. The nigrostriatal pathway (dopaminergic projection from the substantia nigra to the striatum) is involved in motivation for motor movements, and the tuberoinfundibular (hypothalamic dopaminergic neurons to the pituitary axis) pathway regulates hormonal release. Like other neuromodulators, dopamine mediates its effects through different families of receptors: D1-like receptors (D1 and D5) that activate stimulatory G proteins; and D2-like receptors (D2, D3, and D4) that activate inhibitory G protein receptors (Beaulieu & Gainetdinov, 2011). In addition, D1 and D2 heteromeric receptors have distinct downstream signalling pathways and have been implicated in neuropsychiatric disorders (Nestler et al., 2015).

Fear conditioning in rodents given agonists or antagonists for D1 receptors suggests that D1 receptor activity is essential for fear acquisition and consolidation, but that the impact is time dependent (Greba & Kokkinidis, 2000; Inoue et al., 2000). The role of D2 is more complex in fear- and anxiety-related behaviour and extinction. Systemic administration of D2 antagonists enhanced extinction, while local infusion into the BLA and VTA reduced contextual fear expression (de Souza Caetano et al., 2013; Mueller et al., 2010). Dopaminergic systems in the brain pose a complex challenge due to the diversity of receptor families involved and the distinct neural pathways responsible for specific effects. For example, the dorsal VT is excited by reward or reward-associated stimuli, whereas ventral VT dopaminergic neurons are excited by aversive stimuli. Thus, changes in the basal tone of these distinct pathways can potentially influence the perception of environmental stimuli and the generation and termination of responses.

Animal Model to Clinical Translation

It is estimated that anxiety disorders affect up to 20% of the population at some time during their lifetime, and both the personal emotional conflicts and overall health cost to the community are enormous. The treatment of anxiety disorders is complex, consisting of psychotherapy, pharmacotherapy, and behavioural therapy, and while a number of treatments are effective, they are palliative in nature. Pharmacotherapy using benzodiazepines (such as diazepam, Valium), selective serotonin reuptake inhibitors (SSRIs; such as Prozac, fluoxetine), or serotonin–norepinephrine reuptake inhibitors (SNRIs; such as venlafaxine,

Effexor) is commonly employed first (Reinhold, 2015; Starcevic, 2014). Most pharmacological agents are accompanied by a host of side effects, and new methods to treat these disorders are clearly required. These side effects arise from the relatively widespread mode of action of all current anxiolytics and because the mode of therapeutic action is not well understood. Of the compounds currently available, benzodiazepines are rapid acting, and their activity is probably best understood, so we will focus on these compounds as examples.

Benzodiazepines act by positively modulating $GABA_A$ receptors, and benzodiazepine binding sites are expressed in the amygdala at high density (Niehoff & Kuhar, 1983; Richards & Möhler, 1984). It is likely that the anxiolytic actions of these agents are due to their effects on the amygdala (Pesold & Treit, 1994). However, existing benzodiazepines also have potent effects on $GABA_A$ receptors distributed throughout the rest of the central nervous system (CNS) (Sieghart & Sperk, 2002), leading to a range of side effects. Thus, the development of more specific compounds for the treatment of anxiety disorders requires an understanding of the molecular composition of $GABA_A$ receptors and their distributions in specific circuits within the amygdala.

As described above, learning in both fear conditioning and extinction is thought to require synaptic plasticity at glutamatergic synapses to projection neurons in the amygdala (Pape & Paré, 2010; Sah et al., 2008). However, emerging evidence indicates that GABAergic synapses within the amygdala also play key roles in both fear conditioning and extinction (Ehrlich et al., 2009). For example, enhancers of GABAergic inhibition in the BLA interfere with the learning and expression of conditioned fear (Davis, 1979; Harris & Westbrook, 1998), whereas a reduction in GABAergic inhibition has the opposite effect (Tang et al., 2007). Consistent with these findings, inputs to interneurons in the amygdala can also undergo synaptic plasticity (Mahanty & Sah, 1998; Polepalli et al., 2010). Moreover, an emerging body of literature indicates that while fear learning requires synaptic plasticity of inputs mediating CS information to pyramidal neurons in the BLA, extinction is thought to result from potentiation of inputs to ITC neurons, which in turn inhibit the central nucleus, thus reducing fear responses (Paré & Duvarci, 2012). Together, these results show that GABAergic inhibition in the BLA and CeA plays a central role in fear learning.

$GABA_A$ receptors are present in the postsynaptic membrane of inhibitory synapses formed by GABAergic interneurons onto other amygdala neurons. Thus, the actions of anxiolytics such as benzodiazepines result from modulation of local inhibitory circuits in the amygdala (Rudolph & Mohler, 2006). It is likely that the molecular and pharmacological properties of $GABA_A$ receptors present at synapses made by the diverse populations of interneurons in the amygdala are different. For example, within the CeA, GABAergic synapses arising from two different inputs have entirely different biophysical and pharmacological properties. While one of these inputs is potentiated by benzodiazepines, the other is inhibited (Delaney & Sah, 1999, 2001). These findings indicate that neurons in the CeA express $GABA_A$ receptors with different molecular compositions that are targeted to different synapses. As these two inputs are parts of different circuits, modulation of the two receptors will have differential physiological impacts.

$GABA_A$ receptors are heteromeric ligand-gated chloride channels, and 20 different subunits that can assemble to form functional $GABA_A$ receptors have been identified: $\alpha 1$–6, $\beta 1$–4, $\gamma 1$–3, δ, ε, θ, π, and $\rho 1$–3, all of which are products of separate genes (Barnard et al., 1998; Olsen & Tobin, 1990). These subunits assemble as pentamers, and like many other types of ion channel, their biophysical and pharmacological properties are dependent on their subunit stoichiometry (Sieghart & Sperk, 2002). Most $GABA_A$ receptors in the mammalian CNS are thought to contain two α, two β, and one γ subunit, with the most common stoichiometry being α1β2γ2 (Mohler, 2006; Sieghart & Sperk, 2002). High-potency benzodiazepine modulation of the GABA$_A$ receptors requires the presence of γ2 subunits (Mohler, 2006). Recent studies have shown that receptors containing α1 subunits are responsible for the sedative/hypnotic actions of benzodiazepines, while receptors containing α2 subunits mediate their anxiolytic actions (Rudolph & Mohler, 2006). Receptors incorporating α1 and α2 subunits can be distinguished pharmacologically (Atack, 2011; McKernan et al., 2000). In the amygdala, α2, βx, and γ2 subunits are the major GABA$_A$ receptor subunits present in the BLA and CeA (Esmaeili et al., 2009). Interestingly, although γ1 subunits are present throughout the CNS at very low levels (Laurie et al., 1992), they are highly enriched in the CeA (Esmaeili et al., 2009).

Understanding the subunit stoichiometry of GABA receptors within the amygdala therefore provides one target for the development of specific pharmacological treatments for anxiety disorders with reduced side effects. Much effort is therefore being made to identify and understand the molecular nature of GABA receptors at distinct circuits involved in fear and anxiety (Farb & Ratner, 2014).

A second approach to treat anxiety disorders is cognitive behavioural therapy (CBT). In particular, treatment using exposure-based CBT has been found to be very successful in treating phobias, and indeed it is the first therapy of choice. The implementation of CBT is based on the extinction of learnt fear (McNally, 2007). As described above, extinction is a form of learning and requires the activity of NMDA receptors. Thus, infusion of NMDA receptor antagonists into the amygdala blocks fear extinction (Falls et al., 1992) and inhibiting these receptors post-learning blocks consolidation. Thus, activity of NMDA receptors is required for extinction learning, raising the question of whether enhancing the activity of these receptors may enhance extinction. One compound that enhances the activity of NMDA receptors is D-cycloserine (DCS), and indeed delivery of this compound into the amygdala enhanced the extinction of conditioned fear (Ledgerwood et al., 2003). The similarity between extinction and CBT therapy suggested that DCS may also facilitate exposure-based psychotherapy, and indeed, early clinical trials suggest that this may be possible (Davis et al., 2006; Ressler et al., 2004). However, other trials have not confirmed this result (Guastella et al., 2007). NMDA receptors are complex proteins, and the stoichiometry of these receptors is variable in different regions of the amygdala (Delaney et al., 2013; Lopez de Armentia & Sah, 2003). While DCS has been found to potentiate NMDA receptor activity, whether different types of NMDA receptors show differential responses is not known. As with GABA receptors, it seems likely that NMDA receptors with distinct stoichiometries will respond to different agents, raising the possibility that more specific compounds targeted to specific amygdala regions may be more efficient anxiolytics.

Conclusions

In this chapter, we have focused on one animal model that is widely used to probe the neural mechanisms that may underpin anxiety. The fear response, a key behaviour for survival, is highly conserved during evolution, and it is therefore not surprising that we share many features of 'fear' with animals at the cellular, network, and behavioural levels. Rodents are the most commonly used animal models, as their behavioural correlates are well recognized and genetic manipulations and investigations of specific brain circuits are feasible in a cost-efficient way. Different animal models and paradigms have been developed to investigate specific symptoms of human anxiety disorders (Table 13.1).

Table 13.1 Summary of the current understanding of the biology that underpins anxiety-related disorders.

Human anxiety disorder	Clinical features	Circuits and neuromodulatory systems	Paradigms/genetic model	Behavioural measurements	Applications for clinical research
PTSD	Following exposure to a traumatic event develop (1) Anxiety (2) Hyper-arousal (3) Avoidance behaviour (4) Negative cognition	Amygdala–hippocampal–prefrontal networks and HPA axis Serotonergic systems	Pavlovian fear conditioning	Freezing and autonomic response to conditional cue/context	Pharmacology and neural circuitry
			Predator exposure model	1. Avoidance behaviour to anxiogenic stimuli (open arm) 2. Startle response to loud noise – hyperarousal 3. Pairing with different partners in the post-trauma period to mimic social instability	Temporal evolution of PTSD like symptoms
OCD	Recurrent and persistent thoughts → repetitive behaviour	Corticostriatal networks Serotonin and dopaminergic systems	(1) 5-HT1A agonist-induced spontaneous alteration	Preservation of indecision	Pharmacology and circuitry
			(2) D2/D3 antagonist quinpirole-induced compulsive checking model	A 'ritual-like' set of motor tasks at specific locations in an open field	Pharmacology and circuitry of behavioural correlates

Table 13.1 (cont.)

Human anxiety disorder	Clinical features	Circuits and neuromodulatory systems	Paradigms/genetic model	Behavioural measurements	Applications for clinical research
			(3) Spontaneous stereotype in deer mice	Repetitive stereotypic behaviours: vertical jumping, backward somersaulting, and patterned running	Circuitry and genetics
			(4) Signal attenuation	Trained to associate tone with lever press for food reward. Compulsive behaviour occurs when tone presented without reward	Pharmacology and circuitry of behavioural correlates
			(5) Marble-burying behaviour in rodents	Natural behaviour in rodents to bury both harmful and inert objects	Circuits for spontaneous repetitive behaviours
Panic disorder	Abrupt rise of intense fear or discomfort that peak within minutes → increased arousal and sympathetic nervous responses like palpitation, sweating, and shaking	Amygdala, hippocampus, prefrontal cortex, periaqueductal grey, and insula. Serotonergic and noradrenergic transmission systems	Pavlovian fear conditioning Elevated Plus maze	Fear-potentiated startle response	Pharmacological and circuitry
GAD	Excessive anxiety or worry	Amygdala and HPA axis Serotonergic systems	(1) Elevated Plus maze	Avoidance of anxiogenic stimuli	Pharmacological interventions for

Disorder	Clinical feature	Neurobiology	Animal model	Behavioural correlate	Research focus
				(open arm) – avoidance behaviour is sensitive to pharmacological agents acting on GABA and corticotrophin receptors	anxious behaviours
			(2) 5-HT1A-knockout mice	Increased anxious behaviour in Elevated Plus maze – amenable to anxiolytic drugs	Genetic and molecular mechanisms for GAD
				Social status and degree of social affiliation	Interaction of intrinsic and environmental factors in the pathogenesis of anxious behaviour
Social phobia	Excessive fear in one or more social situations	Striatal networks Dopaminergic and serotonergic systems	Social submissiveness in non-human primates		

GAD = generalized anxiety disorder; HPA = hypothalamic–pituitary–adrenal; OCD = obsessive–compulsive disorder; PTSD = post-traumatic stress disorder.

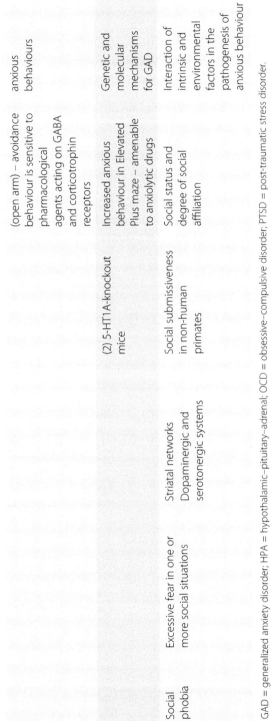

Animal models provide valuable insights into the pathological mechanisms and pathophysiology of many human diseases and disorders. However, it is not currently possible to emulate all of the features of a disease or disorder in an animal model, particularly those with psychological and emotional dimensions. Another core difficulty in developing suitable models for mental disorders lies in the clinical definition used in humans. For example, GAD is defined as excessive worry, which cannot be directly studied in animals. However, it is possible to investigate the neural activity that is associated with these emotional states, providing insight into the biological processes involved in generating emotional responses using a quantifiable physical measure.

As famously stated by evolutionary biologist Theodosius Dobzhansky, 'Nothing in biology makes sense except in the light of evolution'. Fear and anxiety are crucial for the survival of organisms, and their biological substrates and behavioural symptoms have therefore been highly conserved during evolution. They involve densely connected networks between neocortical (prefrontal) and palaeo-cortical structures (amygdala and hippocampus) in the brain – networks that are modulated by projections from evolutionarily older regions in the brainstem. With newer tools, it is possible to dissect specific pathways in animal models, which can be investigated in humans using non-invasive imaging procedures like functional magnetic resonance imaging. Despite their inherent limitations, animal models are essential to understanding the fundamental cellular and molecular mechanisms of fear and anxiety, and they will continue to shed light on new targets for the treatment of anxiety disorders.

Acknowledgements

This work for funded by grants from the National Health and Medical Research Council of Australia (PS) and the Australian Research Council.

References

Abraham, A. D., Neve, K. A. and Lattal, K. M. (2014). Dopamine and extinction: a convergence of theory with fear and reward circuitry. *Neurobiology of Learning and Memory*, **104**, 65–77.

Amano, T., Duvarci, S., Popa, D. and Paré, D. (2011). The fear circuit revisited: contributions of the basal amygdala nuclei to conditioned fear. *Journal of Neuroscience*, **31**, 15481–15489.

Amano, T., Unal, C. T. and Paré, D. (2010). Synaptic correlates of fear extinction in the amygdala. *Nature Neuroscience*, **13**, 489–494.

Ascoli, G. A., Alonso-Nanclares, L., Anderson, S. A., et al. (2008). Petilla terminology: nomenclature of features of GABAergic interneurons of the cerebral cortex. *Nature Reviews Neuroscience*, **9**, 557–568.

Atack, J. R. (2011). GABAA receptor subtype-selective modulators. I. Alpha2/alpha3- selective agonists as non-sedating anxiolytics. *Current Topics in Medical Chemistry*, **11**, 1176–1202.

Azmitia, E. C. and Segal, M. (1978). An autoradiographic analysis of the differential ascending projections of the dorsal and median raphe nuclei in the rat. *Journal of Comparative Neurology*, **179**, 641–667.

Barnard, E. A., Skolnick, P., Olsen, R. W., et al. (1998). International Union of Pharmacology. XV. Subtypes of gamma-aminobutyric acidA receptors: classification on the basis of subunit structure and receptor function. *Pharmacological Reviews*, **50**, 291–313.

Bauer, E. P. (2015). Serotonin in fear conditioning processes. *Behavioural Brain Research*, **277**, 68–77.

Beaulieu, J. M. and Gainetdinov, R. R. (2011). The physiology, signaling, and pharmacology of dopamine receptors. *Pharmacological Reviews*, **63**, 182–217.

Bissiere, S., Humeau, Y. and Luthi, A. (2003). Dopamine gates LTP induction in lateral amygdala by suppressing feedforward inhibition. *Nature Neuroscience*, **6**, 587–592.

Blanchard, D. C. and Blanchard, R. J. (2008). *Handbook of Anxiety and Fear*. Amsterdam: Elsevier.

Blaze, J. and Roth, T. L. (2013). Epigenetic mechanisms in learning and memory. *Wiley Interdisciplinary Reviews. Cognitive Science*, **4**, 105–115.

Burgos-Robles, A., Vidal-Gonzalez, I., Santini, E. and Quirk, G. J. (2007). Consolidation of fear extinction requires NMDA receptor-dependent bursting in the ventromedial prefrontal cortex. *Neuron*, **53**, 871–880.

Campbell, B. M. and Merchant, K. M. (2003). Serotonin 2C receptors within the basolateral amygdala induce acute fear-like responses in an open-field environment. *Brain Research*, **993**, 1–9.

Cassell, M. D., Gray, T. S. and Kiss, J. Z. (1986). Neuronal architecture in the rat central nucleus of the amygdala: a cytological, hodological, and immunocytochemical study. *Journal of Comparative Neurology*, **246**, 478–499.

Ciocchi, S., Herry, C., Grenier, F., et al. (2010). Encoding of conditioned fear in central amygdala inhibitory circuits. *Nature*, **468**, 277–282.

Collingridge, G. L. and Bliss, T. V. P. (1987). NMDA receptors – their role in long-term potentiation. *Trends in Neuroscience*, **10**, 288–293.

Connors, B. W. and Gutnick, M. J. (1990). Intrinsic firing patterns of diverse neocortical neurons. *Trends in Neuroscience*, **13**, 99–103.

Corcoran, K. A. and Quirk, G. J. (2007). Activity in prelimbic cortex is necessary for the expression of learned, but not innate, fears. *Journal of Neuroscience*, **27**, 840–844.

Davis, M. (1979). Diazepam and flurazepam: effects on conditioned fear as measured with the potentiated startle paradigm. *Psychopharmacology (Berlin)*, **62**, 1–7.

Davis, M., Ressler, K., Rothbaum, B. O. and Richardson, R. (2006). Effects of D-cycloserine on extinction: translation from preclinical to clinical work. *Biological Psychiatry*, **60**, 369–375.

Davis, M., Walker, D. L., Miles, L. and Grillon, C. (2010). Phasic vs sustained fear in rats and humans: role of the extended amygdala in fear vs anxiety. *Neuropsychopharmacology*, **35**, 105–135.

de Olmos, J., Hardy, H. and Heimer, L. (1985). Amygdala. In G. Paxinos, ed., *The Rat Nervous System*. Sydney: Academic Press, Australia, pp. 223–334.

De Souza Caetano, K. A., De Oliveira, A. R. and Brandao, M. L. (2013). Dopamine D2 receptors modulate the expression of contextual conditioned fear: role of the ventral tegmental area and the basolateral amygdala. *Behavioural Pharmacology*, **24**, 264–274.

Delaney, A. J. and Sah, P. (1999). GABA receptors inhibited by benzodiazepines mediate fast inhibitory transmission in the central amygdala. *Journal of Neuroscience*, **19**, 9698–9704.

Delaney, A. J. and Sah, P. (2001). Pathway-specific targeting of GABA(A) receptor subtypes to somatic and dendritic synapses in the central amygdala. *Journal of Neurophysiology*, **86**, 717–723.

Delaney, A. J., Sedlak, P. L., Autuori, E., Power, J. M. and Sah, P. (2013). Synaptic NMDA receptors in basolateral amygdala principal neurons are triheteromeric proteins: physiological role of GluN2B subunits. *Journal of Neurophysiology*, **109**, 1391–1402.

Delgado, M. R., Nearing, K. I., Ledoux, J. E. and Phelps, E. A. (2008). Neural circuitry underlying the regulation of conditioned fear and its relation to extinction. *Neuron*, **59**, 829–838.

Dumont, E. C., Martina, M., Samson, R. D., Drolet, G. and Paré, D. (2002). Physiological properties of central amygdala neurons: species differences. *European Journal of Neuroscience*, **15**, 544–552.

Ehrlich, I., Humeau, Y., Grenier, F., Ciocchi, S., Herry, C. and Luthi, A. (2009). Amygdala inhibitory circuits and the control of fear memory. *Neuron*, **62**, 757–771.

Esmaeili, A., Lynch, J. W. and Sah, P. (2009). GABA$_A$ receptors containing gamma1 subunits contribute to inhibitory transmission in the central amygdala. *Journal of Neurophysiology*, **101**, 341–349.

Faber, E. S. L., Callister, R. J. and Sah, P. (2001). Morphological and electrophysiological properties of principal neurons in the rat lateral amygdala *in vitro*. *Journal of Neurophysiology*, **85**, 714–723.

Falls, W. A., Miserendino, M. J. and Davis, M. (1992). Extinction of fear-potentiated startle: blockade by infusion of an NMDA antagonist into the amygdala. *Journal of Neuroscience*, **12**, 854–863.

Fanselow, M. S. and Dong, H. W. (2010). Are the dorsal and ventral hippocampus functionally distinct structures? *Neuron*, **65**, 7–19.

Farb, C. R. and Ledoux, J. E. (1999). Afferents from rat temporal cortex synapse on lateral amygdala neurons that express NMDA and AMPA receptors. *Synapse*, **33**, 218–229.

Farb, D. H. and Ratner, M. H. (2014). Targeting the modulation of neural circuitry for the treatment of anxiety disorders. *Pharmacological Reviews*, **66**, 1002–1032.

Gibson, E. L., Barnfield, A. M. and Curzon, G. (1994). Evidence that mCPP-induced anxiety in the plus-maze is mediated by postsynaptic 5-HT2C receptors but not by sympathomimetic effects. *Neuropharmacology*, **33**, 457–465.

Goosens, K. A. and Maren, S. (2004). NMDA receptors are essential for the acquisition, but not expression, of conditional fear and associative spike firing in the lateral amygdala. *European Journal of Neuroscience*, **20**, 537–548.

Goosens, K. A., Hobin, J. A. and Maren, S. (2003). Auditory-evoked spike firing in the lateral amygdala and Pavlovian fear conditioning: mnemonic code or fear bias? *Neuron*, **40**, 1013–1022.

Gray, J. A. and McNaughton, N. 2000. *The Neuropsychology of Anxiety*. Oxford: Oxford University Press.

Greba, Q. and Kokkinidis, L. (2000). Peripheral and intraamygdalar administration of the dopamine D1 receptor antagonist SCH 23390 blocks fear-potentiated startle but not shock reactivity or the shock sensitization of acoustic startle. *Behavioral Neuroscience*, **114**, 262–272.

Guastella, A. J., Lovibond, P. F., Dadds, M. R., Mitchell, P. and Richardson, R. (2007). A randomized controlled trial of the effect of D-cycloserine on extinction and fear conditioning in humans. *Behaviour Research and Therapy*, **45**, 663–672.

Harris, J. A. and Westbrook, R. F. (1998). Evidence that GABA transmission mediates context-specific extinction of learned fear. *Psychopharmacology (Berlin)*, **140**, 105–115.

Haubensak, W., Kunwar, P. S., Cai, H., et al. (2010). Genetic dissection of an amygdala microcircuit that gates conditioned fear. *Nature*, **468**, 270–276.

Heidbreder, C. A. and Groenewegen, H. J. (2003). The medial prefrontal cortex in the rat: evidence for a dorso-ventral distinction based upon functional and anatomical characteristics. *Neuroscience and Biobehavioral Reviews*, **27**, 555–579.

Held, J. R. (1983). Appropriate animal models. *Annals of the New York Academy of Sciences*, **406**, 13–19.

Herry, C., Ciocchi, S., Senn, V., Demmou, L., Muller, C. and Luthi, A. (2008). Switching on and off fear by distinct neuronal circuits. *Nature*, **454**, 600–606.

Hestrin, S., Nicoll, R. A., Perkel, D. J. and Sah, P. (1990). Analysis of excitatory synaptic action in pyramidal cells using whole-cell recording from rat hippocampal slices. *Journal of Physiology*, **422**, 203–225.

Hitchcock, J. and Davis, M. (1986). Lesions of the amygdala, but not of the cerebellum or red nucleus, block conditioned fear as measured with the potentiated startle paradigm. *Behavioral Neuroscience*, **100**, 11–22.

Humeau, Y., Shaban, H., Bissiere, S. and Luthi, A. (2003). Presynaptic induction of heterosynaptic associative plasticity in the mammalian brain. *Nature*, **426**, 841–845.

Inoue, T., Izumi, T., Maki, Y., Muraki, I. and Koyama, T. (2000). Effect of the dopamine D (1/5) antagonist SCH 23390 on the acquisition of conditioned fear. *Pharmacology, Biochemistry, and Behavior*, **66**, 573–578.

Jasnow, A. M., Ressler, K. J., Hammack, S. E., Chhatwal, J. P. and Rainnie, D. G. (2009). Distinct subtypes of cholecystokinin (CCK)-containing interneurons of the basolateral amygdala identified using a CCK promoter-specific lentivirus. *Journal of Neurophysiology*, **101**, 1494–1506.

Jennings, J. H., Sparta, D. R., Stamatakis, A. M., et al. (2013). Distinct extended amygdala circuits for divergent motivational states. *Nature*, **496**, 224–228.

Kawahara, H., Yoshida, M., Yokoo, H., Nishi, M. and Tanaka, M. (1993). Psychological stress increases serotonin release in the rat amygdala and prefrontal cortex assessed by *in vivo* microdialysis. *Neuroscience Letters*, **162**, 81–84.

Kim, M., Campeau, S., Falls, W. A. and Davis, M. (1993). Infusion of the non-NMDA receptor antagonist CNQX into the amygdala blocks the expression of fear-potentiated startle. *Behavioral and Neural Biology*, **59**, 5–8.

Labar, K. S., Gatenby, J. C., Gore, J. C., Ledoux, J. E. and Phelps, E. A. (1998). Human amygdala activation during conditioned fear acquisition and extinction: a mixed- trial fMRI study. *Neuron*, **20**, 937–945.

Lacivita, E., Leopoldo, M., Berardi, F. and Perrone, R. (2008). 5-HT1A receptor, an old target for new therapeutic agents. *Current Topics in Medical Chemistry*, **8**, 1024–1034.

Lanuza, E., Moncho-Bogani, J. and Ledoux, J. E. (2008). Unconditioned stimulus pathways to the amygdala: effects of lesions of the posterior intralaminar thalamus on foot-shock-induced c-Fos expression in the subdivisions of the lateral amygdala. *Neuroscience*, **155**, 959–968.

Laurent, V. and Westbrook, R. F. (2008). Distinct contributions of the basolateral amygdala and the medial prefrontal cortex to learning and relearning extinction of context

conditioned fear. *Learning & Memory*, **15**, 657–666.

Laurent, V. and Westbrook, R. F. (2009). Inactivation of the infralimbic but not the prelimbic cortex impairs consolidation and retrieval of fear extinction. *Learning & Memory*, **16**, 520–529.

Laurie, D. J., Wisden, W. and Seeburg, P. H. (1992). The distribution of thirteen GABA$_A$ receptor subunit mRNAs in the rat brain. III. Embryonic and postnatal development. *Journal of Neuroscience*, **12**, 4151–4172.

Ledgerwood, L., Richardson, R. and Cranney, J. (2003). Effects of D-cycloserine on extinction of conditioned freezing. *Behavioral Neuroscience*, **117**, 341–349.

Ledoux, J. E., Cicchetti, P., Xagoraris, A. and Romanski, L. M. (1990). The lateral amygdaloid nucleus: sensory interface of the amygdala in fear conditioning. *Journal of Neuroscience*, **10**, 1062–1069.

Lesch, K. P., Bengel, D., Heils, A., et al. (1996). Association of anxiety-related traits with a polymorphism in the serotonin transporter gene regulatory region. *Science*, **274**, 1527–1531.

Lopez de Armentia, M. and Sah, P. (2003). Development and subunit composition of synaptic NMDA receptors in the amygdala: NR2B synapses in the adult central amygdala. *Journal of Neuroscience*, **23**, 6876–6883.

Lopez de Armentia, M. and Sah, P. (2004). Firing properties and connectivity of neurons in the rat lateral central nucleus of the amygdala. *Journal of Neurophysiology*, **92**, 1285–1294.

Lubin, F. D., Gupta, S., Parrish, R. R., Grissom, N. M. and Davis, R. L. (2011). Epigenetic mechanisms: critical contributors to long-term memory formation. *Neuroscientist*, **17**, 616–632.

Mahanty, N. K. and Sah, P. (1998). Calcium-permeable AMPA receptors mediate long-term potentiation in interneurons in the amygdala. *Nature*, **394**, 683–687.

Mahanty, N. K. and Sah, P. (1999). Excitatory synaptic inputs to pyramidal neurons of the lateral amygdala. *European Journal of Neuroscience*, 11, 1217–1222.

Mamiya, N., Fukushima, H., Suzuki, A., et al. (2009). Brain region-specific gene expression activation required for reconsolidation and extinction of contextual fear memory. *Journal of Neuroscience*, 29, 402–413.

Marek, R., Coelho, C. M., Sullivan, R. K., et al. (2011). Paradoxical enhancement of fear extinction memory and synaptic plasticity by inhibition of the histone acetyltransferase p300. *Journal of Neuroscience*, 31, 7486–91.

Maren, S. (2001). Neurobiology of Pavlovian fear conditioning. *Annual Review of Neuroscience*, 24, 897–931.

Maren, S. and Quirk, G. J. (2004). Neuronal signalling of fear memory. *Nature Reviews Neuroscience*, 5, 844–852.

Markram, H., Toledo-Rodriguez, M., Wang, Y., Gupta, A., Silberberg, G. and Wu, C. (2004). Interneurons of the neocortical inhibitory system. *Nature Reviews Neuroscience*, 5, 793–807.

Martina, M., Royer, S. and Paré, D. (1999). Physiological properties of central medial and central lateral amygdala neurons. *Journal of Neurophysiology*, 82, 1843–1854.

Mayford, M., Siegelbaum, S. A. and Kandel, E. R. (2012). Synapses and memory storage. *Cold Spring Harbor Perspectives in Biology*, 4, a005751.

McDonald, A. J. (1982). Neurons of the lateral and basolateral amygdaloid nuclei: a Golgi study in the rat. *Journal of Comparative Neurology*, 212, 293–312.

McDonald, A. J. (1992). Cell types and intrinsic connections of the amygdala. In J. P. Aggleton, ed., *The Amygdala: Neurobiological Aspects of Emotion, Memory and Mental Dysfunction*. New York: Wiley-Liss, pp. 67–96.

McDonald, A. J. (1998). Cortical pathways to the mammalian amygdala. *Progress in Brain Research*, 55, 257–332.

McDonald, A. J. and Mascagni, F. (2001). Colocalization of calcium-binding proteins and GABA in neurons of the rat basolateral amygdala. *Neuroscience*, 105, 681–693.

McKiernan, M. G. and Shinnick-Gallagher, P. (1997). Fear conditioning induces a lasting potentiation of synaptic currents *in vitro*. *Nature*, 390, 607–611.

McKernan, R. M., Rosahl, T. W., Reynolds, D. S., et al. (2000). Sedative but not anxiolytic properties of benzodiazepines are mediated by the GABA(A) receptor alpha1 subtype. *Nature Neuroscience*, 3, 587–592.

McNally, R. J. (2007). Mechanisms of exposure therapy: how neuroscience can improve psychological treatments for anxiety disorders. *Clinical Psychology Review*, 27, 750–759.

McQuade, R. and Sharp, T. (1997). Functional mapping of dorsal and median raphe 5-hydroxytryptamine pathways in forebrain of the rat using microdialysis. *Journal of Neurochemistry*, 69, 791–796.

Milad, M. R. and Quirk, G. J. (2002). Neurons in medial prefrontal cortex signal memory for fear extinction. *Nature*, 420, 70–74.

Miller, K. D., Pinto, D. J. and Simons, D. J. (2001). Processing in layer 4 of the neocortical circuit: new insights from visual and somatosensory cortex. *Current Opinion in Neurobiology*, 11, 488–97.

Millhouse, O. E. (1986). The intercalated cells of the amygdala. *Journal of Comparative Neurology*, 247, 246–271.

Milner, B., Squire, L. R. and Kandel, E. R. (1998). Cognitive neuroscience and the study of memory. *Neuron*, 20, 445–468.

Miserendino, M. J. D., Sananes, C. B., Melia, K. R. and Davis, M. (1990). Blocking of acquisition but not expression of conditioned fear-potentiated startle by NMDA antagonists in the amygdala. *Nature*, 345, 716–718.

Mohler, H. (2006). GABA(A) receptor diversity and pharmacology. *Cell Tissue Research*, 326, 505–516.

Morris, J. S., Frith, C. D., Perrett, D. I., et al. (1996). A differential neural response in the human amygdala to fearful and happy facial expressions. *Nature*, 383, 812–815.

Moser, M. B. and Moser, E. I. (1998). Functional differentiation in the hippocampus. *Hippocampus*, 8, 608–619.

Mueller, D., Bravo-Rivera, C. and Quirk, G. J. (2010). Infralimbic D2 receptors are necessary for fear extinction and extinction-related tone responses. *Biological Psychiatry*, **68**, 1055–1060.

Nestler, E. J., Hyman, S. E. and Malenka, R. (2015). *Molecular Nuropharmacology: A Foundation for Clinical Neuroscience*, 3rd ed. New York: McGraw-Hill.

Nestler, E. J., Walaas, S. I. and Greengard, P. (1984). Neuronal phosphoproteins: physiological and clinical implications. *Science*, **225**, 1359–1364.

Niehoff, D. L. and Kuhar, M. J. (1983). Benzodiazepine receptors: localization in rat amygdala. *Journal of Neuroscience*, **3**, 2091–2097.

Olsen, R. W. and Tobin, A. J. (1990). Molecular biology of GABA$_A$ receptors. *FASEB Journal*, **4**, 1469–1480.

Palomares-Castillo, E., Hernandez-Perez, O. R., Perez-Carrera, D., Crespo-Ramirez, M., Fuxe, K. and Perez De La Mora, M. (2012). The intercalated paracapsular islands as a module for integration of signals regulating anxiety in the amygdala. *Brain Research*, **1476**, 211–34.

Pape, H. C. and Paré, D. (2010). Plastic synaptic networks of the amygdala for the acquisition, expression, and extinction of conditioned fear. *Physiological Reviews*, **90**, 419–463.

Paré, D. and Duvarci, S. (2012). Amygdala microcircuits mediating fear expression and extinction. *Current Opinion in Neurobiology*, **22**, 717–723.

Paré, D. and Smith, Y. (1993). The intercalated cell masses project to the central and medial nuclei of the amygdala in cats. *Neuroscience*, **57**, 1077–1090.

Pavlov, I. P. (1927). *Conditioned Reflexes*, New York: Dover.

Pesold, C. and Treit, D. (1994). The septum and amygdala differentially mediate the anxiolytic effects of benzodiazepines. *Brain Research*, **638**, 295–301.

Pinard, C. R., Mascagni, F. and McDonald, A. J. (2012). Medial prefrontal cortical innervation of the intercalated nuclear region of the amygdala. *Neuroscience*, **205**, 112–124.

Polepalli, J. S., Sullivan, R. K., Yanagawa, Y. and Sah, P. (2010). A specific class of interneuron

mediates inhibitory plasticity in the lateral amygdala. *Journal of Neuroscience*, **30**, 14619–14629.

Power, J. M. and Sah, P. (2008). Competition between calcium-activated K$^+$ channels determines cholinergic action on firing properties of basolateral amygdala projection neurons. *Journal of Neuroscience*, **28**, 3209–3220.

Price, J. L., Russchen, F. T. and Amaral, D. G. (1987). *The Limbic Region. II: The Amygdaloid Complex*. Amsterdam: Elsevier Science.

Quirk, G. J. and Mueller, D. (2008). Neural mechanisms of extinction learning and retrieval. *Neuropsychopharmacology*, **33**, 56–72.

Quirk, G. J., Repa, C. and Ledoux, J. E. (1995). Fear conditioning enhances short-latency auditory responses of lateral amygdaloid neurons: parallel recordings in the freely behaving rat. *Neuron*, **15**, 1029–1039.

Rainnie, D. G., Asprodini, E. K. and Schinnick-Gallagher, P. (1991). Inhibitory transmission in the basolateral amygdala. *Journal of Neurophysiology*, **66**, 999–1009.

Reinhold, J. A. (2015). Pharmacological treatment for generalized anxiety disorder in adults: an update. *Expert Opinion on Pharmacotherapy*, **16**, 1669–1681.

Ressler, K. J., Rothbaum, B. O., Tannenbaum, L., et al. (2004). Cognitive enhancers as adjuncts to psychotherapy: use of D-cycloserine in phobic individuals to facilitate extinction of fear. *Archives of General Psychiatry*, **61**, 1136–1144.

Richards, J. G. and Möhler, H. (1984). Benzodiazepine receptors. *Neuropharmacology*, **23**, 233–242.

Rodrigues, S. M., Schafe, G. E. and Ledoux, J. E. (2004). Molecular mechanisms underlying emotional learning and memory in the lateral amygdala. *Neuron*, **44**, 75–91.

Rogan, M. T., Staubli, U. V. and Ledoux, J. E. (1997). Fear conditioning induces associative long-term potentiation in the amygdala. *Nature*, **390**, 604–607.

Royer, S. and Paré, D. (2002). Bidirectional synaptic plasticity in intercalated amygdala neurons and the extinction of conditioned fear responses. *Neuroscience*, **115**, 455–462.

Royer, S., Martina, M. and Paré, D. (1999). An inhibitory interface gates impulse traffic between the input and output stations of the amygdala. *Journal of Neuroscience*, **19**, 10575–10583.

Rudolph, U. and Mohler, H. (2006). GABA-based therapeutic approaches: GABA$_A$ receptor subtype functions. *Current Opinion in Pharmacology*, **6**, 18–23.

Rumpel, S., Ledoux, J., Zador, A. and Malinow, R. (2005). Postsynaptic receptor trafficking underlying a form of associative learning. *Science*, **308**, 83–88.

Sah, P., Faber, E. S., Lopez de Armentia, M. and Power, J. (2003). The amygdaloid complex: anatomy and physiology. *Physiological Reviews*, **83**, 803–834.

Sah, P., Westbrook, R. F. and Luthi, A. (2008). Fear conditioning and long-term potentiation in the amygdala: what really is the connection? *Annals of the New York Academy of Science*, **1129**, 88–95.

Santini, E., Ge, H., Ren, K., Pena De Ortiz, S. and Quirk, G. J. (2004). Consolidation of fear extinction requires protein synthesis in the medial prefrontal cortex. *Journal of Neuroscience*, **24**, 5704–5710.

Sieghart, W. and Sperk, G. (2002). Subunit composition, distribution and function of GABA(A) receptor subtypes. *Current Topics in Medical Chemistry*, **2**, 795–816.

Slotnick, B. M. (1973). Fear behavior and passive avoidance deficits in mice with amygdala lesions. *Physiology & Behavior*, **11**, 717–720.

Smith, Y., Paré, J. F. and Paré, D. (1998). Cat intraamygdaloid inhibitory network: ultrastructural organization of parvalbumin-immunoreactive elements. *Journal of Comparative Neurology*, **391**, 164–179.

Smith, Y., Paré, J. F. and Paré, D. (2000). Differential innervation of parvalbumin-immunoreactive interneurons of the basolateral amygdaloid complex by cortical and intrinsic inputs. *Journal of Comparative Neurology*, **416**, 496–508.

Sotres-Bayon, F. and Quirk, G. J. (2010). Prefrontal control of fear: more than just extinction. *Current Opinion in Neurobiology*, **20**, 231–235.

Sotres-Bayon, F., Sierra-Mercado, D., Pardilla-Delgado, E. and Quirk, G. J. (2012). Gating of fear in prelimbic cortex by hippocampal and amygdala inputs. *Neuron*, **76**, 804–812.

Spampanato, J., Polepalli, J. and Sah, P. (2011). Interneurons in the basolateral amygdala. *Neuropharmacology*, **60**, 765–773.

Starcevic, V. (2014). The reappraisal of benzodiazepines in the treatment of anxiety and related disorders. *Expert Review of Neurotherapeutics*, **14**, 1275–1286.

Strobel, C., Marek, R. H. G., Sullivan, R. and Sah, P. (2015). Prefrontal and auditory input to intercalated neurons of the amygdala. *Cell Reports*, **10**, 1435–1442.

Tang, H. H., McNally, G. P. and Richardson, R. (2007). The effects of FG7142 on two types of forgetting in 18-day-old rats. *Behavioral Neuroscience*, **121**, 1421–1425.

Tovote, P., Fadok, J. P. and Luthi, A. (2015). Neuronal circuits for fear and anxiety. *Nature Reviews Neuroscience*, **16**, 317–331.

Tully, K. and Bolshakov, V. Y. (2010). Emotional enhancement of memory: how norepinephrine enables synaptic plasticity. *Molecular Brain*, **3**, 15.

Van De Werd, H. J., Rajkowska, G., Evers, P. and Uylings, H. B. (2010). Cytoarchitectonic and chemoarchitectonic characterization of the prefrontal cortical areas in the mouse. *Brain Structure & Function*, **214**, 339–353.

Vertes, R. P. (1991). A PHA-L analysis of ascending projections of the dorsal raphe nucleus in the rat. *Journal of Comparative Neurology*, **313**, 643–668.

Vidal-Gonzalez, I., Vidal-Gonzalez, B., Rauch, S. L. and Quirk, G. J. (2006). Microstimulation reveals opposing influences of prelimbic and infralimbic cortex on the expression of conditioned fear. *Learning & Memory*, **13**, 728–733.

Viviani, D., Charlet, A., Van Den Burg, E., et al. (2011). Oxytocin selectively gates fear responses through distinct outputs from the central amygdala. *Science*, **333**, 104–107.

Wang, Y., Markram, H., Goodman, P. H., Berger, T. K., Ma, J. and Goldman-Rakic, P. S. (2006). Heterogeneity in the pyramidal network of the medial prefrontal cortex. *Nature Neuroscience*, **9**, 534–542.

Washburn, M. S. and Moises, H. C. (1992). Electrophysiological and morphological properties of rat basolateral amygdaloid neurons *in vitro*. *Journal of Neuroscience*, **12**, 4066–4079.

Wei, W., Coelho, C. M., Li, X., et al. (2012). p300/CBP-associated factor selectively regulates the extinction of conditioned fear. *Journal of Neuroscience*, **32**, 11930–11941.

Weisskopf, M. G. and Ledoux, J. E. (1999). Distinct populations of NMDA receptors at subcortical and cortical inputs to principal cells of the lateral amygdala. *Journal of Neurophysiology*, **81**, 930–934.

Weisskopf, M. G., Bauer, E. P. and Ledoux, J. E. (1999). L-type voltage-gated calcium channels mediate NMDA-independent associative long-term potentiation at thalamic input synapses to the amygdala. *Journal of Neuroscience*, **19**, 10512–10519.

Weisstaub, N. V., Zhou, M., Lira, A., et al. (2006). Cortical 5-HT2A receptor signaling modulates anxiety-like behaviors in mice. *Science*, **313**, 536–540.

Woodruff, A. R. and Sah, P. (2007a). Inhibition and synchronization of basal amygdala principal neuron spiking by parvalbumin-positive interneurons. *Journal of Neurophysiology*, **98**, 2956–2961.

Woodruff, A. R. and Sah, P. (2007b). Networks of parvalbumin-positive interneurons in the basolateral amygdala. *Journal of Neuroscience*, **27**, 553–563.

Woodruff, A. R., Monyer, H. and Sah, P. (2006). GABAergic excitation in the basolateral amygdala. *Journal of Neuroscience*, **26**, 11881–11887.

Yokoyama, M., Suzuki, E., Sato, T., Maruta, S., Watanabe, S. and Miyaoka, H. (2005). Amygdalic levels of dopamine and serotonin rise upon exposure to conditioned fear stress without elevation of glutamate. *Neuroscience Letters*, **379**, 37–41.

Zhang, G., Asgeirsdottir, H. N., Cohen, S. J., Munchow, A. H., Barrera, M. P. and Stackman, R. W., Jr. (2013). Stimulation of serotonin 2A receptors facilitates consolidation and extinction of fear memory in C57BL/6J mice. *Neuropharmacology*, **64**, 403–413.

Chapter

14

Late-Life Anxiety
Where to from Here?

Nancy A. Pachana and Gerard J. Byrne

The literature on late-life anxiety has grown exponentially in the last two decades, and a wide array of research questions are being explored by an ever-growing cadre of clinicians and scientists internationally. In fact, in the last decade, there have been several special journal issues devoted to aspects of anxiety in later life – for example, *American Journal of Geriatric Psychiatry* (2011, vol. 19, issue 4), *Journal of Anxiety Disorders* (2013, vol. 27, issue 6), *International Psychogeriatrics* (2015, vol. 27, issue 7), and *Clinical Gerontologist* (2017, vol. 40, issue 3). All have made the point that while our understanding of the etiology, diagnosis, assessment, and treatment of such disorders has grown and continues to increase, there are still many areas requiring further research attention. In addition, experimental techniques to study the biological mechanisms underpinning anxiety continue to grow in sophistication and access. The recent neurocircuitry-based taxonomy of mental disorders, the Research Domain Criteria (RDoC) initiative, may positively influence future research on late-life anxiety (Lenze & Butters, 2016). Measures of physiological, diagnostic, and self-reported symptoms of anxiety specifically as manifested in later life continue to be developed and improved. Increasing numbers of clinical trials of pharmacological and nonpharmacological approaches to the treatment of anxiety, as well as combination therapies, have been published. The costs, in terms of health care systems, economic expenditure, and burden and quality of life, increasingly include or focus on late-life anxiety.

What will the coming decade hold for this important area in geriatric mental health? From which quarters might new advances arise? What questions should further research target? How might diagnosis, assessment, and treatment of anxiety disorders in later life be further tailored and made more precise and effective? This chapter aims to give a brief overview of the topics, issues, and methodologies that we feel demand further inquiry or that offer promise for contributing to our understanding of and interventions for late-life anxiety.

Etiologies: Genetics and Neurophysiology

Genetic studies have found that 30–40% of the variance contributing to the risk of anxiety disorder is heritable (Norrholm & Ressler, 2009), and various specific anxiety disorders have been shown to have similar heritability (Hettema et al., 2005). What is less clear is how the contributions of environmental and genetic factors shift across the lifespan. This question has begun to be tackled. Lee et al. (2016) examined genetic and environmental contributions over time to state anxiety in adults aged 50+ in the Swedish Adoption/Twin Study of Aging. Increasing heterogeneity in later life was reflected in the fact that there was considerable individual variation in the age trajectory of anxiety in this cohort. In individuals in their late 60s, non-shared environmental variance reached its peak and then declined, whereas from age 60 onwards, genetic variance increased at an accelerated pace. There was no evidence in this study for effects of shared environment on late-life anxiety symptoms.

Several longitudinal studies have illuminated factors in early life that may contribute to anxiety later in life, such as childhood physical abuse (Almeida et al., 2012), poverty, parental loss or separation, and low affective support (Zhang et al., 2015). Increasing evidence from epigenetics suggests that sexual and physical abuse may be nonspecific risk factors associated with a broad range of lasting effects on neurophysiology (Kelly-Irving et al., 2013); this remains to be further explored in older populations.

Late-life risk factors for anxiety disorders include female gender, history of depression and/or anxiety, adverse life events, and chronic physical and mental health issues (Chou et al., 2011; Schoevers et al., 2005; Zhang et al., 2015). Protective factors that are amenable to change represent a fertile area for further exploration with regard to late-life anxiety.

Currently, there is little empirical research on the neural circuitry involved in late-life anxiety (Mohlman & Bryant, 2016). However, the extant literature implicates decreased activity in the prefrontal cortex (PFC) in older anxious individuals. The PFC is a component of the response system to emotional cues in the environment, one that experiences declines with increasing age (Andreescu et al., 2011). Recent neuroanatomical studies have demonstrated that anxiety symptoms in community-dwelling cognitively normal individuals were associated with reduced cortical thickness in several areas, an effect that was found to disappear for the most part when adjustments for comorbid depressive symptoms were made (Pink et al., 2017). Indeed, neuropathological and neuroimaging findings from studies of late-life depression continue to outstrip those found for anxiety. Gains in the anxiety literature are appearing, with Andreescu and colleagues (2015) documenting for the first time neural changes following pharmacotherapy in late-life generalized anxiety disorder (GAD), which included greater connectivity between the dorsolateral PFC (dlPFC) and several prefrontal regions.

Perhaps as a signal of the need to think outside the box in terms of the framing of studies of the neural circuitry of late-life anxiety, Kreifelts and colleagues (2017) examined cerebral mediators of social anxiety using functional magnetic resonance imaging, with laughter as a social threat. Their results revealed a central role for the left dlPFC and, in turn, a potential target for future intervention research – and potentially a new line of research in older individuals.

Anxiety as a Symptom or Risk Factor for Neurological Diseases

Psychiatric symptoms may indicate the presence of a variety of disease states, including coronary, endocrine, and neurological disorders, across age ranges, but neurological conditions in particular may feature anxiety as a preclinical symptom or risk factor in later life. Depression has for many years been considered an important differential diagnosis to consider in older persons with cognitive declines and suspected dementia or mild cognitive impairment (MCI) (Collie & Maruff, 2000). A first onset of major depression in later life may also be an early sign of incipient dementia (Boyle et al., 2010). There has been a recent increase in the reporting of anxiety as an important symptom in the early stages of MCI, dementia, and Parkinson's disease (PD). While less is known about anxiety than depression in these disorders, the last decade has seen an increase in research in this area.

Anxiety appears to increase the risk of persons with cognitive difficulties going on to develop dementia. Palmer and colleagues (2007) found that persons with both MCI and anxiety symptoms developed dementia due to Alzheimer's disease (AD) at a much higher rate (83.3%) over time than those with MCI without anxiety (40.9%) and cognitively intact persons (6.1%). Among those with MCI in this study, the 3-year risk of progressing to AD dementia almost doubled with each anxiety symptom reported (relative risk (RR) = 1.8 (95% confidence interval (CI) = 1.2–2.7) per symptom); these results held even after adjusting for baseline cognitive status. However, depression (but not anxiety) predicted later development of dementia in cognitively intact subjects. The authors suggested that these findings demonstrated that anxiety symptoms in MCI may be a response to memory changes, whereas depressive symptoms may be a preclinical sign of AD. However, more recent evidence points more strongly to potential neuropathological pathways linking anxiety and dementia (Lyketsos et al., 2011). In addition, there is evidence of neuropathological ties between dementia and anxiety that include pathological levels of total tau (Visser et al., 2009) and amyloid-β (Pietrzak et al., 2015) in those with significant anxiety who are more likely to progress to dementia.

Anxiety in the presence of cognitive decline as a risk factor for progression to dementia has been demonstrated in large longitudinal studies such as the Cache County Study (Peters et al., 2013). In a recent systematic review and meta-analysis of anxiety as a predictor of cognitive decline and dementia, anxiety was associated with increased risk for cognitive impairment and dementia, with stronger associations for those of a greater age (Gulpers et al., 2016). A similar systematic review and meta-analysis that included both English and Chinese databases also reported that anxiety increases the risk of progression to dementia in people with MCI (Li & Li, 2018). Interestingly, in a study of women over 85 years of age, anxiety predicted progression to dementia but not MCI (Kassem et al., 2018).

Mirza and colleagues (2017) found MCI to increase risk for developing depressive (odds ratio (OR) = 3.13 (95% CI = 1.26–7.77)) and anxiety disorders (OR 2.59 (95% CI = 1.31–5.12)). This research again raises the possibility of common pathological pathways for such psychiatric and cognitive disorders. In the large Swedish Adoption/ Twin Study of Aging, analysis of the temporal order of changes in anxiety and cognition over a 26-year period revealed a complex and bidirectional association, with greater variability for most cognitive performance variables over age compared to anxiety symptoms (Petkus et al., 2017).

Such lines of research are important, as there is the potential that treating psychiatric disorders such as anxiety may delay or prevent the onset of MCI or dementia (Lyketsos et al., 2011). Understanding the causal relationships between anxiety and cognitive functioning in later life has only recently been attempted, but increasing longitudinal data sets, including adults in the latest stages of aging, should continue to shed light on these issues. Further analysis of specific symptoms of anxiety (e.g., agitation), as well as threshold and particularly subthreshold anxiety disorders (as suggested by Tales and Basoudan in their 2016 review of anxiety and cognitive decline and dementia), as risk factors for dementia are also required.

Among older adults with neurological conditions such as PD, anxiety is highly prevalent, while diagnosis of anxiety in these populations is challenging due to considerable overlap of symptoms (Miloyan et al., 2014). Yet the rates of anxiety in PD are impressive: current prevalence of anxiety disorders in PD ranges from 25% to 49%, (Dissanayaka et al., 2010; Leentjens et al., 2011). A recent study showed a potential link between post-traumatic stress disorder (PTSD) and subsequent development of PD (Chan et al., 2017).

Unfortunately, a large proportion of PD patients with anxiety remain undiagnosed and undertreated (Chen & Marsh, 2014). PD-related motor and non-motor symptoms may contribute to anxiety in this group, and understanding these mechanisms (e.g., increased social anxiety due to tremor or risk of falling) may enable more effective diagnosis and treatment. In order to better characterize such PD-specific anxiety symptoms, Dissanayaka and colleagues (2016b) surveyed 90 non-demented PD patients (mean age 67) who were assessed for the presence of 30 PD-related anxiety symptoms derived from the literature, the clinical experience of an expert panel, and the PD Anxiety–Motor Complications Questionnaire (PDAMCQ). PD-specific anxiety symptoms endorsed by more than 25% of the sample included distress, worry, fear, agitation, embarrassment, and social withdrawal due to motor symptoms and PD medication complications. These symptoms were also experienced more commonly in patients meeting Diagnostic and Statistical Manual of Mental Disorders, 4th Edition (DSM-IV) criteria for an anxiety disorder. Such disease-specific inquiries into the precise nature of anxiety experienced as a result of physical or neurological conditions allows for more tailored treatments, including addressing symptoms (such as social withdrawal) that might otherwise be ascribed to age.

Measurement of Anxiety Disorders and Symptomatology

The continued lack of agreement on the incidence and prevalence of anxiety disorders in later life highlights the need for more research in large population cohorts, but also renewed efforts to categorize exactly how anxiety symptoms present at various ages and in a range of health, social, and cultural contexts. Detection of anxiety, whether in the clinical context or in large epidemiological surveys, is made more difficult in later life for a host of reasons, including varying criteria based on the ICD or DSM systems, heterogeneity in expression of anxiety between older individuals, the tendency for both family and health professionals to normalize expressions of anxiety in older individuals, and the need for the development and refinement of age-appropriate measurement tools, particularly for challenging contexts such as residential aged care (Byrne & Pachana, 2010; Mohlman & Bryant, 2016).

Cross-national and comparative studies of anxiety prevalence, incidence, and expression in a variety of cultures and countries is also beginning to bear fruit. An ambitious systematic review and meta-regression of 87 studies across 44 countries found a global prevalence of anxiety disorders at 7.3%; interestingly, this was higher (10.4%) among developed (i.e., Anglo/European) as opposed to developing (i.e., African) countries (5.3%) (Baxter et al., 2013). International use of common inventories to measure late-life anxiety, such as the Geriatric Anxiety Inventory (GAI; Pachana et al., 2007) and the Geriatric Anxiety Scale (GAS; Segal et al., 2010), has enabled more cross-national comparable research on the incidence and prevalence of anxiety disorders, as well as intervention outcome studies. Examinations of the criterion-related validity and discriminant validity of translations of instruments such as the GAS outside the language and country of development, especially as other mood and anxiety assessment tools are developed within specific countries, will be important (Bolghan-Abadi et al., 2013).

Culturally specific responses to such inventories is also worth noting, as when Massena and colleagues (2015) reported on a validation of the GAI (Brazilian Portuguese version), with a higher cut point of 13 (estimated by receiver operating characteristic (ROC) analyses) for their sample than the optimal cut point of 10 (also estimated by ROC analyses) in the original (Australian) development study (Pachana et al., 2007). Massena and colleagues (2015) hypothesized that cultural characteristics, such as a greater 'permissiveness' for anxiety complaints in Brazilian society, may have contributed to this elevated cut point. Further studies to elucidate the culturally specific characteristics of the reporting of anxiety symptoms are needed. However, great care needs to be taken in the adaptation of such screening instruments for use in specific language and cultural contexts (Pachana & Byrne, 2012).

Another area of psychometric exploration with regard to assessment instruments is the development and validation of structured interview guides for their administration. Snow and colleagues (2012) devised such a structured interview guide for the Rating Anxiety in Dementia (RAID; Shankar et al., 1999). Their RAID-SI demonstrated adequate internal consistency and inter-rater reliability, and it offers a structured, standardized interview format that may be helpful when the instrument is administered by less experienced assessors. Further work with other instruments to measure anxiety as well as other cognitive, mood, and behavior parameters is required, particularly for administration in settings (such as long-term care) where assessors may have less experience or training (Pachana et al., 2010).

The assessment (and treatment) of anxiety also has implications for functional independence in later life, with research showing that as many as 20% of drivers aged 55–72 report mild driving anxiety, with 5.5% of this group experiencing moderate to severe driving anxiety (Taylor et al., 2011). Driving anxiety can cause reduced confidence in driving competence (Ragland et al., 2005) and appears to affect more women than men (Gallo et al., 1999). In a recent study (Hempel et al., 2017), driving anxiety was associated with poorer mental health, physical health, and quality of life, over and above the effect of sociodemographic variables. Reduced mobility in older adults can lead to decreases in functionality, affective functioning, and quality of life and thus anxiety in this context may be thought of as excess burden that, if diagnosed and treated, could have significant positive social and health impacts. Driving anxiety has recently been shown to have a significant impact on driving cessation decision-making processes in patients with PD (Turner et al., 2017); driving cessation programs might seek to include assessment, education, and interventions that directly target the detection, treatment, and management of anxiety for patients with PD, as well as for older drivers who may be experiencing driving anxiety.

Additional work in the diagnosis, assessment, and treatment of anxiety disorders for older adults, particularly the oldest old, is required (Laidlaw & Pachana, 2009). Ribeiro and colleagues (2015) examined how sociodemographic, health, functional, and social factors contribute to the presence of clinically significant anxiety symptoms in centenarians recruited from two Portuguese centenarian studies. The main predictors for clinically significant anxiety symptoms (which were found in 45.4% of their sample of 97 centenarians) included worse health perception, higher number of medical conditions, financial concerns, and loneliness.

Further Development of Pharmacological Interventions

There is clinical trial evidence for the short-term efficacy of drugs from a variety of pharmacological classes in the treatment of most types of anxiety disorder in older people. These pharmacological classes include antidepressants, benzodiazepines, antipsychotics, and anticonvulsants. All anxiety disorders except simple phobia appear to respond at least to some extent to pharmacological intervention.

What is missing is evidence for long-term efficacy and safety when drugs are used to treat anxiety in older people. Although anxiety disorders are mainly chronic conditions, drug trials are generally quite brief and are often conducted for only 4–8 weeks, with limited follow-up. Drug trials too often do not enroll participants aged 75 years and over (Mohlman & Bryant, 2016).

Conventional Psychotropic Medication

Several decades of prescriber education, in combination with legislative changes in some countries, have led to changes in benzodiazepine prescribing behavior. However, there remains strong interest in the use of these agents to treat anxiety disorders (e.g., Starcevic, 2014), and there is evidence of their short-term efficacy that is superior to that of antidepressants (e.g., Gomez et al., 2018). The use of benzodiazepines in older people has been attenuated by knowledge of their propensity to cause daytime drowsiness, impaired sleep architecture, cognitive impairment, ataxia, and falls. In the UK, the National Institute for Health and Care Excellence (NICE) guidelines for the treatment of GAD in adults state that benzodiazepines should not be used 'in primary or secondary care except as a short-term measure during crises' (National Institute for Health and Care Excellence, 2011).

Although antidepressants are generally the preferred agents for the drug treatment of anxiety disorders in older adults, they are not always well tolerated, and there is increasing recognition of their adverse effects, including agitation, insomnia, headache, and sexual dysfunction. Upon cessation, antidepressants may be associated with discontinuation symptoms. However, there is evidence that both efficacy and propensity to cause adverse effects may be influenced by genetic polymorphisms (e.g., Lohoff et al., 2013). Thus, in the future, it is possible that pharmacogenomic approaches may allow a more rational and individualized approach to the selection of antidepressants for the treatment of anxiety disorders. Meanwhile, the NICE guidelines support the use of selective serotonin reuptake inhibitor (SSRI) or serotonin–norepinephrine reuptake inhibitor (SNRI) antidepressants as an alternative to an 'individual high intensity psychological intervention' in Step 3 of a four-step escalating sequence of treatments for GAD and in Step 3 of a five-step sequence for long-standing panic disorder (National Institute for Health and Care Excellence, 2011).

Low-potency antipsychotic drugs such as quetiapine show efficacy in the treatment of GAD (Mezhebovsky et al., 2013), but they are not always well tolerated, especially by older people. They cause daytime drowsiness, Parkinsonism, and falls. In some older people, they may cause or exacerbate metabolic syndrome and type 2 diabetes mellitus. Because there appear to be good reasons not to use antipsychotics for the routine treatment of anxiety disorders, large-scale post-marketing studies are needed to assess the safety and tolerability of antipsychotics in older people. The NICE guidelines indicate that antipsychotics should not be used for the treatment of panic disorder or for GAD in primary care (National Institute for Health and Care Excellence, 2011).

Pregabalin and other anticonvulsants warrant further examination in older people with anxiety disorders, although tolerability is likely to be a limiting factor. Generoso et al. (2017) have suggested that pregabalin might be better tolerated than the benzodiazepines in older anxious individuals, but further independent clinical trial evidence is needed on this point. The NICE guidelines indicate that pregabalin can be used in adult patients with GAD who are unable to tolerate SSRIs or SNRIs (National Institute for Health and Care Excellence, 2011).

Despite the availability of findings from several placebo-controlled clinical trials of conventional drugs for anxiety in older people, there are very few studies in which one type of drug is compared with another. As a consequence, the comparative efficacies of drug classes and of individual drugs within a single class are unknown. Long-term comparative drug studies are needed, but they are unlikely to be funded by the pharmaceutical industry.

Phytomedicines

It has been argued that certain substances derived from plants (phytomedicines) may have efficacy in the treatment of anxiety disorders. Savage et al. (2018) conducted a systematic review of plant-derived substances for which they required the following evidence: *in vitro* GABA-modulating activity, animal studies demonstrating an anxiolytic effect, and at least some human clinical trial data. They found evidence for the potential use of the following agents in anxiety states: kava, valerian, pennywort, hops, chamomile, *Ginkgo biloba*, passionflower, ashwagandha, skullcap, and lemon balm. We await methodologically sound and independently replicated clinical trials of these agents in people with anxiety disorders.

Another potential phytomedicine is cannabis. Although cannabis in its usual form – bred to have high levels of psychoactive Δ9-tetrahydrocannabinol (Δ9-THC) – is generally not recommended for the treatment of mental disorders, including anxiety disorders, there has been recent interest in the use of cannabidiol (CBD) extract. CBD is a non-psychotomimetic phytocannabinoid with complex effects on the brain, It exhibits antagonism at CB1 and CB2 receptors and agonism at serotonin 1A receptors. Although it has been proposed that CBD might have anxiolytic properties in humans, the extant clinical trial literature is scant, allowing few conclusions to be drawn. A small, controlled experiment in adults with social anxiety disorder found that CBD attenuated the anxiety response to simulated public speaking (Bergamaschi et al., 2011). With the legalization of the production and use of cannabis and its components becoming more widespread, opportunities now exist for clinical trials of CBD in anxiety disorders.

Novel Agents

Although existing medications used to treat anxiety disorders are either modestly effective or toxic in older people, the search for novel anxiolytic drugs does not appear to be a major focus of the pharmaceutical industry. As new antidepressant drugs are developed, they are generally tested in adults for anxiolytic efficacy. One such antidepressant is vortioxetine, which has been tested in older adults with depression (Nomikos et al., 2017) and has at least some anxiolytic effects (Yee et al., 2018). Another approach is to use drugs to augment psychological interventions. D-Cycloserine (DCS) was extensively trialed in adults and was found to accelerate fear extinction during exposure therapy (Norberg et al., 2008). However, the effects of DCS were time-limited and relatively modest. More research on novel anxiolytic agents and on augmentation agents is needed in order to find drugs that have long-term efficacy and are well tolerated in older people.

Psychosocial Interventions beyond Cognitive Behavioral Therapy

A variety of meta-analyses have supported the use of cognitive behavioral therapy (CBT) for anxiety disorders in later life (e.g., Ayers et al., 2007; Gonçalves & Byrne, 2012; Gould et al.,

2012). More recently, Hall et al. (2016) completed a systematic review, meta-analysis, and meta-regression focusing on older individuals with GAD and the efficacy of CBT to treat uncontrolled and excessive worry, with significant effects shown for CBT compared with wait-list or treatment as usual and nonsignificant effects when compared with active controls. The sum of these reviews to date is that the evidence for the efficacy of CBT in the treatment of anxiety in older adults remains mixed. These persistent findings have spurred interest in exploring other nonpharmacological modes of addressing anxiety in this population.

Acceptance and commitment therapy (ACT) is emerging as an efficacious treatment for emotional distress more generally (Ruiz, 2010), for anxiety disorders (e.g., a randomized controlled trial (RCT) by Roemer et al., 2008), as well as with older adults (Petkus & Wetherell, 2013). The ACT model posits experiential avoidance of distressing internal experiences as being central to the experience of psychopathology, and evidence supports this occurring in later adulthood as well as being amenable to change in this group (Petkus & Wetherell, 2013). A small pilot of ACT by Wetherell and colleagues (2011) comparing ACT and CBT in older patients with GAD found symptoms of worry and depression to improve in the ACT group ($n = 12$), while the CBT group also showed improvement on these dimensions but with more drop-out (5 of 9 completed treatment). Wetherell et al. also note the smaller treatment effects in this trial for older adults as compared to studies in younger persons (e.g., Roemer et al., 2008). A pilot trial of ACT for symptoms of anxiety and depression in nursing home residents demonstrated positive effects for depression (but not anxiety) scores compared to a wait-list control group (Davison et al., 2017). In this trial, as in several ACT studies with older groups, patient satisfaction with this treatment approach was rated highly. Further larger-scale trials of ACT are needed in older patients with GAD and perhaps other anxiety disorders. The utility of combining ACT with CBT, which has shown some promise for older patients with chronic pain (Lunde & Nordhus, 2009), is perhaps another promising direction with respect to the treatment of late-life anxiety.

Mindfulness-based treatment approaches also have a growing evidence base across age groups (e.g., Baer, 2015), for comorbid anxiety and depression in later life (e.g., Labbé et al., 2016), as well as with older populations more generally (Splevins et al., 2009). Mindfulness-based cognitive therapy (MBCT) and mindfulness-based stress reduction (MBSR) as interventions specifically for older adults have been described (Smith, 2004). In a meta-analysis (Fjorback et al., 2011), MBSR was found to be useful in reducing symptoms of stress, anxiety, and depression, but only one study in the review (Morone et al., 2008) focused on older patients (with chronic pain reduction as the aim of treatment). Foulk and colleagues (2014) found positive results with MBCT in older depressed and anxious patients. In a small open trial, Dissanayaka and colleagues (2016a) found that a group mindfulness intervention based on MBSR and tailored for patients with PD resulted in decreased motor and non-motor symptoms, including reductions in symptoms of anxiety. However, larger-scale open trials or RCTs are lacking with regard to mindfulness-based interventions for anxiety, with or without depression, in older populations. Again, results in older anxious patients would support such trials.

The need for trials of combined treatments (i.e., pharmacotherapy and psychotherapy) for older anxious patients has been highlighted in the literature (Lenze & Wetherell, 2011). In one such trial (Wetherell et al., 2013), a sequenced treatment combining pharmacotherapy (escitalopram) and CBT for older adults with GAD resulted in decreased worry, but no decrease in reported anxiety symptoms. Further work in this area is also needed, as such an approach has been shown to hold promise in younger populations (e.g., Cuijpers et al., 2014).

Culturally tailored interventions for late-life anxiety have begun to appear in the literature. Conti and colleagues (2017), citing the need for more trials of interventions with ethnically diverse elders, developed a modular, person-centered approach to CBT for late-life anxiety. Outcomes from a tailored CBT intervention for worry in a small group of older, underserved, mostly ethnic minority persons by Conti and colleagues (2017) showed greater treatment efficacy for Caucasian and Hispanic than African American participants. Demographic factors such as income or education and clinical factors such as homework completion, number of sessions, and depression symptoms did not predict post-treatment scores. The intervention itself was designed to be individually tailored, incorporating spiritual beliefs if deemed appropriate, and developed in consultation with input from Hispanic and African American community leaders. The authors speculate that as-yet unidentified factors may be affecting treatment outcomes and that more research in this area is required. Given the increasing numbers of ethnically diverse patient populations seeking mental health treatment, such research appears warranted.

An exciting new development in the realm of treatment augmentation is virtual reality (VR) technology. Grenier and colleagues (2015) describe how the use of VR may boost efficacy in older populations treated for such conditions as phobias, as aging is associated with declines in the ability to produce vivid mental images. They note that, to date, no studies have tested the efficacy of VR techniques in the treatment of late-life anxiety disorders; however, VR was noted as useful in the treatment of such disorders as phobias and PTSD in adults. VR has been used in older persons and those with PD to assist with gait and balance (e.g., Gallagher et al, 2016). In the course of VR intervention research, much knowledge has been gained with respect to safety, degrees of immersion, and compensation for physical or cognitive limitations. VR may prove to be a fertile ground for assisting in boosting the treatment efficacy of late-life anxiety disorders in the future.

Telehealth and E-Health Approaches

Recent reviews of CBT and ACT have shown that these types of interventions are effective in the treatment of anxiety in older populations (e.g., Ayers et al., 2007; Petkus & Wetherell, 2013). However, in many areas and in many countries, access to mental health professionals, particularly those skilled in interventions with older persons, lags behind increasing proportions of older persons living outside of major metropolitan areas. In some studies, high drop-out rates continue to both stymie researchers and also undermine sample sizes and thus reduce the power of psychotherapy treatment trials of CBT (Wilkinson, 2009) as well as other types of interventions. Barriers to older persons seeking treatment of any kind include mobility issues, treatment costs, stigma associated with mental illness, and desiring practitioners who are conversant with issues in later life (Pepin et al., 2009; Woodward & Pachana, 2009).

A variety of Internet-delivered strategies for the delivery of treatment for psychiatric disorders have been developed, with a view to addressing at least some of these treatment barriers. The use of the Internet as well as access to technology such as computers, tablets, and smartphones has continued to expand and to become more price-competitive. Older adults are also increasing users of the Internet (Pew Research Center, 2014). Thus, such Internet-based solutions to deliver interventions at the place, time, and pace of older adults are appealing, and they are the subject of increasing research.

Internet-delivered CBT (iCBT) is one such approach, delivering online sessions with therapist support coming via the Internet or via telephone (Titov et al., 2011). Cuijpers and colleagues (2009) reported in a recent meta-analysis that iCBT and computerized CBT for anxiety had an effect size that was superior to control conditions (23 studies, Cohen's $d = 1.1$). Brenes et al. (2012) compared telephone-administered CBT with a psychoeducational control for older adults with GAD, panic disorder, or an anxiety disorder not otherwise specified, and they found good reductions in anxiety symptoms as well as ancillary symptoms (e.g., insomnia, worry, quality of life). However, at the 6-month follow-up, only the gains in worry and quality of life remained significant. Zou and colleagues (2012) examined the efficacy of an iCBT program developed to treat anxiety in older adults in an open trial, with all 22 participants completing the trial, and large within-group effect sizes were found at the 3-month follow-up on the Generalized Anxiety Disorder 7-Item Scale (GAD-7; Cohen's $d = 1.03$) and the Depression, Anxiety and Stress Scales – 21 item version (Cohen's $d = 0.98$). Participants in this trial also reported high levels of satisfaction with the program. The potential benefits of such an approach are obvious, with the mean clinical time being 78 minutes in this trial. There is a clear need to follow up the preliminary reports of such trials with larger RCTs and with more detailed health economics cost–benefit analyses.

Telehealth interventions have also been used more broadly to reach older adults for the diagnosis and assessment of mental health issues, as well as the frequently comorbid physical ailments, such as cardiac or pulmonary issues (e.g., Gellis et al., 2012), or cognitive concerns (e.g., Martin-Khan et al., 2010), which can exacerbate – and be exacerbated by – psychiatric issues such as anxiety. However, more efforts are required not just in research, but also in policy and health care practice issues such as appropriate reimbursement, standardized definitions of telehealth-to-home services, and systematic approaches to analyzing cost-effectiveness (Durland et al., 2014).

Conclusions

Anxiety in later life remains a major issue in health care, with low detection and treatment rates, high risk of relapse, and relatively poor public health awareness (Sami & Nilorooshan, 2015). Anxiety disorders such as GAD in later life result in increased disability, decreased quality of life, and significantly increased usage of health care resources – evidence of the significant burden of this disorder in late life (Porensky et al., 2009). Further research on the etiology, diagnosis, assessment, and treatment of late-life anxiety is required in the face of an aging population.

References

Almeida, O. P., Draper, B., Snowdon, J., et al. (2012). Factors associated with suicidal thoughts in a large community study of older adults. *British Journal of Psychiatry*, **201**(6), 466–472.

Andreescu, C., Gross, J. J., Lenze, E., et al. (2011). Altered cerebral blood flow patterns associated with pathologic worry in the elderly. *Depression and Anxiety*, **28**, 202–209.

Andreescu, C., Sheu, L. K., Tudorascu, D., et al. (2015). Emotion reactivity and regulation in late-life generalized anxiety disorder: functional connectivity at baseline and post-treatment. *The American Journal of Geriatric Psychiatry*, 23(2), 200–214.

Ayers, C. R., Sorrell, J. T., Thorp, S. R. and Wetherell, J. L. (2007). Evidence-based psychological treatments for late-life anxiety. *Psychology and Aging*, **22**, 8–17.

Baer, R. A., ed. (2015). *Mindfulness-based Treatment Approaches: Clinician's Guide to Evidence Base and Applications*. Cambridge, MA: Academic Press.

Baxter, A. J., Scott, K. M., Vos, T. and Whiteford, H. A. (2013). Global prevalence of anxiety disorders: a systematic review and meta-regression. *Psychological Medicine*, **43**, 897–910.

Bergamaschi, M. M., Queiroz, R. H., Chagas, M. H., et al. (2011). Canabidiol reduces the anxiety induced by simulated public speaking in treatment-naïve social phobia patients. *Neuropsychopharmacology*, 36(6), 1219–1226.

Bolghan-Abadi, M., Segal, D. L., Coolidge, F. L. and Gottschling, J. (2013). Persian version of the Geriatric Anxiety Scale: translation and preliminary psychometric properties among Iranian older adults. *Aging & Mental Health*, 17(7), 896–900.

Boyle, L. L., Porsteinsson, A. P., Cui, X., King, D. A. and Lyness, J. M. (2010). Depression predicts cognitive disorders in older primary care patients. *Journal of Clinical Psychiatry*, 71, 74–79.

Brenes, G. A., Miller, M. E., Williamson, J. D., McCall, W. V., Knudson, M. and Stanley, M. A. (2012). A randomized controlled trial of telephone-delivered cognitive–behavioral therapy for late-life anxiety disorders. *American Journal of Geriatric Psychiatry*, 20(8), 707–716.

Byrne, G. J. and Pachana, N. A. (2010). Anxiety and depression in the elderly: do we know any more? *Current Opinion in Psychiatry*, 23 (6), 504–509.

Chan, Y. L. E., Bai, Y. M., Hsu, J. W., et al. (2017). Post-Traumatic Stress Disorder and risk of Parkinson's Disease: a nationwide longitudinal study. *American Journal of Geriatric Psychiatry*, 25(8), 917–923.

Chen, J. J. and Marsh, L. (2014). Anxiety in Parkinson's disease: identification and management. *Therapeutic Advances in Neurological Disorders*, 7, 52–59.

Chou, K. L., Mackenzie, C. S., Liang, K. and Sareen, J. (2011). Three-year incidence and predictors of first-onset of DSM-IV mood, anxiety, and substance use disorders in older adults: results from Wave 2 of the National Epidemiologic Survey on Alcohol and Related Conditions. *Journal of Clinical Psychiatry*, 72, 144–155.

Collie, A. and Maruff, P. (2000). The neuropsychology of preclinical Alzheimer's disease and mild cognitive impairment. *Neuroscience & Biobehavioral Reviews*, 24(3), 365–374.

Conti, E. C., Barrera, T. L., Amspoker, A. B., et al. (2017). Predictors of outcomes for older adults participating in Calmer Life, a culturally tailored intervention for anxiety. *Clinical Gerontologist*, 40(3), 172–180.

Cuijpers, P., Marks, I. M., van Straten, A., Cavanagh, K., Gega, L. and Andersson, G. (2009). Computer-aided psychotherapy for anxiety disorders: a meta-analytic review. *Cognitive Behavior Therapy*, 38(2), 66–82.

Cuijpers, P., Sijbrandij, M., Koole, S. L., Andersson, G., Beekman, A. T. and Reynolds, C. F. (2014). Adding psychotherapy to antidepressant medication in depression and anxiety disorders: a meta-analysis. *World Psychiatry*, 13(1), 56–67.

Davison, T. E., Eppingstall, B., Runci, S. and O'Connor, D. W. (2017). A pilot trial of acceptance and commitment therapy for symptoms of depression and anxiety in older adults residing in long-term care facilities. *Aging & Mental Health*, 21(7), 766–773.

Dissanayaka, N., Idu Jion, F., Pachana, N. A., et al. (2016a). Mindfulness for motor and non-motor dysfunctions in Parkinson's disease. *Parkinson's Disease*, 2016, 7109052.

Dissanayaka, N. N. W., O'Sullivan, J. D., Pachana, N. A., et al. (2016b). Disease specific anxiety symptomatology in Parkinson's disease. *International Psychogeriatrics*, 28(7), 1153–1163.

Dissanayaka, N. N., Sellbach, A., Matheson, S., et al. (2010). Anxiety disorders in Parkinson's disease: prevalence and risk factors. *Movement Disorders*, 25, 838–845.

Durland, L., Interian, A., Pretzer-Aboff, I. and Dobkin, R. D. (2014). Effect of telehealth-to-home interventions on quality of life for individuals with depressive and anxiety disorders. *Smart Homecare Technology and Telehealth*, 2, 105–119.

Fjorback, L. O., Arendt, M., Ørnbøl, E., Fink, P. and Walach, H. (2011). Mindfulness-based stress reduction and mindfulness-based cognitive therapy – a systematic review of randomized controlled trials. *Acta Psychiatrica Scandinavica*, 124(2), 102–119.

Foulk, M. A., Ingersoll-Dayton, B., Kavanagh, J., Robinson, E. and Kales, H. C. (2014). Mindfulness-based cognitive therapy with older adults: an exploratory study. *Journal of Gerontological Social Work*, **57**(5), 498–520.

Gallagher, R., Damodaran, H., Werner, W. G., Powell, W. and Deutsch, J. E. (2016). Auditory and visual cueing modulate cycling speed of older adults and persons with Parkinson's disease in a Virtual Cycling (V-Cycle) system. *Journal of Neuroengineering and Rehabilitation*, **13** (1), 77.

Gallo, J. J., Rebok, G. W. and Lesikar, S. E. (1999). The driving habits and patterns of adults aged 60 years and older. *Journal of the American Geriatrics Society*, **47**, 335–341.

Gellis, Z. D., Kenaley, B., McGinty, J., Bardelli, E., Davitt, J. and Ten Have, T. (2012). Outcomes of a telehealth intervention for homebound older adults with heart or chronic respiratory failure: a randomized controlled trial. *The Gerontologist*, **52**(4), 541–552.

Generoso, M. B., Trevizol, A. P., Kasper, S., Cho, H. J., Cordeiro, Q. and Shiozawa, P. (2017). Pregabalin for generalized anxiety disorder: an updated systematic review and meta-analysis. *International Clinical Psychopharmacology*, **32**(1), 49–55.

Gomez, A. F., Barthel, A. L. and Hofmann, S. G. (2018). Comparing the efficacy of benzodiazepines and serotonergic anti-depresants for adults with generalized anxiety disorder: a meta-analytic review. *Expert Opinion on Pharmacotherapy*, **19**(8), 883–894.

Gonçalves, D. C. and Byrne, G. J. (2012). Interventions for generalized anxiety disorder in older adults: systematic review and meta-analysis. *Journal of Anxiety Disorders*, **26**(1), 1–11.

Gottschalk, M. G. and Domschke, K. (2017). Genetics of generalized anxiety disorder and related traits. *Dialogues in Clinical Neuroscience*, **19**(2), 159–168.

Gould, R. L., Coulson, M. C. and Howard, R. J. (2012). Efficacy of cognitive behavioral therapy for anxiety disorders in older people: a meta-analysis and meta-regression of randomized controlled trials. *Journal of the American Geriatrics Society*, **60**(2), 218–229.

Grenier, S., Forget, H., Bouchard, S., et al. (2015). Using virtual reality to improve the efficacy of cognitive–behavioral therapy (CBT) in the treatment of late-life anxiety: preliminary recommendations for future research. *International Psychogeriatrics*, **27** (7), 1217–1225.

Gulpers, B., Ramakers, I., Hamel, R., Köhler, S., Voshaar, R. O. and Verhey, F. (2016). Anxiety as a predictor for cognitive decline and dementia: a systematic review and meta-analysis. *American Journal of Geriatric Psychiatry*, **24**(10), 823–842.

Hall, J., Kellett, S., Berrios, R., Bains, M. K. and Scott, S. (2016). Efficacy of cognitive behavioral therapy for generalized anxiety disorder in older adults: systematic review, meta-analysis, and meta-regression. *American Journal of Geriatric Psychiatry*, **24** (11), 1063–1073.

Hempel, M. E., Taylor, J. E., Connolly, M. J., Alpass, F. M. and Stephens, C. V. (2017). Scared behind the wheel: what impact does driving anxiety have on the health and well-being of young older adults? *International Psychogeriatrics*, **29**(6), 1027–1034.

Hettema, J. M., Prescott, C. A., Myers, J. M., Neale, M. C. and Kendler, K. S. (2005). The structure of genetic and environmental risk factors for anxiety disorders in men and women. *Archives of General Psychiatry*, **62**, 182–189.

Kassem, A. M., Ganguli, M., Yaffe, K., et al. (2018). Anxiety symptoms and risk of dementia and mild cognitive impairment in the oldest old women. *Aging & Mental Health*, **22**(4), 474–482.

Kelly-Irving, M., Mabile, L., Grosclaude, P., Lang, T. and Delpierre, C. (2013) The embodiment of adverse childhood experiences and cancer development: potential biological mechanisms and pathways across the life course. *International Journal of Public Health*, **58**, 3–11.

Kreifelts, B., Brück, C., Ethofer, T., et al. (2017). Prefrontal mediation of emotion regulation in social anxiety disorder during laughter perception. *Neuropsychologia*, **96**, 175–183.

Labbé, M., Nikolitch, K., Penheiro, R., et al. (2016). Mindfulness-based cognitive therapy in the treatment of late-life anxiety and depression – a pilot study. *Canadian Geriatrics Journal*, **19**(3), 127–128.

Laidlaw, K. and Pachana, N. A. (2009). Aging, mental health, and demographic change. *Professional Psychology: Research and Practice*, **40**(6), 601–608.

Lee, L. O., Gatz, M., Pedersen, N. L. and Prescott, C. A. (2016). Anxiety trajectories in the second half of life: genetic and environmental contributions over age. *Psychology and Aging*, **31**(1), 101–113.

Leentjens, A. F., Dujardin, K., Marsh, L., Martinez-Martin, P., Richard, I. H. and Starkstein, S. E. (2011). Symptomatology and markers of anxiety disorders in Parkinson's disease: a cross-sectional study. *Movement Disorders*, **26**, 484–492.

Lenze, E. J. and Butters, M. A. (2016). Consequences of anxiety in aging and cognitive decline. *American Journal of Geriatric Psychiatry*, **24**(10), 843–845.

Lenze, E. J. and Wetherell, J. L. (2011). Anxiety disorders: new developments in old age. *American Journal of Geriatric Psychiatry*, **19**(4), 301–304.

Li, X. X. and Li, Z. (2018). The impact of anxiety on the progression of mild cognitive impairment to dementia in Chinese and English data bases: a systematic review and meta-analysis. *International Journal of Geriatric Psychiatry*, **33**(1), 131–140.

Lohoff, F. W., Aquino, T. D., Narasimhan, S., Multani, P. K., Eemad, B. and Rickels, K. (2013). Serotonin receptor 2A (HTR2A) gene polymorphism predicts treatment response to venlafaxine XR in generalized anxiety disorder. *Pharmacogenomics Journal*, **13**(1), 21–26.

Lunde, L. H. and Nordhus, I. H. (2009). Combining acceptance and commitment therapy and cognitive behavioral therapy for the treatment of chronic pain in older adults. *Clinical Case Studies*, **8**(4), 296–308.

Lyketsos, C. G., Carrillo, M. C., Ryan, J. M., et al. (2011). Neuropsychiatric symptoms in Alzheimer's disease. *Alzheimer's & Dementia*, **7**(5), 532–539.

Martin-Khan, M., Wootton, R. and Gray, L. (2010). A systematic review of the reliability of screening for cognitive impairment in older adults by use of standardised assessment tools administered via the telephone. *Journal of Telemedicine and Telecare*, **16**(8), 422–428.

Massena, P. N., de Araujo, N. B., Pachana, N. A., Laks, J. and de Padua, A. C. (2015). Validation of the Brazilian Portuguese version of Geriatric Anxiety Inventory – GAI-BR. *International Psychogeriatrics*, **27**(7), 1113–1119.

Mezhebovsky, I., Magi, K., She, F., Datto, C. and Eriksson, H. (2013). Double-blind randomized study of extended release quetiapine fumarate (quetiapine XR) monotherapy in older patients with generalized anxiety disorder. *International Journal of Geriatric Psychiatry*, **28**(6), 615–625.

Miloyan, B., Byrne, G. J. and Pachana, N. A. (2014). Age-related changes in generalized anxiety disorder symptoms. *International Psychogeriatrics*, **26**(4), 565–572.

Mirza, S. S., Ikram, M. A., Bos, D., Mihaescu, R., Hofman, A. and Tiemeier, H. (2017). Mild cognitive impairment and risk of depression and anxiety: a population-based study. *Alzheimer's & Dementia*, **13**(2), 130–139.

Mohlman, J. and Bryant, C. (2016). Anxiety in later life. In S. K. Whitbourne, ed., *The Encyclopedia of Adulthood and Aging*. New York: Wiley-Blackwell, pp. 73–85.

Morone, N. E., Greco, C. M. and Weiner, D. K. (2008). Mindfulness meditation for the treatment of chronic low back pain in older adults: a randomized controlled pilot study. *Pain*, **134**, 310–319.

National Institute for Health and Care Excellence (2011) Generalised anxiety disorder and panic disorder in adults: management (NICE Clinical Guideline No. 113). Last updated June 2018. www.nice.org.uk/guidance/cg113 (last accessed 21 January 2019).

Nomikos, G. G., Tomori, D., Zhong, W., Affinito, J. and Palo, W. (2017) Efficacy, safety, and tolerability of vortioxetine for the treatment of major depressive disorder in patients aged 55 years or older. *CNS Spectrum*, **22**(4), 348–362.

Norberg, M. M., Krystal, J. H. and Tolin, D. F. (2008). A meta-analysis of d-cycloserine and the facilitation of fear extinction and exposure therapy. *Biological Psychiatry*, **63** (12), 1118–1126.

Norrholm, S. D. and Ressler, K. J. (2009). Genetics of anxiety and trauma-related disorders. *Neuroscience*, **164**, 272–287.

Pachana, N. A. and Byrne, G. J. A. (2012). The Geriatric Anxiety Inventory: international use and future directions. *Australian Psychologist*, **47**(1), 33–38.

Pachana, N. A., Byrne, G. J., Siddle, H., Koloski, N., Harley. E. and Arnold, E. (2007). Development and validation of the Geriatric Anxiety Inventory. *International Psychogeriatrics*, **19**, 103–114.

Pachana, N. A., Helmes, E., Byrne, G. J. A., Edelstein, B. A., Konnert, C. A. and Pot, A. M. (2010). Screening for mental disorders in residential aged care facilities. *International Psychogeriatrics*, **22** (7), 1107–1120.

Palmer, K., Berger, A. K., Monastero, R., Winblad, B., Bäckman, L. and Fratiglioni, L. (2007). Predictors of progression from mild cognitive impairment to Alzheimer disease. *Neurology*, **68**(19), 1596–1602.

Pepin, R., Segal, D. L. and Coolidge, F. L. (2009). Intrinsic and extrinsic barriers to mental health care among community-dwelling younger and older adults. *Aging & Mental Health*, **13**(5), 769–777.

Peters, M., Rosenberg, P., Steinberg, M., et al. (2013). Neuropsychiatric symptoms as risk factors for progression from CIND to dementia: the Cache County Study. *American Journal of Geriatric Psychiatry*, **21**(11), 1116–1124.

Petkus, A. J. and Wetherell, J. L. (2013). Acceptance and commitment therapy with older adults: rationale and considerations. *Cognitive and Behavioral Practice*, **20**(1), 47–56.

Petkus, A. J., Reynolds, C. A., Wetherell, J. L., Kremen, W. S. and Gatz, M. (2017). Temporal dynamics of cognitive performance and anxiety across older adulthood. *Psychology and Aging*, **32**(3), 278–292.

Pew Research Center (2014). Older Adults and Technology Use. www.pewinternet.org/2014/04/03/older-adults-and-technology-use/ (last accessed 5 August 2020).

Pietrzak, R. H., Lim, Y. Y., Neumeister, A., et al. (2015). Amyloid-β, anxiety, and cognitive decline in preclinical Alzheimer disease: A multicenter, prospective cohort study. *Jama psychiatry*, **72**(3), 284–291.

Pink, A., Przybelski, S. A., Krell-Roesch, J., et al. (2017). Cortical thickness and anxiety symptoms among cognitively normal elderly persons: The Mayo Clinic study of aging. *Journal of Neuropsychiatry and Clinical Neurosciences*, **29**(1), 60–66.

Porensky, E. K., Dew, M. A., Karp, J. F., et al. (2009). The burden of late-life generalized anxiety disorder: effects on disability, health-related quality of life, and healthcare utilization. *American Journal of Geriatric Psychiatry*, **17**(6), 473–482.

Ragland, D. R., Satariano, W. A. and MacLeod, K. E. (2005). Driving cessation and increased depressive symptoms. *Journal of Gerontology*, **60A**, 399–403.

Ribeiro, O., Teixeira, L., Araujo, L., Afonso, R. M. and Pachana, N. A. (2015). Predictors of anxiety in centenarians: health, economic factors and loneliness. *International Psychogeriatrics*, **27**(7), 1167–1176.

Roemer, L., Orsillo, S. M. and Salters-Pedneault, K. (2008). Efficacy of an acceptance-based behavior therapy for generalized anxiety disorder: evaluation in a randomized controlled trial. *Journal of Consulting and Clinical Psychology*, **76**(6), 1083–1089.

Ruiz, F. J. (2010). A review of acceptance and commitment therapy (ACT) empirical evidence: correlational, experimental psychopathology, component and outcome studies. *Revista Internacional de Psicología y Terapia Psicológica*, **10**(1), 125–162.

Sami, M. B. and Nilforooshan, R. (2015). The natural course of anxiety disorders in the elderly: a systematic review of longitudinal trials. *International Psychogeriatrics*, **27**(07), 1061–1069.

Savage, K., Firth, J., Stough, C. and Sarris, J. (2018). GABA-modulating phyomedicines for anxiety: a systematic review of preclinical and clinical evidence. *Phytotherapeutic Research*, **32**(1), 3–18.

Schoevers, R. A., Deeg. D. J., van Tilburg, W. and Beekman, A. T. (2005). Depression and generalized anxiety disorder: co-occurrence and longitudinal patterns in elderly patients. *American Journal of Geriatric Psychiatry*, **13**, 31–39.

Segal, D. L., June, A., Payne, M., Coolidge, F. L. and Yochim, B. (2010). Development and initial validation of a self-report assessment tool for anxiety among older adults: the Geriatric Anxiety Scale. *Journal of Anxiety Disorders*, **24**(7), 709–714.

Shankar, K. K., Walker, M., Frost, D. and Orrell, M. W. (1999). The development of a valid and reliable scale for rating anxiety in dementia (RAID). *Aging & Mental Health*, **3**(1), 39–49.

Smith, A. (2004). Clinical uses of mindfulness training for older people. *Behavioural and Cognitive Psychotherapy*, **32**(4), 423–430.

Snow, A. L., Huddleston, C., Robinson, C., et al. (2012). Psychometric properties of a structured interview guide for the rating for anxiety in dementia. *Aging & Mental Health*, **16**(5), 592–602.

Splevins, K., Smith, A. and Simpson, J. (2009). Do improvements in emotional distress correlate with becoming more mindful? A study of older adults. *Aging & Mental Health*, **13**(3), 328–335.

Starcevic, V. (2014). The reappraisal of benzodiazepines in the treatment of anxiety and related disorders. *Expert Review of Neurotherapeutics*, **14**(11), 1275–1286.

Tales, A. and Basoudan, N. (2016). Anxiety in old age and dementia-implications for clinical and research practice. *Neuropsychiatry (London)*, **6**(4), 142–148.

Taylor, J. E., Alpass, F., Stephens, C. and Towers, A. (2011). Driving anxiety and fear in young older adults in New Zealand. *Age and Ageing*, **40**, 62–66.

Titov, N., Dear, B. F., Schwencke, G., et al. (2011). Transdiagnostic internet treatment for anxiety and depression: a randomised controlled trial. *Behaviour Research and Therapy*, **49**(8), 441–452.

Turner, L. M., Liddle, J. and Pachana, N. A. (2017). Parkinson's disease and driving cessation: a journey influenced by anxiety. *Clinical Gerontologist*, **40**(3), 220–229.

Visser, P. J., Verhey, F. R., Knol, D. L., et al. (2009). Prevalence and prognostic value of CSF markers of Alzheimer's disease pathology in patients with subjective cognitive impairment or mild cognitive impairment in the DESCRIPA study: a prospective cohort study. *Lancet Neurology*, 8, 619–627.

Wetherell, J. L., Liu, L., Patterson, T. L., et al. (2011). Acceptance and commitment therapy for generalized anxiety disorder in older adults: a preliminary report. *Behavior therapy*, **42**(1), 127–134.

Wetherell, J. L., Petkus, A. J., White, K. S., et al. (2013). Antidepressant medication augmented with cognitive–behavioral therapy for generalized anxiety disorder in older adults. *American Journal of Psychiatry*, **170**(7), 782–789.

Wilkinson, P. (2009). Cognitive behavioural therapy with older adults: enthusiasm without the evidence? *The Cognitive Behaviour Therapist*, **2**, 75–82.

Woodward, R. and Pachana, N. A. (2009). Attitudes towards psychological treatment among older Australians. *Australian Psychologist*, **44**(2), 86–93.

Yee, A., Ng, C. G. and Seng, L. H. (2018) Vortioxetine treatment for anxiety disorder: a meta-analysis study. *Current Drug Targets*, **19**(12), 1412–1423.

Zhang, X., Norton, J., Carriere, I., Ritchie, K., Chaudieu, I. and Ancelin, M. L. (2015). Risk factors for late-onset generalized anxiety disorder: results from a 12-year prospective cohort (the ESPRIT study). *Translational Psychiatry*, **5**(3), e536.

Zou, J. B., Dear, B. F., Titov, N., et al. (2012). Brief Internet-delivered cognitive behavioral therapy for anxiety in older adults: a feasibility trial. *Journal of Anxiety Disorders*, **26**(6), 650–655.

Index

Acceptance and Commitment
Therapy (ACT)
cross-cultural issues, 71
future research, 233
as novel treatment
model, 180
Parkinson's disease, late-life
anxiety and, 148
Acculturation, late-life anxiety
and, 14
Activity, Balance, Learning and
Exposure (ABLE)
treatment, fear of falling
and, 178
Adjusting to Chronic
Conditions Using
Education, Support, and
Skills (ACCESS),
179–180
Adverse effects of
pharmacological
treatment, 193–194
Agoraphobia
clinical assessment of late-
life anxiety and, 86–87
DSM-5 and, 87
Agoraphobic Cognitions
Questionnaire (ACQ), 87
Alcohol use disorder
co-morbidity of anxiety
and, 4
subthreshold late-life anxiety
and, 46
Alcohol Use Disorder and
Associated Disabilities
Interview (AUDADIS),
11, 13
Alerting, 98
Almeida, O. P., 15–16
Alpidem, 198
Alprazolam, 198
Alzheimer's disease
amyloid-beta deposition
and, 125
apolipoprotein E ε4 and, 123
cardiovascular disease
(CVD) and, 125
cognitive behavioural
therapy (CBT) and, 52

cognitive functioning
and, 117
genetic factors in, 123
neuropsychiatric anxiety
and, 120–121
American College of Sports
Medicine, 72
American Heart
Association, 72
*American Journal of Geriatric
Psychiatry*, 226
American Psychiatric
Association. *See*
Diagnostic and Statistical
Manual of Mental
Disorders (DSM-5)
American Society of Clinical
Oncology (ASCO), 167
Ames, D., 11
Amputation, subacute settings
and late-life anxiety, 158
Amygdala
anxiety and, 1, 205
attention bias and, 109–110
blastolateral group
(BLA), 207
centromedial group (CeA),
207, 208
cognitive functioning
and, 123
mediation of fear learning
and extinction in, 209–210
neuromodulation of fear and
anxiety circuits, 211
neurons in, 207–208
Parkinson's disease, late-life
anxiety and, 145
Pavlovian fear conditioning
and, 206
physiology of, 207–208
Amyloid-beta deposition,
Alzheimer's disease
and, 125
Andreas, S., 12
Animal models of fear and
anxiety
amygdala, mediation of fear
learning and extinction in,
209–210

anxiety compared, 206
cognitive behavioural
therapy (CBT), fear
conditioning and
extinction and, 214
defined, 205
gamma-aminobutyric acid
(GABA) system, fear
conditioning and
extinction and,
213–214
hippocampus, mediation of
fear learning and
extinction in, 210–211
neuromodulation of fear and
anxiety circuits,
211–212
overview, 7, 205–206,
214–218
Pavlovian fear conditioning,
206–207
prefrontal cortex, mediation
of fear learning and
extinction in,
210–211
Anterior cingulate
anxiety and, 1
attention and, 97–98
Parkinson's disease, late-life
anxiety and, 145
Anticonvulsants
future research, 231
overview, 200
pregabalin, 200, 231
treatment of late-life anxiety
with, 200
Antidepressants. *See also
specific drug*
buspirone, 200
future research, 231
generalized anxiety disorder
(GAD) and, 174
hyponatraemia and, 196
monoamine oxidase
inhibitors (MAOIs), 196
overview, 195–196
selective serotonin reuptake
inhibitors (SSRIs),
146, 196

Antidepressants (cont.)
serotonin and noradrenaline
(norepinephrine)
reuptake inhibitors
(SNRIs), 196
suicide and, 196
tricyclic antidepressants
(TCAs), 72, 196
Antipsychotics
overview, 199
quetiapine, 199, 231
treatment of late-life anxiety
with, 199
Anxiety and Related Disorders
Interview Schedule-5
(ADIS-5), 81
Anxiety disorders not
otherwise specified
(ADNOS)
Parkinson's disease and, 140,
141–142
subthreshold late-life anxiety
and, 33, 51–52
Anxiety in Cognitive
Impairment and
Dementia (ACID), 87–88
Anxiety Sensitivity Index
(ASI), 87
Anxiety Status Inventory (ASI),
Parkinson's disease and
late-life anxiety and, 142
Apolipoptotein E ε4, 123–124
Ashwagandha, 201, 232
Asnaani, A., 14
Åström, M., 157
Attention bias, depression and
late-life anxiety and
age difference, effect of, 107
alerting and, 98
amygdala and, 109–110
anterior cingulate and,
97–98
anxiety and, 101–108
attention bias modification
(ABM) training, 111
bottom-up process in
attention, 97–98
co-morbidity of late-life
anxiety and depression
and, 109, 110
depression and, 108–109
empirical evidence of,
101–106
executive function and, 98
fear of falling and, 107–108
four-stage process, 99

functional connectivity in
default mode network
(DMN) and, 110
functional magnetic
resonance imaging (fMRI)
and, 107, 110
future research, 111–112
generalized anxiety disorder
(GAD) and, 107, 111
integrated model, 110
meditation and, 111
neurophysiology of, 109–110
neuropsychology of,
109–110
orientating and, 98
overview, 97
pharmacological treatment,
110–111
positivity effect and, 100
prefrontal cortex and, 107,
109–110
psychosocial treatment,
110–111
research findings, 101–106
state anxiety and, 101
threat and, 99, 109, 111
time and, 99
top-down process in
attention, 97–98
trait anxiety and, 101–107
worry and, 107
Attention Control
Theory (ACT)
cognitive functioning
and, 120
depression and late-life
anxiety and, 99
subthreshold late-life anxiety
and, 49
Attention Process Training II
(APT), executive
dysfunction and, 178
Australian National Survey of
Mental Health, 4, 22
Avoidant-vigilant
response, 101
Ayers, C. R., 129

Bachelor-level lay providers
(BLPs), 182
Bar-Haim, Y., 99, 109, 110
Basoudan, N., 228
Baxter, A. J., 11, 66
Beaudreau, Sherry A., 6,
118, 128
Beck, A. T., 98–99

Beck Anxiety Inventory (BAI)
clinical assessment of late-
life anxiety and, 83, 87
diagnosis of late-life anxiety
and, 24
overview, 4
Parkinson's disease and late-
life anxiety and, 142, 147
Behavioural observations, 88
Benzodiazepines (BZDs)
ceasing use of, 195
cross-cultural issues, 72
future research, 231
gamma-aminobutyric acid
(GABA) system and,
197, 213
generalized anxiety disorder
(GAD) and, 174
Parkinson's disease, late-life
anxiety and, 146
subthreshold late-life anxiety
and, 51
treatment of late-life anxiety
with, 197–198
Z-drugs versus, 198
Beta-blockers, 200–201
Bower, Emily, 6, 85
Braam, A. W., 44
Bradley, B., 99, 109
Brain-derived neurotrophic
factor (BDNF)
cognitive functioning and,
123–124
Parkinson's disease, late-life
anxiety and, 145
Brenes, G. A., 235
Breslau, J., 14
Bryant, Christina, 5, 11, 25
Buddhism, 71
Burden of disease due to
anxiety, 3, 11
Burden of Disease Study, 11
Buspirone
antidepressants versus, 200
sertraline versus, 196
treatment of late-life anxiety
with, 199–200
Byers, A. L., 12
Byrne, Gerard, 5, 6, 7
BZD. See Benzodiazepines
(BZDs)

Calmer Life model, 180–181
Campbell, G., 25
Cannabidiol (CBD), 232
Cannabis, 232

Canuto, A., 12, 16
Cardiovascular disease (CVD)
  Alzheimer's disease and, 125
  clinical assessment of late-
    life anxiety and, 90
  cognitive behavioural
    therapy (CBT) and, 52
  cognitive functioning
    and, 125
  subthreshold late-life
    anxiety, co-morbidity
    with, 50
Care settings, late-life anxiety
  across
  home-based care (See Home-
    based care, late-life
    anxiety in)
  long-term care (See Long-
    term care, late-life
    anxiety in)
  overview, 6, 157
  palliative care settings (See
    Palliative care settings,
    late-life anxiety in)
  subacute settings (See
    Subacute settings, late-life
    anxiety in)
Case formulation, 27
CBT. See Cognitive
    behavioural
    therapy (CBT)
Chamomile, 201, 232
Childhood
  anxiety and, 2
  cognitive functioning
    and, 123
Chou, K. L., 13, 15, 16
Chronic obstructive
    pulmonary disease
    (COPD)
  clinical assessment of late-
    life anxiety and, 89
  cognitive behavioural
    therapy (CBT) and, 52
  in subacute settings, 158
  subthreshold late-life
    anxiety, co-morbidity
    with, 50
Chronic pain, co-morbidity
  with subthreshold late-life
    anxiety, 51
Citalopram, 196
Clark, L. A., 98
Clinical assessment of late-life
    anxiety
  agoraphobia and, 86–87

Agoraphobic Cognitions
  Questionnaire (ACQ), 87
Anxiety and Related
  Disorders Interview
  Schedule-5 (ADIS-5), 81
Anxiety in Cognitive
  Impairment and
  Dementia (ACID), 87–88
Anxiety Sensitivity Index
  (ASI), 87
Beck Anxiety Inventory
  (BAI), 83, 87
behavioural observations, 88
cardiovascular disease
  (CVD) and, 90
chronic obstructive
  pulmonary disease
  (COPD) and, 89
cognitive functioning and,
  126–128
dementia and, 87–88
diabetes and, 89–90
diagnosis and, 79–80
diversity differences in, 90
ecological momentary
  assessment (EMA), 88–89
experience and, 79–80
fear of falling and, 85
Fear of Falling
  Questionnaire (FFQ), 85
Fear Survey Schedule-II
  (FSS-II), 85
gender differences in, 90
generalized anxiety disorder
  (GAD) and, 84
Generalized Anxiety
  Disorder Severity Scale
  (GADSS), 82
Geriatric Anxiety Inventory
  (GAI), 83
Geriatric Anxiety Scale
  (GAS), 83–84
Hamilton Anxiety Rating
  Scale (HAM-A), 82
in home-based care, 161–162
informant reports, 88
information used in, 80
Liebowitz Social Anxiety
  Scale (LSAS), 85–86
in long-term care, 165
Mini-International
  Neuropsychiatric
  Interview (MINI), 81–82
Mobility Inventory (MI), 87
Montreal Cognitive
  Assessment (MoCA), 128

Older Adult Social
  Evaluative Scale
  (OASES), 86
overview, 6, 79, 90–91
in palliative care settings, 167
panic disorder and, 86–87
Panic Disorder Severity
  Scale, 82
Parkinson's disease and, 89,
  142–143
Patient-Reported Outcomes
  Measurement
  Information System
  (PROMIS), 84
Penn State Worry
  Questionnaire (PSWQ),
  84–85
pharmacological treatment,
  prior to, 193
phobias and, 85
physical illness and,
  89–90
physiological measures, 88
presentation and, 79–80
Rating Scale for Anxiety in
  Dementia (RAID), 87
St. Louis University Mental
  Status (SLUMS)
  Examination, 128
self-reports and, 82
setting, relevance of, 80–81
social anxiety disorder and,
  85–86
Social Interaction Anxiety
  Scale (SIAS), 86
Social Phobia and Anxiety
  Inventory (SPAI), 86
Social Phobia Scale (SPS), 86
Structured Clinical Interview
  for DSM-5 Disorders
  (SCID), 81
technology, use of, 88–89
Clinical Gerontologist, 226
Clinical interviews, 24
Cognitive behavioural
  therapy (CBT)
  Alzheimer's disease and, 52
  cardiovascular disease
    (CVD) and, 52
  chronic illness and,
    179–180
  chronic obstructive
    pulmonary disease
    (COPD) and, 52
  cognitive functioning
    and, 129

(CBT) (cont.)
combination with
pharmacological
treatment, 174, 201
cross-cultural issues, 71
dementia and, 179
executive dysfunction
and, 178
fear conditioning and
extinction and, 214
fear of falling and, 52, 178
future research, 232–233
generalized anxiety disorder
(GAD) and, 6, 173
hoarding disorder and, 177
Internet-delivered cognitive
behavioural therapy
(iCBT), 182, 234–235
meta-analytic evaluation of,
173–174
modular approaches, 180
overview, 5, 6
panic disorder and, 173
Parkinson's disease
and late-life anxiety and,
52, 146–148, 174, 179
pharmacological treatment
versus, 201
post-traumatic stress
disorder (PTSD) and, 176
sertraline versus, 196
subthreshold late-life anxiety
and, 51–53
telephone-based treatment,
181–182
traditional efficacy trials,
173–175
younger populations
compared, 174
Cognitive bias. *See* Attention
bias, depression and
late-life anxiety and
Cognitive Debt, 120
Cognitive functioning, late-life
anxiety and
Alzheimer's disease and, 117
amygdala and, 123
apolipoptotein E ε4 and,
123–124
Attention Control
Theory, 120
biological models generally,
121, 126
brain-derived neurotrophic
factor (BDNF) and,
123–124

cardiovascular disease
(CVD) and, 125
childhood and, 123
clinical assessment of late-
life anxiety and, 126–128
clinical implications
generally, 126
cognitive behavioural
therapy (CBT) and, 129
Cognitive Debt, 120
complex cognitive
abilities, 118
cortisol and, 124
depression and, 119
early-life experience and, 123
evolutionary basis for
anxiety, 122
gamma-aminobutyric acid
(GABA) system and, 124
generalized anxiety disorder
(GAD) and, 117, 118–119
genetic factors in anxiety,
122–124
hippocampus and, 123, 124
hormones and, 124
hyperthyroidism and, 125
hypothalamic–pituitary–
adrenal (HPA) axis
and, 124
hypothyroidism and, 125
Mindfulness-based Stress
Reduction (MBSR)
and, 130
Montreal Cognitive
Assessment (MoCA), 128
negative effects,
118–119, 121
neuropsychiatric anxiety,
120–121
neurotransmitters and, 124
overview, 6, 117, 131
Parkinson's disease and, 125
pharmacological treatment
and, 130
prefrontal cortex and,
123, 124
problem-solving therapy
(PST) and, 129–130
Processing Efficiency
Theory, 120
St. Louis University Mental
Status (SLUMS)
Examination, 128
sexual abuse and, 123–124
specific cognitive
abilities, 118

studies of, 117–118
thyroid disease and, 125
treatment generally,
128–129
twin studies and, 122–123
worry and, 119
Cognitive impairment
psychotropic drugs, use of in
presence of, 194
risk factor, anxiety as,
227–228
subthreshold late-life
anxiety, co-morbidity
with, 48–49
symptom, anxiety as, 227
Collaborative Psychiatric
Epidemiology Survey
(CPES), 14
Community–academic
partnership models, 182
Co-morbidity of anxiety. *See
also specific disease*
findings of studies, 16
other conditions, 16
overview, 3–4
pharmacological treatment
and, 191
Complementary medicine, 201
Composite International
Diagnostic Interview
(CIDI), 11, 13, 24, 27
Confucianism, 67
Contextual, Adult Lifespan
Theory for Adapting
Psychotherapy (CALTAP)
model, 20, 24, 28–29
Conti, E. C., 234
Conventional treatment of
anxiety, 4–5
COPD. *See* Chronic obstructive
pulmonary disease
(COPD)
Cortisol, cognitive functioning
and, 124
Coyne, J. C., 26
Craddock, N., 21
Creamer, M., 22
Creighton, A. S., 13
Cross-cultural issues in late-life
anxiety
Acceptance and
Commitment Therapy
(ACT) and, 71
benzodiazepines (BZDs)
and, 72
Buddhism and, 71

cognitive behavioural
  therapy (CBT) and, 71
Confucianism and, 67
cultural syndrome, 68
culture defined, 63
culture-specific disorders, 68
death anxiety and, 70
diagnosis and, 26–27,
  68–69
display rules and, 67
epidemiology and, 13–14
exercise and, 72
family and, 71–72
future research, 72–73
Geriatric Anxiety Inventory
  (GAI) and, 69
Hospital Anxiety and
  Depression Scale (HADS)
  and, 69
immigration and, 69–70
Mandala of Health and,
  64–65
mindfulness-based
  interventions and, 71
non-Western cultures, 63
overview, 5–6, 63,
  72–73
perception of mental
  disorders, 65–66
pharmacological treatment
  and, 72
presentation of symptoms
  and, 67–68
prevalence of anxiety and,
  66–67
protective factors and, 69–70
psychosocial treatment and,
  70–72
relaxation and, 71
religious explanation for
  mental disorders, 65
risk factors and, 69–70
screening and, 68–69
stigma and, 65–66
supernatural explanation for
  mental disorders, 65
Taoism and, 71
tricyclic antidepressants
  (TCAs) and, 72
Western cultures, 63
Zen Buddhism and, 71
Cuijpers, P., 235
Cultural syndrome, 68
Culture-specific disorders, 68
CVD. See Cardiovascular
  disease (CVD)

Daily functioning, effect of
  subthreshold late-life
  anxiety on, 45–46
Darwin, Charles, 1, 205
Davies, K. N., 25
Davison, T. E., 13
D-Cycloserine (DCS), 232
Death anxiety, cross-cultural
  issues in late-life anxiety
  and, 70
Decline of anxiety with age, 3
Deep brain stimulation (DBS)
  treatment, 142
Dementia
  clinical assessment of late-
    life anxiety and, 87–88
  cognitive behavioural
    therapy (CBT) and, 179
  co-morbidity with late-life
    anxiety, 16, 23
  long-term care, co-
    morbidity with late-life
    anxiety in, 164–165
  mindfulness-based
    interventions and, 179
  psychosocial treatment,
    178–179
  risk factor, anxiety as,
    227–228
  subthreshold late-life
    anxiety, co-morbidity
    with, 48–49
  symptom, anxiety as, 227
Demeyer, I., 101
Depression, Anxiety and Stress
  Scale (DASS-21),
  Parkinson's disease and
  late-life anxiety and, 147
Depression, late-life
  anxiety and
  attention bias and (See
    Attention bias, depression
    and late-life anxiety and)
  Attention Control Theory
    (ACT) and, 99
  cognitive functioning
    and, 119
  cognitive theories and,
    99–100
  findings of studies, 16
  information processing
    model and, 99
  maladaptive schemas and,
    98–99
  mirtazapine and, 197
  nortriptyline and, 197

overview, 4, 6
socioemotional selectivity
  theory (SST) and, 100
subthreshold late-life anxiety
  and, 47
tripartite model of, 98
De Raedt, R., 101
Diabetes, clinical assessment of
  late-life anxiety and,
  89–90
Diagnosis of late-life anxiety
  age range as challenge of, 21
  Beck Anxiety Inventory
    (BAI), 24
  best practice in, 27–29
  CALTAP model, 20, 24,
    28–29
  case formulation, 27
  challenges of, 21–24
  clinical assessment
    of late-life anxiety and,
    79–80
  clinical interviews and, 24
  Composite International
    Diagnostic Interview
    (CIDI), 24, 27
  cross-cultural issues in,
    26–27, 68–69
  dementia, co-morbidity with
    as challenge of, 23
  detection and recognition of
    symptoms as challenge of,
    21–22
  differential presentation as
    challenge of, 22
  fear of falling as challenge
    of, 23
  future directions, 29
  generalized anxiety disorder
    (GAD), 29
  Geriatric Anxiety Inventory
    (GAI), 24–25
  Geriatric Depression Scale
    (GDS), 24
  GMS/AGECAT System,
    25, 27
  Hamilton Anxiety Rating
    Scale (HAM-A), 24
  Hospital Anxiety and
    Depression Scale (HADS),
    24–25, 26
  importance of, 20–21
  overview, 5, 20, 29
  physical illness, co-
    morbidity with as
    challenge of, 22–23

Diagnosis (cont.)
Rating Scale for Anxiety in Dementia (RAID), 24
screening instruments, 24–26
self-reports, problems with, 20–21
shortcomings of existing diagnostic criteria, 3
stigma as challenge of, 22
Structured Clinical Interview for DSM-5 Disorders (SCID), 27
Diagnostic and Statistical Manual of Mental Disorders (DSM-5)
agoraphobia and, 87
anxiety defined, 205
anxiety disorders not otherwise specified (ADNOS) and, 140
changes to, 23–24
clinical assessment of late-life anxiety and, 79
cultural syndrome, 68
hoarding disorder, 161–162
late-life anxiety and, 20
methodological issues, 10–11
OCD and, 2, 23
post-traumatic stress disorder (PTSD) and, 176
PTSD and, 2, 23
Structured Clinical Interview for DSM-5 Disorders (SCID), 81
Western cultural bias in, 63
Diagnostic Interview Schedule (DIS), 13
Diefenbach, G. J., 68
Diffusion tensor imaging (DTI), Parkinson's disease and late-life anxiety and, 145
Dimensional measurement of anxiety, 2–3
Disability-adjusted life-years (DALYs), 3
Display rules, 67
Dissanayaka, N., 6, 228, 233
Diversity differences in clinical assessment of late-life anxiety, 90
Dobkin, R. D., 147
Dobzhansky, Theodosius, 218
Donepezil, 200

Dopamine dysregulation syndrome (DDS), 142
Dopamine withdrawal syndrome (DWAS), 142
Dreeben, Samuel, 6
Driving anxiety, 230
Drugs. See Pharmacological treatment of late-life anxiety
DSM-5. See Diagnostic and Statistical Manual of Mental Disorders (DSM-5)
Duloxetine, 197

Early-life experience
anxiety and, 2
cognitive functioning and, 123
future research, 227
Ecological momentary assessment (EMA), 88–89
Edelstein, Barry, 6, 85, 88
e-Health, 234–235
Eldreth, D. A., 107
enhanced community care (ECC), 181, 182
Enquête sur la Santé des Aînés (ESA) Study, 13
Epidemiology of late-life anxiety
acculturation and, 14
cultural differences and, 13–14
findings of studies, 11
methodological issues, 10–11
nursing homes and, 13
overview, 5, 10, 16
population-based incidence estimates, 13
population-based prevalence estimates, 12–13
Escitalopram
combination with cognitive behavioural therapy (CBT), 201
treatment of late-life anxiety with, 196–197
ESPRIT Study, 15
Evolutionary basis for anxiety, 122
Executive dysfunction
Attention Process Training II (APT) and, 178

cognitive behavioural therapy (CBT) and, 178
psychosocial treatment of, 178
Executive function, 98
Exercise, cross-cultural issues, 72
Eysenck, M. W., 120

Family
cross-cultural issues, 71–72
palliative care and, 167
Fan, A. Z., 90
Fear and anxiety. See Animal models of fear and anxiety
Fear of falling
Activity, Balance, Learning and Exposure (ABLE) treatment and, 178
attention bias and, 107–108
clinical assessment of late-life anxiety and, 85
cognitive behavioural therapy (CBT) and, 52, 178
diagnosis of late-life anxiety, as challenge of, 23
prevalence of, 177
psychosocial treatment, 177–178
subthreshold late-life anxiety and, 45
Fear of Falling Questionnaire (FFQ), 85
Fear Survey Schedule-II (FSS-II), 85
Flint, A. J., 21
Foulk, M. A., 233
Fox, L. S., 101, 107
Functional magnetic resonance imaging (fMRI)
anxiety and, 1
attention bias and, 107, 110
future research, 227
Parkinson's disease, late-life anxiety and, 145
Future research
Acceptance and Commitment Therapy (ACT), 233
anticonvulsants, 231
antidepressants, 231
attention bias, 111–112
benzodiazepines (BZDs), 231
cannabidiol (CBD), 232

cognitive behavioural
therapy (CBT), 232–233
conventional psychotropic
medication, 231–232
cross-cultural issues in late-
life anxiety, 72–73
early-life experience, 227
e-Health, 234–235
fMRI, 227
genetic factors, 226–227
incidence of late-life anxiety,
229–230
late-life experience, 227
mindfulness-based
interventions, 233
neural circuitry, 227
novel agents, 232
overview, 226, 235
pharmacological treatment
of late-life anxiety, 202,
230–231
phytomedicines, 232
prefrontal cortex, 227
prevalence of late-life
anxiety, 229–230
psychosocial treatment of
late-life anxiety, 182–183
race, late-life anxiety
and, 234
risk factor, anxiety as,
227–229
subthreshold late-life
anxiety, 53–54
symptom, anxiety as, 227
telehealth, 234–235
virtual reality (VR)
technology, 234

GAD. *See* generalized anxiety
disorder (GAD)
GAI. *See* Geriatric Anxiety
Inventory (GAI)
Galantamine, 200
Galphimia, 201
Gamma-aminobutyric acid
(GABA) system
benzodiazepines (BZDs)
and, 197, 213
cognitive functioning
and, 124
fear conditioning and
extinction and, 213–214
pharmacological treatment
and, 189
pregabalin and, 200
Z-drugs and, 198

Gatz, M., 226–227
Gender differences in clinical
assessment of late-life
anxiety, 90
Generalized anxiety
disorder (GAD)
alpidem and, 198
alprazolam and, 198
antidepressants and, 174
attention bias and, 107, 111
benzodiazepines (BZDs)
and, 174
clinical assessment of late-
life anxiety and, 84
cognitive behavioural
therapy (CBT) and, 6, 173
cognitive functioning and,
117, 118–119
co-morbidity of, 4
diagnosis of, 29
duloxetine and, 197
escitalopram and, 196–197
ketazolam and, 198
nortriptyline and, 197
onset of, 4
in palliative care settings, 166
Parkinson's disease and,
139–140
risk factors, 15
subthreshold late-life anxiety
and, 44, 46, 48
telephone-based treatment,
181–182
venlafaxine and, 197
Generalized Anxiety Disorder
Severity Scale
(GADSS), 82
Genetic factors
in Alzheimer's disease, 123
in anxiety, 1–2
cognitive functioning and,
122–124
future research, 226–227
Parkinson's disease, late-life
anxiety and, 145–146
Geriatric Anxiety
Inventory (GAI)
clinical assessment of late-
life anxiety and, 83
cross-cultural issues, 69
culturally specific responses,
229–230
diagnosis of late-life anxiety
and, 24–25
long-term care and, 165
overview, 4, 229

Parkinson's disease, late-life
anxiety and, 143
pharmacological treatment,
measurement of effect, 192
Geriatric Anxiety Scale (GAS)
clinical assessment of late-
life anxiety and, 83–84
long-term care and, 165
overview, 4, 229
pharmacological treatment,
measurement of effect, 192
Geriatric Depression Scale
(GDS), 24
Geriatric Resources for
Assessment and Care of
Elders (GRACE)
model, 175
Gingko biloba, 201, 232
GMS/AGECAT system, 11, 13,
14, 25, 27
Gould, Christine, 6
Grenier, Sébastien, 5,
50, 234
Grigsby, A. B., 89–90
Group psychodrama,
Parkinson's disease and
late-life anxiety and, 148
Guy's/Age Concern Survey, 11

HADS. *See* Hospital Anxiety
and Depression Scale
(HADS)
Hall, J., 232–233
Haller, J., 200
Hamilton Anxiety Rating Scale
(HAM-A)
buspirone and, 200
clinical assessment of late-
life anxiety and, 82
diagnosis of late-life anxiety
and, 24
duloxetine and, 197
overview, 4
oxazepam and, 198
Parkinson's disease, late-life
anxiety and, 142, 147
pharmacological treatment,
measurement of effect, 192
pregabalin and, 200
quetiapine and, 199
sertraline and, 196
Hantke, Nathan, 6
Hatzdimitriadou, E., 66
Headaches, co-morbidity with
subthreshold late-life
anxiety, 51

Hearing impairment, co-morbidity with subthreshold late-life anxiety, 51
Hendriks, G. J., 201
Herbal medicines, 201
Hinton, D. E., 13–14
Hippocampus
  anxiety and, 1, 205
  cognitive functioning and, 123, 124
  mediation of fear learning and extinction in, 210–211
  neuromodulation of fear and anxiety circuits, 211
  Pavlovian fear conditioning and, 206
  physiology of, 208–209
Hoarding disorder
  cognitive behavioural therapy (CBT) and, 177
  diagnostic features, 177
  home-based care and late-life anxiety and, 161–162
  prevalence of, 177
  psychosocial treatment, 177
Hofmann, S. G., 13–14
Home-based care, late-life anxiety in
  clinical assessment of late-life anxiety and, 161–162
  hoarding disorder in, 161–162
  home-based primary care (HBPC) programmes, 160
  need for care, 160–161
  pharmacological treatment in, 164–165
  psychosocial treatment in, 165, 182
  relaxation in, 162
  types of services, 160–161
home-based primary care (HBPC) programmes, 160
Hopko, D. R., 85
Hops, 201, 232
Hormones, cognitive functioning and, 124
Hospital Anxiety and Depression Scale (HADS)
  co-morbidity and, 16
  cross-cultural issues, 69
  diagnosis of late-life anxiety and, 24–25, 26

Parkinson's disease, late-life anxiety and, 142, 147
  risk factors, 15–16
Hosseini, Charissa, 5–6, 14
Howard, R. J., 120
Hwang, W. C., 71
Hyperthyroidism, cognitive functioning and, 125
Hyponatremia, antidepressants and, 196
Hypothalamic–pituitary–adrenal (HPA) axis
  anxiety and, 1, 2
  cognitive functioning and, 124
Hypothyroidism, cognitive functioning and, 125

Immigration, cross-cultural issues, 69–70
Improving Mood – Promoting Access to Collaborative Treatment (IMPACT) model, 175
Impulse control disorders (ICDs), 142
Incidence of late-life anxiety
  future research, 229–230
  population-based estimates, 13
Informant reports, 88
Information processing model, depression and late-life anxiety and, 99
Institute of Medicine (IOM), 175, 182
Insula, anxiety and, 1
International Classification of Diseases, 10th Revision (ICD-10)
  culture-specific disorders, 68
  methodological issues, 10–11
  OCD and, 2
  PTSD and, 2
  Western cultural bias in, 63
International Psychogeriatrics, 226
Internet-delivered cognitive behavioural therapy (iCBT), 182, 234–235

Jackson, H., 11
Jimenez, D. E., 66, 90
Journal of Anxiety Disorders, 226

Kang, H.-J., 13, 15
Karlsson, B., 22
Kava, 201, 232
Ketazolam, 198
Kissane, D. W., 13
Knight, B. G., 20, 27, 101, 107, 108–109
Kogan, J. N., 85, 88
Kok, Brian, 6
Kraepelien, M., 147
Kreifelts, B., 227
Kwangju Study, 13, 15

Lee, K., 65, 66
Lee, L. O., 101, 226–227
Lemon balm, 201, 232
Lenze, E. J., 130
Letamendi, A. M., 67–68
Li, S., 66
Liebowitz Social Anxiety Scale (LSAS)
  clinical assessment of late-life anxiety and, 85–86
  Parkinson's disease, late-life anxiety and, 142
Limbic system, anxiety and, 1
Lin, Xiaoping, 5–6, 14
Lithium, 200
Longitudinal Aging Study Amsterdam, 11, 16
Long-term care, late-life anxiety in
  characteristics of, 163
  clinical assessment of late-life anxiety and, 165
  continuum of care, 162–163
  dementia, co-morbidity with, 164–165
  Geriatric Anxiety Inventory (GAI) and, 165
  Geriatric Anxiety Scale (GAS) and, 165
  long-term care defined, 162–163
  patient experience, 163
  pharmacological treatment, 190, 194–195
  research findings, 164

Ma, Vanessa, 6
Mackenzie, C. S., 15
MacLeod, C., 99
Majercsik, E., 200
Mandala of Health, 64–65
Marchant, N. L., 120
Marques, L., 67

Massena, P. N., 69, 229–230
Maters, G. A., 69
Mathews, A., 99
McBride, Shalagh, 6
McKee, D. R., 88
MDS-UPDRS – Anxiety Item, Parkinson's disease and late-life anxiety and, 142
Medicare Skilled Home Care Program (US), 160
Medication. *See* Pharmacological treatment of late-life anxiety
Meditation, attention bias and, 111
Memantine, 200
MentDis_ICF65+ Study, 14, 16
Menza, M., 145
Mezhebovsky, I., 199
Mindfulness-based Cognitive Therapy (MBCT), 233
Mindfulness-based interventions
cross-cultural issues, 71
dementia and, 179
future research, 233
Parkinson's disease, late-life anxiety and, 148
subthreshold late-life anxiety and, 52
Mindfulness-based Stress Reduction (MBSR)
cognitive functioning and, 130
future research, 233
as novel treatment model, 180
Mini International Neuropsychiatric Interview (MINI), 11, 81–82
Mirtazapine, 197
Mirza, S. S., 228
Mobility Inventory (MI), 87
Mogg, K., 99, 109
Mohlman, J., 100, 107
Monoamine oxidase inhibitors (MAOIs), 196
Montreal Cognitive Assessment (MoCA), 128
Mynors-Wallis, L., 21

National Comorbidity Survey Replication (NCS-R), 12, 14, 90

National Guideline Clearinghouse (US), 24–25
National Institutes of Health (US), 84
Nègre-Pagès, L., 49
NESARC-II Study, 12–13, 15, 16
NESARC-III Study, 3–4
Neuropsychiatric anxiety, 120–121
Neuropsychiatric Inventory – Anxiety subscale (NPI-Anxiety)
neuroticism and, 2
Parkinson's disease, late-life anxiety and, 142
Neuroticism, anxiety and, 2
Neurotransmitters
cognitive functioning and, 124
Parkinson's disease, late-life anxiety and, 144–145
Nguyen, H., 111
NMDA receptors, 214
Noiret, N., 108
Norandrenergic locus ceruleus, 145
Nortriptyline, 197
Novel agents, 232
Nursing homes, prevalence estimates of late-life anxiety in, 13

Obsessive-compulsive disorder (OCD)
anxiety and, 2
DSM-5 and, 23
O'Hara, R., 118
Okai, D., 147
Older Adult Social Evaluative Scale (OASES), 86
Omnibus Budget Reconciliation Act (US), 194
Onset of anxiety, 4
Orientating, 98
Osteoporosis, co-morbidity with subthreshold late-life anxiety, 51
Oxazepam
ceasing use of, 195
treatment of late-life anxiety with, 198

Pachana, Nancy, 5, 7
Palliative care settings, late-life anxiety in
anxiety as symptom, 166
caregivers and, 167
clinical assessment of late-life anxiety and, 167
exacerbation of anxiety, 166–167
family and, 167
generalized anxiety disorder (GAD) and, 166
overview, 165–166
palliative care defined, 165
panic disorder and, 166
pharmacological treatment, 167
post-traumatic stress disorder (PTSD) and, 166
psychosocial treatment, 167
Palmer, K., 121, 227–228
Panic disorder
clinical assessment of late-life anxiety and, 86–87
cognitive behavioural therapy (CBT) and, 173
in palliative care settings, 166
Panic Disorder Severity Scale, 82
Parker, G., 26
Parkinson's disease, late-life anxiety and
Acceptance and Commitment Therapy (ACT) and, 148
amygdala and, 145
anterior cingulates and, 145
anxiety disorders not otherwise specified (ADNOS) and, 140, 141–142
Anxiety Status Inventory (ASI) and, 142
Beck Anxiety Inventory (BAI) and, 142, 147
benzodiazepines (BZDs) and, 146
brain-derived neurotrophic factor (BDNF) and, 145
characteristics of anxiety, 143, 144
clinical assessment of late-life anxiety and, 89, 142–143

Parkinson's disease (cont.)
cognitive behavioural
therapy (CBT) and, 52,
146–148, 174, 179
cognitive functioning
and, 125
co-morbidity, 16
deep brain stimulation
(DBS) treatment, 142
Depression, Anxiety and
Stress Scale (DASS-21)
and, 147
diffusion tensor imaging
(DTI) and, 145
dopamine dysregulation
syndrome (DDS) and, 142
dopamine withdrawal
syndrome (DWAS)
and, 142
functional magnetic
resonance imaging (fMRI)
and, 145
future research, 149
generalized anxiety disorder
(GAD) and, 139–140
genetic factors and,
145–146
Geriatric Anxiety Inventory
(GAI) and, 143
group psychodrama and, 148
Hamilton Anxiety Rating
Scale (HAM-A) and,
142, 147
Hospital Anxiety and
Depression Scale (HADS)
and, 142, 147
impulse control disorders
(ICDs) and, 142
Liebowitz Social Anxiety
Scale (LSAS) and, 142
MDS-UPDRS – Anxiety
Item and, 142
mindfulness-based
interventions and, 148
movement disorder,
Parkinson's disease as, 139
Neuropsychiatric
Inventory – Anxiety
subscale (NPI-Anxiety)
and, 142
neurotransmitters and,
144–145
norandrenergic locus
ceruleus and, 145
onset of anxiety, 143, 144
overview, 6, 139, 149

Parkinson's Disease Anxiety
Scale (PAS) and, 143
paroxetine and, 146
Patient Education Program
Parkinson's (PEPP)
and, 148
pharmacological
treatment, 146
positron emission
tomography (PET)
and, 145
prevalence of anxiety, 139
prevalence of Parkinson's
disease, 139
psychosocial treatment,
146–148
rating scales and, 142–143
risk factor, anxiety as,
228–229
selective serotonin reuptake
inhibitors (SSRIs) and, 146
serotonergic raphe nucleus
and, 145
sertraline and, 146
single-photon emission
computed tomography
(SPECT) and, 145
Spielberger State Trait
Anxiety Inventory (STAI)
and, 142, 147
striatal dopamine
transporter (DAT) density
and, 145
subthreshold late-life
anxiety, co-morbidity
with, 49
subtypes of anxiety,
139–140
symptoms of anxiety,
140–141
Zung Self-Rated Anxiety
Scale (SAS) and, 142
Parkinson's Disease Anxiety
Scale (PAS), 143
Paroxetine
ceasing use of, 195
Parkinson's disease and late-
life anxiety and, 146
Parslow, R., 22
Passionflower, 201, 232
Patient Education Program
Parkinson's (PEPP),
Parkinson's disease and
late-life anxiety and, 148
Patient-Reported Outcomes
Measurement

Information System
(PROMIS), 84
Pavlovian fear conditioning,
206–207
PD Anxiety-Motor
Complications
Questionnaire
(PDAMCQ), 228
Pedersen, N. L., 226–227
Penn State Worry
Questionnaire (PSWQ),
84–85, 201
Pennywort, 201, 232
Perry, G., 123
Perumal, Bhagvathi, 7
PET. See Positron emission
tomography (PET)
Petersen, R. B., 123
Petkus, Andrew J., 6, 111
Pharmacological treatment of
late-life anxiety. See also
specific drug
adverse effects, 193–194
antidepressants (See
Antidepressants)
antipsychotics (See
Antipsychotics)
attention bias, 110–111
ceasing use of psychotropic
medication, 195
clinical assessment of late-
life anxiety prior to, 193
clinical context of, 190
clinical trials, lack of, 195
cognitive behavioural
therapy (CBT) versus, 201
cognitive functioning
and, 130
cognitive impairment, in
presence of, 194
combination with cognitive
behavioural therapy
(CBT), 174, 201
combination with
psychosocial treatment,
174, 201
co-morbidity and, 191
complementary
medicine, 201
conventional psychotropic
medication, 231–232
cross-cultural issues, 72
future research, 202,
230–231
gamma-aminobutyric acid
(GABA) system and, 189

Geriatric Anxiety Inventory
(GAI) and, 192
Geriatric Anxiety Scale
(GAS) and, 192
Hamilton Anxiety Rating
Scale (HAM-A) and, 192
in home-based care, 164–165
limitations of evidence, 195
in long-term care, 190,
194–195
measurement of treatment
effect, 191–192
novel agents, 232
overview, 5, 6, 189, 202–000
in palliative care settings, 167
Parkinson's disease, late-life
anxiety and, 146
pharmacodynamic
considerations, 190–191
pharmacokinetic
considerations, 190–191
phytomedicines, 201, 232
polypharmacy, 191
post-traumatic stress
disorder (PTSD), 176
pro re nata (as needed), 192
psychiatric visits, 190
psychological impact of,
192–193
psychosocial treatment
versus, 201
rationale for drug use,
189–190
subthreshold late-life
anxiety, 51
PhD-level providers
(PLPs), 182
Phobias
clinical assessment of late-
life anxiety and, 85
Social Phobia and Anxiety
Inventory (SPAI), 86
Social Phobia Scale (SPS), 86
subthreshold late-life anxiety
and, 44–45
Physiological measures, 88
Phytomedicines, 201, 232
Polypharmacy, 191
Poon, C. Y., 108–109
Positivity effect, 100
Positron emission
tomography (PET)
anxiety and, 1
neuroticism and, 2
Parkinson's disease, late-life
anxiety and, 145

Post-traumatic stress disorder
(PTSD)
anxiety and, 2
cognitive behavioural
therapy (CBT) and, 176
DSM-5 and, 23, 176
in palliative care settings, 166
pharmacological
treatment, 176
prevalence of, 176
psychosocial treatment,
176–177
in veterans, 176–177
Prefrontal cortex
anxiety and, 205
attention bias and, 107,
109–110
cognitive functioning and,
123, 124
future research, 227
mediation of fear learning
and extinction in, 210–211
neuromodulation of fear and
anxiety circuits, 211
Pavlovian fear conditioning
and, 206
physiology of, 208
Pregabalin, 200, 231
Prescott, C. A., 226–227
Prevalence of late-life anxiety
cross-cultural issues and,
66–67
future research, 229–230
Parkinson's disease and, 139
population-based prevalence
estimates, 12–13
subthreshold late-life
anxiety, 33–45
Price, R. B., 100, 107
Problem-solving therapy
(PST), cognitive
functioning and,
129–130
Processing Efficiency Theory,
49, 120
Protective factors
cross-cultural issues in late-
life anxiety and, 69–70
for late-life anxiety, 14–16
in subacute settings, 157
Psoinos, M., 66
Psoriatic arthritis, co-
morbidity with
subthreshold late-life
anxiety, 51
Psychiatric visits, 190

Psychosocial treatment of
late-life anxiety
Acceptance and
Commitment Therapy
(ACT) (*See* Acceptance
and Commitment
Therapy (ACT))
Adjusting to Chronic
Conditions Using
Education, Support, and
Skills (ACCESS),
179–180
attention bias, 110–111
bachelor-level lay providers
(BLPs), 182
Calmer Life model, 180–181
chronic illness and, 179–180
cognitive behavioural
therapy (CBT) (*See*
Cognitive behavioural
therapy (CBT))
combination with
pharmacological
treatment, 174, 201
community–academic
partnership models, 182
cross-cultural issues, 70–72
dementia and, 178–179
enhanced community care
(ECC), 181, 182
executive dysfunction
and, 178
fear of falling, 177–178
future research, 182–183
Geriatric Resources for
Assessment and Care of
Elders (GRACE)
model, 175
hoarding disorder, 177
in home-based care, 165,
182
Improving Mood –
Promoting Access to
Collaborative Treatment
(IMPACT) model, 175
Internet-delivered cognitive
behavioural therapy
(iCBT), 182, 234–235
limitations of efficacy
trials, 175
mindfulness-based
interventions (*See*
Mindfulness-based
interventions)
modular approaches, 180
need for new models, 175

Psychosocial (cont.)
novel delivery options,
181–182
novel treatment models,
180–181
overview, 5, 6, 173, 182–183
in palliative care settings, 167
Parkinson's disease, late-life
anxiety and, 146–148
pharmacological treatment
versus, 201
PhD-level providers
(PLPs), 182
post-traumatic stress
disorder (PTSD), 176–177
relaxation (See Relaxation)
religion and/or spirituality
(R/S), 180–181
subthreshold late-life
anxiety, 51–53
telephone-based treatment,
181–182
traditional efficacy trials,
173–175
Vida Calma, 181
Psychotropic medication. See
Pharmacological
treatment of late-life
anxiety
PTSD. See Post-traumatic
stress disorder (PTSD)

Quetiapine, 199, 231

Race, late-life anxiety and, 234
Ramos, Katherine, 6
Rating Scale for Anxiety in
Dementia (RAID), 4, 24,
25–26, 87, 230
Rating scales for anxiety
overview, 4
Parkinson's disease, late-life
anxiety and, 142–143
Relaxation
cross-cultural issues, 71
in home-based care, 162
subthreshold late-life anxiety
and, 51–53
Religion and/or spirituality (R/
S), 180–181
Religious explanation for
mental disorders, 65
Research Domain Criteria
(RDoC), 226
Reynolds, C. F., 12–13
Ribeiro, O., 69, 230

Richer, Marie-Josée, 5
Risk factors
anxiety as risk factor for
other conditions, 227–229
cross-cultural issues in late-
life anxiety and, 69–70
for generalized anxiety
disorder (GAD), 15
for late-life anxiety, 4,
14–16
in subacute settings, 157
Rivastigmine, 200
Robinaugh, D. J., 67
Rodrigues, R., 123
Rodriguez, Rachel, 6
Rumination, 45

Sah, Pankaj, 7
St John's wort, 201
St. Louis University Mental
Status (SLUMS)
Examination, 128
Salem witch trials, 65
Savage, K., 232
Schuurmans, J., 196, 201
Selective serotonin reuptake
inhibitors (SSRIs)
overview, 196
Parkinson's disease and
late-life anxiety and, 146
Self-reports
clinical assessment of late-
life anxiety and, 82
problems with, 20–21
Serotonergic raphe nucleus,
Parkinson's disease and
late-life anxiety and, 145
Serotonin and noradrenaline
(norepinephrine)
reuptake inhibitors
(SNRIs), 196
Sertraline
buspirone versus, 196
cognitive behavioural
therapy (CBT) versus, 196
Hamilton Anxiety Rating
Scale (HAM-A) and, 196
Parkinson's disease and
late-life anxiety and, 146
treatment of late-life anxiety
with, 196
Sexual abuse, cognitive
functioning and, 123–124
Shead, Veronica, 6
Short Anxiety Screening Test
(SAST), 4, 24, 25

The Sign of Four (Conan
Doyle), 79
Single-photon emission
computed tomography
(SPECT), Parkinson's
disease and, 145
Skullcap, 201, 232
Sleep, effect of subthreshold
late-life anxiety on, 45
Snow, A. L., 230
Social anxiety disorder, clinical
assessment of late-life
anxiety and, 85–86
Social Interaction Anxiety
Scale (SIAS), 86
Social Phobia and Anxiety
Inventory (SPAI), 86
Social Phobia Scale (SPS), 86
Socioemotional selectivity
theory (SST) and, 100
Spielberger State Trait Anxiety
Inventory (STAI),
Parkinson's disease and
late-life anxiety and,
142, 147
Stanley, Melinda, 6
Steiner, A. R., 111
Stress disorders, anxiety and, 2
Striatal dopamine transporter
(DAT) density,
Parkinson's disease
and, 145
Strokes, subacute settings and
late-life anxiety, 157
Structured Clinical Interview
for DSM-5 Disorders
(SCID), 27, 81
Structured interview
guides, 230
Subacute settings, late-life
anxiety in
amputation and, 158
avoidance strategies, 158
chronic obstructive
pulmonary disease
(COPD) and, 158
communication, importance
of, 159
control, limitations on, 158
discharge and, 158
pain management and, 158
personal values and goals,
importance of, 159
pre- or early admission,
importance of, 159
protective factors in, 157

risk factors in, 157
routine, importance of, 159
strokes and, 157
subacute setting defined, 157
trust, importance of, 159
Subthreshold late-life anxiety
alcohol consumption and, 46
anxiety disorders not
otherwise specified
(ADNOS) and, 33, 51–52
Attention Control Theory
(ACT) and, 49
benzodiazepines (BZDs)
and, 51
cardiovascular disease
(CVD), co-morbidity
with, 50
chronic obstructive
pulmonary disease
(COPD), co-morbidity
with, 50
chronic pain, co-morbidity
with, 51
cognitive behavioural
therapy (CBT) and, 51–53
cognitive impairment, co-
morbidity with, 48–49
daily functioning, effect on,
45–46
dementia, co-morbidity
with, 48–49
depression, co-morbidity
with, 47
evolution over time, 44, 48
fear of falling and, 45
future research, 53–54
generalized anxiety disorder
(GAD) and, 44, 46, 48
headaches, co-morbidity
with, 51
hearing impairment, co-
morbidity with, 51
medication and, 46
need for mental health
services and, 46
osteoporosis, co-morbidity
with, 51
overview, 5, 33, 53–54
Parkinson's disease and, 49
pharmacological treatment
of, 51
phobias and, 44–45

physical illness,
co-morbidity with, 51
prevalence of, 33–45
psoriatic arthritis,
co-morbidity with, 51
psychosocial treatment of,
51–53
relaxation and, 51–53
rumination and, 45
sleep, effect on, 45
vision impairment, co-
morbidity with, 51
well-being, effect on,
45–47
Suicide, antidepressants
and, 196
Supernatural explanation for
mental disorders, 65
Swedish Adoption/Twin Study
of Aging, 226–227, 228

Tales, A., 228
Taoism, 71
Technology, use of in clinical
assessment of late-life
anxiety, 88–89
Telehealth, 234–235
Telephone-based treatment,
181–182
10/66 Study, 14
Thyroid disease, cognitive
functioning and,
125
Tricyclic antidepressants
(TCAs)
cross-cultural issues, 72
overview, 196
Troeung, L., 147
Twin studies, cognitive
functioning and,
122–123

Uchino, B. N., 88
United States Census, 163

Valerian, 201, 232
van Sonderen, E., 26
Veazey, C., 147
Venlafaxine, 197
Veterans Health
Administration, 176–177
Vida Calma, 181

Vietnam Era Twin Study of
Aging, 122
Vietri, J., 100
Virtual reality (VR)
technology, 234
Vision impairment, co-
morbidity with
subthreshold late-life
anxiety, 51

Watson, D., 98
Well-being, effect of
subthreshold late-life
anxiety on, 45–47
Wetherell, Julie, 6, 71, 111, 178,
201, 233
Williams, A. M.,
107–108
Williams, J. M. G., 99
World Health Organization
(WHO), 163, 165
Worry
attention bias and, 107
cognitive functioning
and, 119

Years of life lived with
disability (YLDs), 3,
11, 205
Years of life lost due to
premature mortality
(YLLs), 3
Young, W. R.,
107–108

Z-drugs
benzodiazepines (BZDs)
versus, 198
gamma-aminobutyric acid
(GABA) system and,
198
treatment of late-life anxiety
with, 198
Zeilmann, C. A., 72
Zen Buddhism, 71
Zhang, X., 15
Zou, J. B., 235
Zung Self-Rated Anxiety
Scale (SAS),
Parkinson's disease
and late-life anxiety,
142